Disease and Medicine in India

A Historical Overview

edited by Deepak Kumar

T0323731

Disease and Medicine in India

A Historical Overview

edited by Deepak Kumar

Indian History Congress

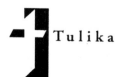 Tulika

Published by **Tulika Books**
35A/1 (ground floor), Shahpur Jat, New Delhi 110 049, India

© Indian History Congress

First published in India 2001

Reprint 2012

ISBN: 978-93-82381-05-1

Designed by Ram Rahman, typeset in Minion at Tulika
Print Communication Services, New Delhi, and printed at
Chaman Enterprises, 1603 Pataudi House, Daryaganj,
Delhi 110 006

To the memory of
DEBIPRASAD CHATTOPADHYAYA
and
SRINIVASA AMBIRAJAN

Contents

CONTENTS

MODERN INDIA

Preface

The Indian History Congress has been endeavouring to pay special attention to fields where historians need to interact with their colleagues in the physical and other sciences. One such field is the history of health conditions and the progress of medicine in India. There was, accordingly, a special panel organized at the 61st session of the Indian History Congress at Kolkota, 1–3 January 2001, on this subject. The present volume contains papers presented at the panel, edited by our distinguished colleague, Professor Deepak Kumar, who chaired the panel, and who now contributes an important introduction.

A collection of papers cannot admittedly provide connected history. On the other hand, it does what is difficult for a general textbook: to look in depth at individual aspects and investigate nooks and corners. The volume will hopefully provide some of the essential building blocks out of which a fuller history of disease and medicine in India can be reconstructed.

This effort could not have been made without generous support from two major donors: Sir Dorabji Tata Trust, whose Director Mr R.M. Lala also took a very kindly interest in the success of our panel, and CIPLA, under its visionary Director, Mr M.K. Hamied. We are also grateful to the Indian Council of Medical Research and the Hamdard National Foundation for their grants.

Professor Deepak Kumar has been most considerate not only in agreeing to be the editor but also in meeting my various requests cheerfully.

As with other matters concerned with the Indian History Congress, Professor Irfan Habib provided inestimable help at every stage of the present undertaking. To say more would be superfluous.

The Bibliography for the volume has been prepared by Ms

Radha Gayatri and Mr Dhrub Kumar Singh, Research Scholars at Jawaharlal Nehru University, New Delhi, to whom our thanks are due.

The papers were processed by Mr Muneeruddin Khan at Aligarh, from the stage of pre-circulation to the final press copy. Mr Arshad Ali has kept all our records and accounts.

Many thanks are due to Mr Rajendra Prasad and Ms Indira Chandrasekhar for undertaking, on behalf of Tulika, to publish this volume despite the short period that the Indian History Congress has been able to allow them.

My successor Professor Ramakrishna Chatterji, the present Secretary of the Indian History Congress, has given me wholehearted cooperation in completing the task that the Indian History Congress had assigned to me while I held the same office. Professor S.P. Verma, who was Treasurer of the Indian History Congress during my term as Secretary, bore all the further financial responsibility this venture has involved with stoical fortitude. Needless to say, I am very grateful to both of them.

And now the reader is invited to see what Professor Deepak Kumar and his fellow-contributors (including the undersigned with a short piece) have to offer.

Aligarh   SHIREEN MOOSVI

Social History of Medicine

Some Issues and Concerns

Deepak Kumar

The historical study of science enjoys two great advantages over studies of contemporary science; it encourages the study of long-term developmental processes that require decades or centuries to detect and it permits the more confident identification of figures and episodes associated with scientific progress.[1]

Historical dynamics affect us and our times as much as they did our ancestors. These dynamics have influenced and have, in turn, been influenced by our quest for truth and reality, our fascination for tools, and our search for food, health and better living. Where does this concern take us? The History of Science, Technology and Medicine (HSTM) is a path neither untrodden nor very frequented, yet it is worth several visits and revisits.[2] Its significance, especially from a socio-cultural perspective, cannot be ignored. It always occupied a special place in Indian history through the ages. Centuries ago Said al-Andalusi (1029–70), in his *Tabaqat al-Uman* (probably the first work on the history of science in any language), referred to India as the first nation which cultivated the sciences.[3] In ancient India, medical men, in spite of their scripture-orientation, insisted on the supreme importance of direct observation of natural phenomena and on the technique of rational processing of empirical data. The *Charakasamhita*, an ancient medical text, says, 'To one who understands, knowledge of nature and love of humanity are not two things but one.'[4] Nothing illustrates better the links between science and society.

Ours is an age of biology. The range and 'quantum' of its applications are truly breathtaking: cloning, genome, and now the prospect of 'bio-wars'! On the more positive side, during the last one hundred and fifty years or so, much work has been done on disease, its vectors, vaccines, etc. New paradigms have been laid, and we are in the midst of a 'genetic revolution'. Not surprisingly, many historians have now turned to medical history. Earlier we had some studies on the Indian medical tradition as part of philosophical and cultural enquiries (Indology?).[5] Now, even scholars of modern Indian history have taken to it in a big way.[6] Several works have appeared on medicine in politics and the politics of medicine.[7] At a micro-level, anthropologists and sociologists have contributed a great deal. Comparative or prosopographical studies of medical men can be equally instructive.[8] The social history of medicine is no less significant a field than the social history of science or technology. And it should be possible to add to them a cultural dimension as well.

It has always been fashionable to talk about 'mainstream' thought, 'mainstream' society, and even 'mainstream' history, though not many bother to think about what constitutes the mainstream or whether it really exists. A recent work sets as its primary goal the need to 'mainstream' the history of medicine. The author explains:

> Mainstreaming takes a historical subspeciality, like the history of medicine, lifts it out of the confining limits of a disciplinary channel, and refloats it in broader historical currents. Doing so requires us to write medical history in new ways. No longer is an epic or romantic story of spectacular breakthroughs and embattled pioneers enough.[9]

The 'mainstreaming' goal may sound ambitious or, biologically speaking, even chimerical, but the diagnosis is correct and valid. In an era of biology, the history of medicine can no longer afford to remain Whiggish or iatocentric. At the same time, care should be taken not to swing to the other extreme. Not everything is socially or culturally constructed; the role of individuals and specific requirements should not be ignored.[10] It is possible to think of and attempt a balance between social constructivism and historical relativism. In the Indian context this is even more important.

The present volume is a small step in this direction. Being a collection of essays, it has its limitations. No single volume can encapsulate more than two millennia, i.e. from Indus to Indira Gandhi. Nevertheless, a better job could have been done. The first millennium could attract only two essays; the second has sixteen. I wish we could find a Zysk, Zimmermann or Meulenbeld among contemporary

Indian scholars.[11] The late Debiprasad remains an exception. For medieval times there are five fine contributions from the Aligarh scholars. For the colonial period there is no shortage of either data or scholars; so some dimensions could be probed in detail. In this rather brief introduction, I do not intend to summarize them; instead, I shall use this opportunity to share some doubts and concerns as a student of Indian history, especially of the colonial period.

Doubts and Questions

It is generally agreed that the Indian universe has been complex, pluralistic and hierarchical. Unlike in the Cartesian world-view, here nature and culture, subject and object were never seen in an adversarial mould.[12] Pluralism was recognized but at the core there remained a quest for synthesis and a holistic understanding. This trend is manifest especially in the Indian medical thought and system. Again, it is this trend which takes even *yukti-vyapashraya bheshaja* (rational medicine) into the mirth and mire of metaphysics.[13] How does it take place? From magico–religious beginnings to rationalistic therapeutics and then back to decadence—it must be a fascinating journey. Or is it possible to think of another trajectory? If not, what were the factors responsible for the ups and downs? Was it because of the priestly class and the *varnashrama* hierarchy? The priests would naturally have been interested in supernaturalism and the mystification of nature. Why did the medical men bow to them?[14] Were there other options? Linear, hagiographical accounts or even philosophical explanations do not suffice. We need critical sociological enquiries, as shown by Debiprasad Chattopadhyay.[15]

We require a similar exercise for medieval times. Be it for Ayurveda, i.e. the knowledge or science (*veda*) of longevity (*ayus*), or the Yunani (Graeco–Arab) system, socio-historical explanations would probably be more rewarding and relevant than metaphysical ones. For example, how were the Mutazilites (who based their arguments on reason but without contradicting Quranic observations) gradually replaced by the fatalistic Asharites who repudiated rational thought? Al Haytham's ideas and experiments in optics later degenerated into metaphysical debates. Why could the experimental rigour of a Sushruta or an Al Hytham not be institutionalized? As a perceptive scholar explains: 'A society oriented towards fatalism, or one in which an interventionist deity forms part of the matrix of causal connections, is bound to produce fewer individuals inclined to probe the unknown with the tools of science.'[16]

To this was added a highly divisive caste system very peculiar to South Asian society. Caste led to the ruinous separation of theory from practice, of mental work from manual work.[17] Faith and caste were to prove a fatal combination. In late medieval times, this was compounded by an enormous intellectual (cultural?) failure on the part of the ruling class.[18] Abul Fazl, a reliable witness to the Mughal era, mourned 'The blowing of the heavy wind of *taqlid* (tradition) and the dimming of the lamp of wisdom . . . the door of "how" and "why" has been closed, and questioning and enquiry have been deemed fruitless and tantamount to paganism.'[19]

Apart from the above-mentioned concerns of a general and societal nature, one may also ask certain specific questions, as Roy Porter does in the context of late medieval England.[20] How was healing practised and who practised it? How was disease perceived? Medical anthropologists have looked into magico–religious rites, rituals and shamans. Can these be contextualized historically? Who were the grassroot healers? How did professionalism emerge? What were the contours of medical pluralism? How can one chart the interaction between the great and little traditions in terms of folk medicine and ethno-history?[21] Disease histories are many but we may need to look at them from the patients' eyes.[22] How did the sick evaluate doctors? As Nadeem Rezavi's paper in this volume enquires, was a physician's position just that of a client bound to his patrons in expectation of a respectable income, or did a general demand exist for his services among various sections of the society? How did the many distinct and competing practitioners relate to each other? This question was put in sharp focus when modern medicine entered new lands riding the colonial wave. Colonialism required bodies to travel from one place to another and this influenced the relations between the bodies and the pathogens. Moreover, the colonizing bodies were naturally anxious about their fragility either in the face of larger natural and social environments or in relation to other bodies (indigenous or foreign) that constituted an implicit threat.[23] What were the epidemiological consequences? What were the concerns for sanitation and for public health? Then, how 'public' was public health?[24] Colonial expansion strengthened the alliance between science and the state and the concept of state science/medicine emerged. How did it function; what was its impact? Is there anything specifically colonial about colonial medicine? To this we will return a little later, after a look at the pre-colonial heritage.

Pre-colonial Medicine: Its Texts and Practices

As mentioned earlier, medicine has always been a significant part of the Indian heritage. Flourishing about 2000 BC, the architectural design of Harappa does point to a conscious concern for public health and sanitation. Does the fabled Great Bath of Mohenjodaro (like the Roman bath) refer to hydropathy as a therapeutic measure? Unfortunately, very little is known of the Indus people. The *Atharvaveda* was probably the first repository of ancient Indian medical lore and these were later transmitted through the *Brahmana* texts. It was magico–religious in nature and incantations (*mantras*) were frequently resorted to.[25] Ayurveda as 'the science of (living to a ripe) age', sans *mantras*, appeared around Buddha's time. The concept of humours or *doshas* which is central in Ayurveda, is nowhere seen in the Vedic literature. Nor does it reflect Hippocratic or Galenic thinking. Ayurveda's emphasis on humoral 'balance', moderation, etc., seems closer to Buddha's 'Middle Path'. Disease causation in Ayurveda is not only because of humoral 'imbalance' (*vaishamya*) but due to a variety of reasons like weather, food, emotional agitation, sins from past life, and even 'sins against wisdom' (*prajna paradha*).[26] Its protagonists may have been inaccurate in their knowledge of human physiology but they were extremely good at plant morphology, its medical functions and therapeutics. Thakur's paper in this volume refers to surgery becoming synonymous with rationality. Both Charaka and Sushruta placed emphasis on direct observation. But unfortunately their texts and later commentaries have no anatomical or surgical illustrations. It is difficult to see how such techniques as rhinoplasty could have persisted purely textually.[27] In any case, Ayurveda remains a living and fertile area of research and interpretations.

The scenario became even more interesting when Islamic medical men introduced the Galenic tradition. There gradually appeared a hybrid Muslim–Hindu system known as the *Tibb*. They differed in theory, but in practice both traditions seem to have interacted and borrowed from each other. A fine example of this interaction is *Ma'din al-shifa-i-Sikandarshahi*, AD 1512, which was authored by Miyan

Bhuwah.[28] He leaned heavily on Sanskrit sources and thought that the Greek system was not suitable for the Indian constitution and climate. From the Islamic side, the concept of *arka* entered Ayurveda. Several Sanskrit medical texts were translated into Arabic and Persian, but instances of Islamic works being translated into Sanskrit are rare. The eighteenth century is significant for the appearance of two Sanskrit texts, *Hikmatprakasa* and *Hikmatparadipa,* which refer to the Islamic system and use numerous Arabic and Persian medical terms.[29] The concept of individual case studies and hospitals (*bimaristans*) also came from the Unani practioners.[30] In 1595 Quli Shah built a huge *Dar us-Shifa* (House of Cures) in Hyderabad.[31] During the reign of Muhammad Shah (1719–48) a large hospital was constructed in Delhi, and its annual expenditure was more than Rs 300,000. Numerous medical texts, mostly commentaries, were written during this century; for example, Akbar Arzani's *Tibb i-Akbari* (1700), Jafar Yar Khan's *Talim i-Ilaj* (1719–25), Madhava's *Ayurveda Prakasha* (1734), and the *Bhaisajya Ratnavali* of Govind Das. A Christian Mughal, Dominic Gregory, wrote the *Tuhafatul Masiha* (1749), which, along with descriptions of diseases, anatomy and surgery, contains important notes in Persian and Portuguese on alchemy and the properties of various plants, along with drawings of instruments and, interestingly, a horoscope.[32] An outstanding physician of this century, Mirza Alavi Khan, wrote seven texts, of which *Jami ul-Jawami* is a masterpiece, embodying all the branches of medicine then known in India.[33] Another great physician during the period of Shah Alam II (1759–1806) was Hakim Sharif Khan, who wrote ten important texts and enriched Unani medicines and indigenous Ayurvedic herbs.[34] Some works were unique and ahead of their time. For example, Nurul Haq's *Ainul Hayat* (1691) is a rare Persian text on the plague, and Pandit Mahadeva's *Rajasimha-sudhasindhu* (1787) refers to cowpox and inoculation.[35]

A number of European physicians visited Mughal India. Francois Bernier, Niocolao Manucci, Garcia d'Orta and John Ovington wrote extensively on Indian medical practices. The western medical episteme was not radically different from that of Indian physicians; both were humoral. But their practices differed greatly. Neither was able to develop a comprehensive theory of disease causation, but there seems to have been general agreement that Indian diseases were environmentally determined and should be treated by Indian methods. The Europeans, however, continued to look at Indian practices with curiosity and disdain.[36] They preferred bloodletting, whereas the *vaidyas* prescribed urine analysis and urine therapy. But in the use of drugs the Europeans and Indians learned from each other, as testified to by the works of van Rheede, Sassetti and d'Orta.[37] The Europeans introduced new plants in India that were gradually incorporated into the Indian pharmacopoeia. They brought venereal diseases such as syphilis, which was noticed as early as the sixteenth century by Bhava Misra, a noted *vaidya* in Benaras, who called it *firangi roga* (disease of the Europeans). Indian diseases received graphic description in Ovington's travelogue.[38] The best account of smallpox and the Indian method of variolation was given by J.Z. Holwell in 1767. To him this method, although quasi-religious, still appeared 'rational enough and well-founded'.[39] The travellers depicted Indian medical practices more as craft and as governed by caste rules and wrapped in supersition. Yet they could not help admiring the wonder called rhinoplasty (on which modern plastic surgery is founded), nor could they deny the efficacy of Indian drugs. The Indians, for their part, did not completely insulate themselves from 'other' practices. As the interaction grew in the eighteenth century, the *vaidyas* even took to bleeding in a large number of cases. Yet, while the European medical men gradually moved, thanks to the works of Vesalius and Harvey, from a humoral to a chemical or mechanical view of the body, the Indians remained faithful to their texts.[40]

The Colonial Watershed

Western medical discourse occupied an extremely important place in the colonization of India. It functioned in several ways: as an instrument of control which would swing between coercion and persuasion as the exigencies demanded, and as a site for interaction and often resistance. In its former role it served the state and helped ensure complete dominance. The European doctors who accompanied every naval despatch from Europe emerged as powerful interlocutors (for both political and cultural purposes). They not only looked after the sick aboard ships and on land, but were also the first to report on the flora, fauna, resources and cultural practices of the new territory. They were surgeon–naturalists and adventure–scientists, roles in which they felt superior in their encounters with the medical practices of other peoples, although, intermittently, they did show respect for the latter.[41]

Increasingly, however, the colonial doctors developed into a cultural force. They began to redefine what they saw in terms of their own training and perceptions. Their work encompassed not only the understanding and possible conquest of new diseases but also the extension of western cultural values to the non-western world. Gradual assimilation or synthesis was not on their agenda.

The colonial discourse on medicine was mediated not only by considerations of political economy but also by several other factors. The polity, biology, ecology, the circumstances of material life and new knowledge, interacted and produced this discourse. The emergence of tropical medicine at the turn of the last century is to be seen in this light. It may be argued that tropical medicine itself was a cultural construct, 'the scientific step-child of colonial domination and control'.[42] In the now-burgeoning literature, terms like tropical medicine, imperial medicine and colonial medicine are often used interchangeably. But they have specific connotations. Tropical medicine and imperial medicine emphasize the tropics and the empire as units of analysis, while colonial medicine stresses the colony. Each may attract different sets of questions. In tropical medicine these were: what ought to be the determining factor—climate, race, geography, or all of these taken together? What was carried over from the old medicine of tropical civilizations into the new tropical medicine? What attempts were made outside Europe to reconcile the older discourse of body humors and environmental miasmas with the new language of microbes and germs?

As for the use of the prefix colonial, post-colonial theorists have tried to challenge, even reject, the binary division between the colonizer and the colonized. A recent work talks of the 'tensions of empire' based on the universalizing claims of European ideology and the limitations faced by the rulers.[43] This is a smart subterfuge. The meaning of 'colonial' is neither elusive nor shifting. What makes colonization real is that even in its rejection there is an implicit acceptance of the standards set by the colonizer.[44] Interestingly enough, a medical historian has described colonialism as 'literally a health hazard'.[45] But to dismiss the colonial doctors reductively as the handmaidens of colonialism or capitalism would also be to ignore a more complex, and more interesting, reality.[46] The doctors had to assume multiple roles. They had little choice. Still, one can ask, what role did the 'peripherals' play? Could a synergetic relationship develop between the core and the periphery? These questions assume special significance when viewed against four centuries of the Europeans' 'struggles' in the 'torrid zones', and their transition from early explorers, travellers and traders to becoming conquerors and ultimate arbiters of the trampled tropics. Earlier the 'tropical discourse' was viewed through its pioneers; now issues and dichotomies have been given primacy.[47] However, these still abound in metropolitan theorizations and do not include the study of indigenous (non-settler) societies through their own literature and practitioners.

It is not difficult to see the close relationship between the micro-parasites and the macro-parasites (i.e. the colonizers). Control over one was crucial to the success of the other. Yet, some scholars argue that its role in the 'stabilization of colonial rule was far more limited'. This role was conditioned and constricted by the values, opinions and opposition of the indigenous society and the ground realities of a colonial economy.[48] This is a valid but limited argument. Parasitology had given many colonizers (especially those with lofty utilitarian views) a sense of purpose and a practical programme. It enabled and emboldened the colonizer, and sustained by this new will, the microscope supplanted the sword.[49] Given the political will, it was possible to move and deliver. Haffkine (a vaccine pioneer, 1860–1930) could show charts of success when he had political support, and he flopped the moment it was withdrawn.

In the given scenario of complete hegemonization, the possibilities of inter-cultural interactions were rather limited. The indigenous systems felt so marginalized that they sought survival more in resistance than in collaboration. Total acceptance of new knowledge sometimes did mean total rejection of the old. Under such pressure some of the 'old' withdrew into their own shell. Yet, the majority of Indians favoured revival and synthesis. There were several areas in which the western and indigenous systems could have collaborated but did not. The former put emphasis on the cause of the disease, the latter on *nidana* (treatment). Microbes and microscopes constituted the new medical spectacle. But the *vaidyas* put emphasis on the power of resistance in the human body. 'The improvement of the *kshetra* (body of the patient) is far more important than the microbe and its destruction.'[50] The westerners were forced to take cognizance of indigenous drugs, and the *vaidyas* took to anatomy, ready delivery of medicines, quick relief and so forth. But the comparison ends here. As a recent critique argues, they were inclined to borrow but could not 'create a dialogue between the two epistemies'.[51] Borrowed knowledge seldom develops into organic knowledge. This was true also of the hundreds of doctors produced annually by the government medical colleges. In the melée, some really good opportunities were lost. All guns were targeted at the government: 'Let the government renounce its special care for English medicines. When fought on equal fields we can see the valour of this unscientific system. Then only we can understand whether native medicine is relevant to science and how far the science of English medicine is magnificent.'[52]

Such criticisms were never taken seriously by the practioners of western medicine. Perhaps they were too sure of their competence and superiority. They continued to ridicule the 'other'. As a professor of physiology at Lucknow wrote: 'The financing of Unani and Ayurvedic institutes by Government in the hope of finding some soul of goodness in them is precisely on a par with the same Government financing archery clubs to find out the possibilities of the bow and arrow in modern warfare.'[53]

In the midst of claims and counter-claims, we probably need to desist from building disciplinary enclaves, be it from the colonizer's perspective or from an inward-looking nationalist viewpoint.[54] Critical contextualism may give us better insights. I hope the papers presented here stand this test.

Permit me to end on a personal note. This volume is dedicated to the memory of two distinguished scholars, Debiprasad Chattopadhyay and Srinivasa Ambirajan. They differed greatly—one a Marxist philosopher, the other a liberal economist—yet both emphasized and practised critical contextualism. Academically I owe a great deal to them.

This volume would not have been possible without the affectionate supervision of Professor Irfan Habib and Professor Shireen Moosvi. My students Radha Gayathri, Dhrub Kumar Singh and Savitri Das Sinha gave critical comments and added to the bibliography.

Notes and References

1 B. Gholson et al. (eds), *Psychology of Science: Contributions to Metascience*, Cambridge, 1989, p. 442.

2 Deepak Kumar, 'Science and Society in Colonial India: Exploring an

Agenda', Presidential Address, Modern India Section, *Proceedings of the Indian History Congress*, Aligarh, 2000, pp. 434–55.

3 M.S. Khan, 'Qadi Said-al-Aludalusi's Account of Ancient Indian Sciences and Culture', *Journal of The Pakistan Historical Society*, XLV, 1997, pp. 1–31.

4 Debiprasad Chattopadhyay, *Science and Society in Ancient India*, Calcutta, 1977, p. 7.

5 Bhagvat Singjee, *Aryan Medical Science*, 1895, rpt, Delhi, 1993; U.C. Dutt and G. King, *The Materia Medica of the Hindus*, Calcutta, 1922; Shiv Sharma, *The System of Ayurveda*, 1929, rpt, Delhi, 1993; J. Filliozat, *La Doctrine Classique de la medicine indienne*, translated by Dev Raj Chanana, Delhi, 1964; P.V. Sharma, *History of Medicine in India*, New Delhi, 1992.

6 Apart from intrinsic interest, this trend owes a great deal to the funds and facilities provided by the Wellcome Trust, London.

7 In the Indian context the important ones are: Poonam Bala, *Imperialism and Medicine in Bengal: A Socio-Historical Perspective*, New Delhi, 1991; David Arnold, *Colonizing the Body: State Medicine and Epidemic Disease in Nineteenth Century India*, Delhi, 1993; Mark Harrison, *Public Health in British India, 1854–1914*, Cambridge, 1994; Anil Kumar, *Medicine and the Raj*, New Delhi, 1998; Biswamoy Pati and Mark Harrison (eds), *Health, Medicine and Empire: Perspectives on Colonial India*, New Delhi, 2001.

8 Bruno Latour, *The Pasteurization of France*, Massachusetts, 1988; Deepak Kumar, 'Colony under a Microscope: The Medical Works of W.H. Haffkine', *Science, Technology and Society*, IV, 2, 1999, pp. 239–71.

9 Mary Lindemann, *Medicine and Society in Early Modern Europe*, Cambridge, 1999, p. 1.

10 A very recent example of a personalized and romantic account of medical history in the Indian context is K. Rajsekharan Nair, *Evolution of Modern Medicine in Kerala*, Trivandrum, 2001.

11 K.G. Zysk, *Asceticism and Healing in India*, Delhi, 1991, and *Medicine in the Veda*, Delhi, 1996; F. Zimmermann, *The Jungle and the Aroma of Meat: An Ecological Theme in Hindu Medicine*, Berkeley, 1987; Zysk, Meulenbeld, Wujastyk (eds), *Studies on Indian Medical History*, Groningen, 1987.

12 Ole Brunn and Arnae Kalland (eds), *Asian Perceptions of Nature*, London, 1995.

13 R.C. Majumdar's enthusiastic account of Ayurveda is an example. See D.M. Bose et al. (eds), *A Concise History of Science in India*, New Delhi, 1971, pp. 213–62.

14 This question is relevant for our own time as well. If a particular political dispensation imposes astro-medicine, should our medical institutions accept it?

15 D. Chattopadhyay, *Science and Society*.

16 Pervez Hoodbhoy, *Islam and Science: Religious Orthodoxy and the Battle for Rationality*, London, 1991, p. 120.

17 'The intellectual portion of the community being thus withdrawn from

active participation in the arts, the how and why of phenomena—the coordination of cause and effect—were lost sight of—the spirit of enquiry gradually died out. Her [India's] soil was rendered morally unfit for the birth of a Boyle, a Descartes, or a Newton.' P.C. Ray, *History of Hindu Chemistry*, II, Calcutta, 1909, p. 195.

[18] Athar Ali, 'The Eighteenth Century: An Interpretation', *Indian Historical Review*, 1–2, 1979, pp. 175–86.

[19] Quoted in Irfan Habib, 'Capacity of Technological Change in Mughal India', in A. Roy and A.K. Bagchi, *Technology in Ancient and Medieval India*, Delhi, 1986, pp. 12–13.

[20] Roy Porter, *Disease, Medicine and Society in England 1550–1860*, Cambridge, 1993, p. 2.

[21] D.V. Hart, *Bmisayan Filipino and Malayan Humoral Pathologies: Folk medicine and ethno-history in South East Asia*, Data Paper No. 76, Cornell University, Ithaca.

[22] Elaborating on the history of tuberculosis, a new work has called for a new kind of history of disease that proceeds 'from the perspective of the patient' rather than the doctor. For details see, Shiela Rothman, *Living in the Shadow of Death: Tuberculosis and the Social Experience of Illness in American History*, New York, 1994.

[23] Alan Bewell, *Romanticism and Colonial Disease*, Baltimore, 1999, p. 24.

[24] C. Hamlin, *Public Health and Social Justice in the Age of Chadwick: Britain 1800–1854*, Cambridge, 1998, pp. 1–14.

[25] K.G. Zysk, 'Mantra in Ayurveda: A study of the use of magico-religious speech in ancient India', in Alper Harvey (ed.), *Understanding the Mantra*, New York, 1985.

[26] Dominik Wujastyk, *The Roots of Ayurveda*, New Delhi, 1998, pp. 1–38.

[27] Ibid.

[28] The manuscript was first printed by Nawal Kishore Press, Lucknow, in 1877.

[29] G.J. Meulenbeld, 'The Many Faces of Ayurveda', *Journal of the European Ayurvedic Society*, 4, 1995, pp. 1–9.

[30] S.H. Askari, 'Medicines and Hospitals in Muslim India', *Journal of Bihar Research Society*, 43, 1957, pp. 7–21.

[31] D.V. Subba Reddy, 'Dar-us-Shifa built by Sultan Muhammad Quli: The first Unani teaching hospital in Deccan', *Indian Journal of History of Medicine*, II, 1957, pp. 102–05.

[32] A. Rahman (ed.), *Science and Technology in Medieval India: A Bibliography of Source Materials in Sanskrit, Arabic and Persian*, New Delhi, 1982, p. 57.

[33] R.L. Verma and N.H. Keswani, 'Unani Medicine in Medieval India: Its Teachers and Texts', in N.H. Keswani (ed.), *The Science of Medicine in Ancient and Medieval India*, New Delhi, 1974, pp. 127–42.

[34] Hakim Abdul Hameed, *Exchanges between India and Central Asia in the Field of Medicine*, New Delhi, 1986, p. 41.

[35] A. Rahman (ed.), *Science and Technology in Medieval India*, p. 165.

[36] A European traveller, Edward Ives (1755–57) thus writes of the Indian belief

that 'man was divided into two or three hundred thousand part; ten thousand of which were made up of veins, ten thousand of nerves; seventeen thousand of blood, and a certain number of bones, choler, lymph, etc. And all this was laid down without form or order, either of history, disease or treatment.' Quoted in H.K. Kaul, *Travellers India: An Anthology*, Delhi, 1979, p. 299.

[37] For details see John M.de Figueredo, 'Ayurvedic Medicine in Goa according to European sources in the sixteenth and seventeenth centuries', *Bulletin of History of Medicine*, 58, 2, 1984, pp. 225–35.

[38] A. Neelmeghan, 'Medical Notes in John Ovington's Travelogue', *Indian Journal of History of Medicine*, VII, 1962, pp. 12–21.

[39] J.Z. Holwell, *An account of the manner of innoculating for the small pox in the East Indies*, London, 1767, p. 24.

[40] M.N. Pearson, 'The Thin End of the Wedge: Medical Relativities as a Paradigm of Early Modern Indian–European Relations', *Modern Asian Studies*, 29, 1, 1995, pp. 141–70.

[41] Variolation, for example, impressed them most. Dharampal (ed.), *Indian Science and Technology in the Eighteenth Century: Some Contemporary European Accounts*, Delhi, 1971, pp. 141–63.

[42] Lenore Manderson, *Sickness and the State: Health and Illness in Colonial Malaya 1870–1940*, Cambridge, 1996, pp. 10–14.

[43] F. Cooper and A.L. Stoler (eds), *Tensions of Empire: Colonial Cultures in a Bourgeois World*, Berkeley, 1997, p. xi.

[44] B. Surendra Rao, 'The "Modern" in Modern Indian History', Presidential Address, Modern Indian History Section, *Indian History Congress Proceedings*, Calcutta, 2001, p. 22.

[45] Donald Denoon, *Public Health in Papua New Guinea*, Cambridge, 1889, p. 52.

[46] Heather Bell, *Frontiers of Medicine in the Anglo-Egyptian Sudan, 1899–1940*, Oxford, 1999, p. 10.

[47] David Arnold (ed.), *Warm Climates and Western Medicine: The Emergence of Tropical Medicine 1500–1900*, Amsterdam, 1996.

[48] Mark Harrison, *Public Health in British India*, pp. 228–34.

[49] Warwick Anderson, 'Laboratory Medicine as a Colonial Discourse', *Critical Inquiry*, 18, pp. 506–29.

[50] *Dhanwantari* (Malayalam), 4 February 1925, pp. 133–35; see also G. Srinivasa Murti, *The Science and the Art of Indian Medicine*, Madras, 1948, pp. 139–42.

[51] K.N. Panikkar, 'Indigenous Medicine and Cultural Hegemony: A Study of the Revitalization Movement in Keralam', *Studies in History*, 8, 2, 1992, pp. 283–307.

[52] *Dhanwantari*, 18 October 1920, p. 146.

[53] *Indian Medical Gazette*, 62, 1927, p. 223.

[54] Warwick Anderson, 'Where is the Postcolonial History of Medicine', *Bulletin of History of Medicine*, 72, 1998, pp. 522–30.

Pre-Modern India

Disease, Surgery and Health in the Harappan Civilization

Suraj Bhan and K.S. Dahiya

Until recently, health was generally understood as the absence of disease or infirmity. Medical science has gradually realized that poverty and related social conditions like poor sanitation are a major cause of ill health. Studies have shown that people's health improves remarkably when the basic requisites of good health such as nutrition, safe drinking water, hygiene and sanitation become available to them and when the conditions of stress and violence are controlled. Important technical advances in medical science to control infectious diseases and social efforts to extend medical coverage, as in the use of 'barefoot doctors' in China, the Mexican health workers' programme under David Werner and the Jamkhed programme in India, have also been credited with remarkable improvements in public health.

In the absence of the decipherment of the Harappan script, there is no direct means of knowing the Harappans' state of knowledge about medicine and health. Health conditions in the Harappan civilization can be inferred from two categories of data that may be designated as (a) cultural evidence and (b) biological evidence. The cultural data throw light on the concept and access of the Harappans to nutrition, safe drinking water, and hygienic and civic facilities. They give evidence of the preventive health measures adopted by the Harappans as early as *c.* 250–1900 BC. Biological evidence from the excavated Harappan sites can help us trace diseases or infirmities prevalent during those times and the curative measures taken, including surgery. The skeletal evidence can be further supplemented by traces of herbal plants, minerals, instruments, etc., used for treatment. Attempts of a symbolic and ritualistic nature are hardly meaningful, since these do not enhance our understanding of the growth of medical ideas and practices in history.

3

Cultural Evidence on Hygienic/Sanitary Conditions and Nutrition

The Harappan civilization represents a historical stage (*c.* 2500–1900 BC) characterized by the growth of urbanization in the Copper–Bronze Age tradition. It is distinguished by a hierarchy of settlements ranging from urban centres (the largest being 200 hectares in area) to rural villages and camp-sites. Large-scale excavations at more than two dozen urban sites have revealed different features in terms of time and space. The major cities are found divided into two portions, the citadel and the fortified lower town in the Indus valley, and an acropolis and the lower town within fortification walls in Gujarat and Kutch. Both parts of the cities are well planned with wide streets and public drainage and soakage systems. We have wells and/or water-storage tanks (in Gujarat and Kutch),[1] and find separate baths and kitchens in houses connected with the public drains and soakage jars. Some of the houses were equipped with privies. The cities thus reveal a high level of civic and hygienic standards within their walls. Greater care in these matters is found in the citadel and acropolis areas than in other parts of the cities.

Similar attention to hygiene, however, does not appear to have been paid to the outskirts of the cities, to control pollution. The cemeteries and brick-and-pottery kilns were located just outside the cities. The clay dug for the manufacture of bricks and pottery on an extensive scale must have left behind large pits and ponds, resulting in the stagnation of rain water.[2] The public drains also possibly discharged into the moats or ponds outside the citadel, acropolis or lower towns.[3] The disposal of cowdung and night soil, the general habit of answering calls of nature in the open, and the disposal of carcasses of dead animals outside the towns must have further polluted the environs of the cities. The hygienic conditions could also have been affected by recurring floods in the rivers, leaving behind swamps and stagnating waters in ponds and pools, ideal breeding ground for mosquitoes and flies.[4]

Diet and Nutrition

The Harappan civilization was sustained by a relatively advanced stage of agriculture marked by the use of the plough and artificial irrigation. The peasants cultivated both the *rabi* and *kharif* crops, growing wheat, barley, millet, pulses, oil-seeds, etc.[5] The dis-covery of granaries and bins speak of storage by peasants to meet scarcities. People supplemented their diet by keeping cattle, fishing, hunting and gathering wild plants, fruits and roots. Their meat intake depended heavily on domesticated cattle, as 50 per cent of the bones recovered from the cities were of domesticated cattle. Wild fruit included the jujube. The foodgrains were milled with the help of grind-ing stones. Food was cooked in *tandoors* and ovens in earthen and copper utensils. So far as we can judge from the evidence at urban sites, it appears that the Harappans ate soft (i.e. well-cooked and/or ground) food.

Biological Evidence on Disease, Surgery and Health

Skeletal remains constitute a major source of information on diseases that affected the Harappans. Early studies of skeletal biology mainly concentrated on the racial features of the skeletons even though the notion of race was abandoned by population geneticists and syste-matic biologists over seventy years ago.[6] Biological anthropologists too have discarded it since the 1960s.

Recently, biological studies have been undertaken to answer a number of questions which can, indeed, be answered from the archaeological record.[7] The new questions asked include: distribution of individuals by age and sex; the health status, nutrition and stature of individuals; the kinds of diseases from which people suffered; the marks of occupational stress (MOS) resulting from habitual physical activities, both behavioural activities and labour practices.

General Health

Not much attention was paid in the early work on the skeletal evidence in respect of matters like sex ratio and life expectancy among different age groups and the living stature ratio between sexes. How-ever, evidence from the excavations at Harappa, Mohenjodaro, Lothal and Kalibangan in the last three decades has thrown some light on such questions.

Sex ratio

The sex ratio determined on the basis of skeletons recovered from Harappa in 1987–88 must be regarded as tentative. The reason is that only 34 of the skeletons recovered happened to be complete, and 7 of these revealed no certain gender characteristics. Kennedy has identified 10 as males and 17 as females out of the 27 reliable skeletons.[8] This gives the proportion of 37 per cent males and 63 per cent females.

Life expectancy

The 34 skeletons studied from Harappa (1987–88 excavation) yield the following ages at death:[9]

Young adults (16–35 years)	18	(53%)
Middle-aged adults (36–55 years)	11	(33%)
Children (3.5–12 years)	1	(3%)
Infants (below 3.5 years)	2	(6%)
Adults of uncertain age	2	(6%)

The validity of the life expectancy of the Harappan population from the limited data needs to be further substantiated by more studies. The present evidence suggests the highest mortality rate among young adults (16–35 years).

Physical stature

The stature attained by the Harappans has been studied by B.K. Chatterjee (1973).[10] It has been calculated on the basis of the formulae propounded by Manouvrier and Karl Pearson, using skeletons at Harappa of 75 adult males, 92 adult females, 7 juveniles, and 49 infants and children. The gender differences in the living statures established by the study are as under:

(i) Male height	1837–1519 mm	
Average height	1674.84 mm	
(ii) Female height	1636–1463 mm	
Average height	1545.61 mm	

Another 8 skeletons from Lothal were studied by Chatterjee and Kumar. These comprised 4 males and 4 females. Sarkar studied 20 skeletons. He identified among them an overwhelming majority of male adults (15). They too belonged to the age group of 20–30 years.[11]

Disease

Disease describes the physical condition of the individual which causes some discomfort and hinders the normal functioning of the body. Its recognition, diagnosis and treatment varies from culture to culture. Although few, studies made from this angle have brought forth evidence related to dental diseases, deformity, paralysis, arthritis, arrested growth, malaria, delivery death and trauma. A brief account of the same is given here.

Dental pathology

We have very little information on the dental health of the Harappans from earlier excavations. The primary, secondary and isolated dental samples from Cemetery R–37 at Harappa excavated during 1987–88 have been studied by John R. Lukacs of the University of California.[12]

The most frequent dental disorder, according to this study, is gross linear enamel hypoplasia, found in 72.2 per cent of 36 individuals. Hypercementosis (4.9 per cent) was the least frequent condition. Other dental afflictions include: (1) abscesses, 18.4 per cent; (2) exposure of the pulp chamber, 17.1 per cent; (3) antemortem tooth loss, 31.7 per cent; (4) calculus, 42.5 per cent; (5) dental caries, 43.6 per cent; and (6) alveolar resorption, 52.6 per cent.

Sex differences in the dental health of the Harappans are most prominent in antemortem tooth loss and hypoplasia. The teeth of males and females exhibit similar rates of caries throughout the dentition. In one case a female skeleton showed exceptional high frequency of caries in the maxillary anterior teeth (incisors and canines). This deviation from the normal pattern of the number of caries in the anterior teeth suggests important dietary differences based on sex or occupational specialization. The main conclusions of the study by Lukacs are as follows:

(i) The dental pathology profile at Harappa conforms to an agricultural mode of subsistence with use of soft food.

(ii) Gross enamel hypoplasia is the most common dental disease and hypercementosis the least common.

(iii) Dental caries are observed in 43.6 per cent of the individuals examined.

(iv) Antemortem tooth loss (AMTL), calculus (mineralization of bacterial plaque) and alveolar resorption reveal moderate incidence.

(v) Dental caries analysed by tooth-count method revealed a rate of 6.8 per cent.

(vi) Dental diseases such as enamel hypoplasia, AMTL, caries and pulp exposure reveal different rates for the two sexes.

Arrested growth

Three cases of arrested growth in childhood were found from the excavation at Harappa (1987–88) under radiographic observations of long bones.[13] R.H. Meadow has suggested that the halting of growth lines on the bones results from malnutrition or acute illness.

Arthritis

It is the most common condition, generally occurring in the spine and joints of the knee, hands and feet, and normally associated with old age. Several cases of severe arthritis in the neck including fusion of adjacent elements have been identified in the skeletons from Harappa (1987–88). This is thought to be the result of unusual stress on the neck vertebrae, possibly on account of heavy loads carried on the head as in the case of coolies.

Deformities

The study of skeletons from Kalibangan by A.K. Sharma has brought to light some evidence of skeletal deformities.[15] According to him the skeleton of a 30-year-old crippled man revealed bones of the left hand, radius and ulna marked by pathological deformities. The carpals and meta-carpals were badly twisted outwards to the left. The left hand radius and ulna were smaller than their counterparts in the right hand. The flanges of the left foot were represented by only rudimentary bones riding over each other.

Paralysis

A.K. Sharma has reported a skeleton dumped carelessly upside down in a crouching position from the Kalibangan cemetery. The grave yielded three pots as funerary goods. According to Sharma, the position of the limbs and the torso suggests that it was a case of paralysis where rigor mortis had set in before the body was buried in the grave.

Delivery death

The skeleton of a young female (21–25 years) with an infant under her lower right leg was found from Harappa (1987–88). The long bone-length of the infant indicates that 'it was very young, perhaps a newborn'. The circumstantial evidence suggests a mother–child relationship between the two and a case of delivery death.[16]

Malaria

There is no direct evidence for the incidence of malaria. Yet studies by Dutta and Kennedy have an important bearing on the problem. A case of chronic anaemia syndrome resulting in bilateral thinning of parietal bones in a Harappan skeleton was pointed out by Dutta in 1969. A re-investigation of the skeletons from Mohenjodaro by K.A.R. Kennedy revealed varying degrees of porotic hyperostosis modification among several skeletons. Further studies of skeletal evidence from other urban sites show that 25 per cent of the total Harappan data examined by him in 1964, 1977 and 1980 bore porotic hyperostosis deformity in both sexes and all ages. According to Kennedy this suggests the presence of either thalassemia or sicklaemia or both categories of disease. The condition relates to inheritance of abnormal haemoglobins. Kennedy further pointed out that the diagnosis of the above pathological variables among the Harappans has an implication for the incidence of malaria there.[17]

Incidence of malaria in the Harappan civilization has also been inferred from the circumstantial evidence of sanitary conditions in the outskirts of cities which provided breeding ground for the mosquito and the fly. The prevalence of conditions conducive to the spread of malaria must have increased owing to the deterioration of civic standards in the later phase of Mohenjodaro and other cities. The intermittent recurrence of abnormal floods[18] must have resulted in swamps and bodies of stagnant water in the pits dug for clay needed for bricks and pottery. Carelessness in the discharge of the public drains outside the citadel, acropolis or city, and any failure to maintain the irrigation channels could have added to the deterioration of hygienic conditions. The problem may have been further aggravated by the disposal of cowdung, night-soil, etc., outside the cities. Such a social and environmental situation would have created the necessary conditions for the incidence of water- and vector-borne diseases like malaria.

The study of skeletal evidence from Harappa (1987–88 excavation) through microscopic and radiographic examinations reveals low incidence of traumatic injuries and chronic infectious diseases, and absence of malignant neoplastic diseases. A scaphocephalic skull revealed developmental abnormality. But there were no cases of rickets, scurvy or anaemia, which result from malnutrition, among the population of the city.

Trauma

Violence perpetrated on the human body resulting in death can be recognized by traces left on the bones in the form of cut-marks, fractures, removal of bone at cranial base, and decapitation of skulls and cervical vertebrae. Excavations at Mohenjodaro by Sir John Marshall and Mackay brought to light 37 skeletons of men, women and children lying helter-skelter in rooms, streets, lanes, courtyards or staircases within the habitation area. There was no evidence of any ceremonial disposal of the dead. The circumstances led Marshall to suggest sudden death owing to plague or famine as the cause of this unusual phenomenon.[19] Mackay assigned the skeletons from his excavation to the Late Indus period and postulated a military attack leading to the slaughter of the residents trying to escape.[20] The physical anthropologists Sewell and Guha, and Guha and Basu, studied the physical characteristics of these skeletons and supported the thesis of a traumatic end of these residents by identifying cut-marks and fractures on their bones.[21] Wheeler used these findings to suggest that Mohenjodaro suffered a sacking by invaders, followed by a massacre of its residents in Late Harappan times.[22]

The thesis of a traumatic end of the people at Mohenjodaro was challenged by Dales after the site was re-excavated by him in 1964.[23] He found that all the skeletons at Mohenjodaro, though lying haphazardly, did not come from the same temporal and cultural context. Nor were the skeletons associated with any arms or armour that would imply physical assault.

The biological evidence from Mohenjodaro has also been re-examined by K.A.R. Kennedy to evaluate signs of traumatic stress, etc., on bones.[24] Kennedy found only two cases of trauma, one being Skeleton 10 of the Marshall series and the other Skeleton DK 7411 (Male 27) of the Mackay series, which could have caused death.

Although Dales and Kennedy have been able to rule out the possibility of a single massacre of people at Mohenjodaro, they have not been able to explain satisfactorily the unceremonial disposal of bodies of men, women and children, at least two of whom bear telltale marks of trauma on their bodies. Besides, one need not expect markings on skeletons in all cases of traumatic death. Death by damage of soft tissues and excessive bleeding, strangulation and cardiac arrest due to fright, cannot be ruled out. Even in cases of head injury, death can take place without fracture of the skull bones because of injury to the brain.

Surgery

Although several types of diseases have been identified from skeletal biology, there is very limited data on their treatment. The only certain evidence on curative health is in respect of trephining or trepanation.

Trephining

This was possibly one of the earliest forms of surgical operations on the skull. In the operation, a piece of calvarium was removed from the human skull without damaging the blood vessels, meninges and the brain. The practice was quite widespread in prehistoric times. Indigenous medicine-men still practise it in several parts of the world. Trephination involves a high degree of technical skill. The number of survivals after trephination attests the competence of the surgeons.

The prevalence of trephining in the Neolithic Age in France was detected by Paul Broca, a famous French physical anthropologist of the nineteenth century. It was occasionally performed by the early Danubians, around c. 3000 BC. The people of the Battle Axe culture of France (c. 2000 BC) practised it frequently. Other Neolithic peoples of Europe are also reported to have practised it. Its rarity later may be partly because in the Later Bronze Age and the La Tene period, after the practice of cremation came into vogue, skeletons could not survive. The practice however survived, as is evidenced by the fact that Hippocrates (c. 460–377 BC) recommended trephination for head injuries.

In India, the technique of trephining surgery is known from the historical Buddhist and Ayurvedic literature. The earliest biological evidence for this comes from Lothal and Kalibangan and so goes back to the Harappan culture. At Lothal the evidence comes from the skeleton of an 8–9-year-old child. The skull of the child seems to have been pierced by an instrument to cut a hole into it. In the absence of any trace of healing at the bone ends, it seems the child could not have survived long after the surgical operation.[25] The trephining at Kalibangan is attested by the skull of a child buried in the cemetery.[26] The skull revealed two holes joined by a black line. Does this suggest the process of insensitization of the veins by branding them with a heated metal object before undertaking the operation? The head of the child happened to be unusually large. This may be due to excessive accumulation of fluid in the brain cells, causing it to swell.

Conclusions

It bears repeating that we have no archaeological and biological evidence on the total life-conditions of the Harappan civilization in the absence of horizontal excavations of village and camp sites. Thus, our picture of the civilization has an urban bias. Our study of disease, surgery and health pertains only to urban Harappan centres. But even here our information on the social background of the diseased with special reference to class and gender is limited. The lack of relevant information from the graveyards denies us the opportunity to know about the social status of the affected people. How women were physically treated has yet to be studied from the Harappan remains. The re-examination of the Mohenjodaro skeletons by K.A.R. Kennedy shows that Skeletons 1 and 10 of the Marshall series bear evidence of blows on the skulls of the women, and could be taken as evidence of brutal treatment. The fact that the stature of Harappan females is distinctly shorter than that of the males may also reflect disparity in the nutrition of the two sexes.

Much has been written on the measures taken by urban authorities in Harappan towns with regard to sanitation and hygiene, clean drinking water and a pollution-free environment within the citadels and cities. They also took steps to meet natural calamities by storing grain in large granaries for the ruling class at least, if not for the urban population as a whole. But there is little evidence on curative health except for the evidence on surgery, which too is limited to trephining. We can say, however, that the Harappans did not know the technique of tooth-filling. Lastly, it may be pointed out that sole reliance on skeletal remains for understanding the health-conditions of a people has its own limitations. What is further needed is analysis of other categories of evidence, such as study of nutrition, instruments and data on herbal medicines, along with the social factors affecting individuals' health.

Notes and References

1 The tank at Lothal was identified as a dockyard. (S.R. Rao, *Lothal: A Harappan Port Town (1955–62)*, Vol. I, New Delhi, 1979, pp. 123–36.) A number of serious archaeologists have challenged this view and identified the structure as a tank. See L. Leshnick, 'The Harappan Port at Lothal: Another View', *American Anthropologist*, 70, No. 5, 1968, pp. 911–22; Suman Pandya, 'Lothal dockyard hypothesis and sea level changes', in *Ecology and Archaeology of Western India*, Delhi, 1977, pp. 99–103. For the tank at Dholavira, see R.S. Bisht, 'Dholavira and Banawali', *Puratattva*, No. 29, 1998–99, pp. 14–32.

2 A similar phenomenon could be seen on the outskirts of the cities and towns until recently, before modern brick kilns (*bhathhas*) appeared.

3 The public drainage at Lothal discharged outside the acropolis on the north as well as to the south. A similar phenomenon is noticed at Mohenjodaro and several other sites.

4 R.E.M. Wheeler, *The Indus Civilization*, 3rd edn, Cambridge, 1968, p. 129.

5 S. Ratnagar, 'An Aspect of Harappan Agricultural Production', in *Studies in History*, 2, 1986, pp. 137–53; Vishnu Mitre and R. Savithri, 'Food Economy of the Harappans', in G.L. Possehl (ed.), *Harappan Civilization: A Contemporary Perspective*, New Delhi, 1982, pp. 205–21.

6 K.A.R. Kennedy, Brian E. Hamphill and John R. Luckacs, 'Bring Back the Bones: The Hard Evidence', in *Man and Environment*, XXV, 1, 2000, p. 105.

7 G.L. Possehl, *Indus Age: The Beginnings*, New Delhi, 1999, pp. 27–35.

8 K.A.R. Kennedy and Nancy Lovell, 'Morphology, diet and pathology', *Pakistan Archaeology*, pp. 94–106.

9 Ibid.

10 B.K. Chatterjee and G.D. Kumar, 'Oesteometric Variations of Human Skeletal Remains since Neolithic and Chalcolithic Periods of Indian Subcontinent', in *Indian Museum Bulletin*, Calcutta, 1981, pp. 31–38.

11 S.R. Rao, *Lothal: A Harappan Port Town*, pp. 137–69.

12 John R. Luckacs, 'Dental Paleopathology and Agricultural Intensification in South Asia: New Evidence from Bronze Age Harappa', *American Journal of Physical Anthropology*, Vol. 20, 1991; and Hemphil, Lukacs and Kennedy, 'Biological Adaptations and Affinities of Bronze Age Harappans', in Richard H. Meadow (ed.), *Harappa Excavations 1986–90: A multi-disciplinary approach to 3rd millennium urbanism*, 1991, pp. 137–81.

13 R.H. Meadow (ed.), *Harappa Excavations*, pp. 185–262. S.R. Walimbe and P.B. Gambhir, 'Harris Lines: An Indicator of Physiological stress', *Man and Environment*, XV, 2, 1990, pp. 63–69.

14 A.K. Sharma, 'The Harappa Cemetery at Kalibangan: A Study', in G.L. Possehl, *Harappan Civilization*, pp. 297–99.

15 Ibid., p. 298.

16 *Pakistan Archaeology*, 24, Karachi, 1989, pp. 91–93: Fig. 34, 194a and 194b.

17 K.A.R. Kennedy, 'Trauma and Disease in the Ancient Harappans', in B.B.

Lal and S.P. Gupta (eds), *Frontiers of Indus Civilization*, pp. 425–36.

[18] R.E.M. Wheeler, *The Indus Civilization*, p. 129.

[19] Sir John Marshall (ed.), *Mohenjodaro and the Indus Civilization*, I, 1931, pp. 79–81, 107–08, 184–85, 222–23.

[20] E.J.H. Mackay, *Further Excavations at Mohenjodaro*, I, 1937, pp. 116–18.

[21] R.B.S. Sewell and B.S. Guha, 'Human Remains', in John Marshall (ed.), *Mohenjodaro and the Indus Civilization*, II, pp. 599–684; B.A. Guha and B.C. Basu, 'Report on the Human Remains Excavated at Mohenjodaro, in 1928–29', in E.J.H. Mackay (ed.), *Further Excavations at Mohenjodaro*, I, pp. 613–38.

[22] Sir Mortimer Wheeler, *The Indus Civilization*, 3rd edn, Cambridge, 1968.

[23] G.F. Dales, 'The Mythical Massacre at Mohenjodaro', *Expedition*, 6, 1964, pp. 36–43.

[24] K.A.R. Kennedy, 'Trauma and Disease in the Ancient Harappans', pp. 425–36.

[25] S.R. Rao, *Lothal: A Harappan Port Town*, pp. 145–46.

[26] B.B. Lal, *The Earliest Civilization in South Asia*, Delhi, 1997, pp. 218–19.

Surgery in Early India

A Note on the Development of Medical Science

Vijay Kumar Thakur

The science of medicine in early India, unlike the other primitive sciences—phonetics (*shiksha*), grammar (*vyakarana*), etymology (*nirukta*), metrics (*chandas*), calendrical astronomy (*jyotisha*), and even geometry, in the restricted sense of being a part of ritual technique (*kalpa*)—that originated in the priestly circles, thus carrying with them the birth-pangs of anti-secularism and facing almost insurmountable constraints in developing towards science proper, is marked by a momentous transmutation quite early in its life from magico-religious therapeutics to rational therapeutics, that is, in the terminology of the famous medicine-man Charaka himself, from *daiva-vyapashraya bheshaja* to *yukti-vyapashraya bheshaja*. To the modern mind this laboured departure of the medical science from the all-pervasive dominant ecclesiastical tradition may not seem to be a very significant development, but even a minimal insight into the dynamics of power and the nature of the prevailing ideology of those times brings into bold relief the revolutionary nature of the profession vis-à-vis the orthodox milieu in which it was rooted. The hegemonic regime of mysticism, ritualism and religion, sanctified by powerful priestly corporations and ideologically sustained by the contemporary brahmanical law-givers, came to be inadvertently questioned by the doctors in their quest for a scientific base for their profession. This was sacrilege, an attack on the very constructed belief system from which the hierarchical society drew its sustenance. The established order and its protagonists, not incidentally therefore, start condemning the doctors right from the time of the *Yajurveda*. In fact the doctors had to pay a heavy price for their fight for scientific knowledge in an age dominated by religious orthodoxy and intense ideological involution—from a respectable position in the Rigvedic society, they were downgraded to the status of

15

shudras by the beginning of the early historical period. Despite this official condemnation and ritual degradation, the medicine-men kept the torch of a scientific–rational spirit burning in early India. The surgeons deserve special credit on this count because, unlike the physicians, they sought to interfere with and alter the anatomical structure that was 'divinely ordained', and for this they could not take recourse to any linguistic camouflage. This distance between the physician and the surgeon in early India is brought to the fore in the course of a comparative analysis of the formulations of Charaka, the physician, and Sushruta, the surgeon. Despite both the compilations having similar contents, analogous divisions and corresponding theoretical and practical ideas, it is the *Sushrutasamhita* that is surprisingly free from the priestly bias superimposed on medicine. 'Charaka, in his writings, has a combined role of moralist, philosopher, and above all a physician; whereas, Sushruta has tried to cast off whatever shackles of priestly domination remained at his time, and created an atmosphere of independent thinking and investigation, which later characterized the Greek medicine.'[1]

The scientific quest for knowledge and the expanding horizon of the medical profession is well articulated in the compilation of a series of texts directly touching upon this theme. The process, which began with the *Yajurveda* and the *Atharvaveda*, though in the garb and under the spell of religious orthodoxy, matured by the time the *Charakasamhita* came to be compiled during the early centuries of the Christian era. The text, which enjoyed great prestige in antiquity, was edited by Dridhabala, a resident of Kashmir in the ninth century AD, and it is in this form that it has come down to us. The significance of the text is borne out by the number of commentaries that it attracted—the eleventh century commentary of Chakrapanidatta entitled the *Charaka-tatparya-tika*, the twelfth century commentary of Hari Chandra, Jaijjata's commentary entitled the *Nirantar-padvyakhya*, Shiva Das's *Charaka-tattva-pradipika*, and Gangadhara's *Jalpa-kalpa-taru* (AD 1879). The original Sanskrit text was translated into Arabic way back at the beginning of the eighth century, and its Arabic name *Sharaka Indianus* finds mention in the Latin translations of Avicenna (Ibn-Sina), Avenzoar (Ibn-Zuhr) and Averroes (Ibn-Rushd). The *Fihrst* (completed in AD 987) refers to a Persian rendering of the *Charakasamhita* and its subsequent translation into Arabic. It is a simple and indubitable argument, therefore, to posit the influence of the Indian system of medicine on both the Arabic and the western systems.

The *Sushrutasamhita*, our main source of knowledge about surgery and anaesthesia, has an uncertain chronology and a second-hand structured format. The text, originally known as the *Shalya-tantra*, was inflated and an *Uttaratantra* was appended to it. The Indian tradition credits Nagarjuna (whose identity remains uncertain) with the reconstruction of the text. Like the *Charakasamhita*, this text too enjoyed great authority and was translated into Arabic as the *Kitab-Shaw-Shoon-a-Hindi* or the *Kitab-i-Susrud* in the eighth century. Subsequently it was translated into Latin and German and it did exercise a meaningful influence on the development of the surgical traditions of these areas. The *Ashtanga Samgraha* and the *Ashtanga Hridaya Samgraha*, both composed by Vagabhata in the seventh century, carry forward the tradition of Sushruta. While the *Ashtanga Samgraha* dwells on both medicine and surgery, the *Ashtanga Hridaya Samgraha* is more concerned with surgical and anaesthetic issues. The two texts underline a distinct improvement in medical knowledge over the *Samhitas* of Charaka and Sushruta. The *Ashtanga Hridaya* attracted as many as eleven commentaries in the indigenous intellectual tradition. The *Nava Nitaka* or the *Bower Manuscript*, referred to by different authorities between the tenth and sixteenth centuries, was possibly compiled in the fourth to fifth centuries under Buddhistic influence, and is essentially a book of prescriptions. The *Bhelasamhita*, the *Chikitsha Kalika* and the *Kashyapasamhita*, all of uncertain authorship and chronology, have a similar content-tenor. The *Roga-Vinishchaya* of Madhavakara, a text of the ninth to tenth centuries, however, makes a departure by describing diseases in their entirety. A contemporary text of the Jaina tradition, the *Kalyana Karaka*, compiled by Ugraditya-charya, concentrated on dietetics and the structure and functions of the body. The concept of *nadipariksha* (pulse examination) was first enunciated in a twelfth-century text, the *Sarangadharasamhita*. A host of other treatises—some lost and some extant—were also composed, and the process continued to enrich the indigenous branch of medical science till the establishment of the colonial hegemony and the consequent evolution of the mechanism of colonial ideological and cultural dominance over Indians.

The developments in surgery, unlike in most of the other branches of primitive science, had the advantage of praxis. Very early in the day, Indian surgeons realized that it was basically futile to go about their work without gaining a sound knowledge of the human anatomy, and that for this there was no substitute to direct observation by dissecting the dead bodies. The *Sushrutasamhita* points out,

> The different parts or members of the body—including the skin—cannot be correctly described by one who is not versed in anatomy. Hence anyone desirous of acquiring a thorough knowledge of anatomy should prepare a dead body and carefully observe, by dissecting it, and examine its different parts. For a thorough knowledge can only be acquired by comparing the accounts given in the *Shastras* (authoritative works on the subject) with direct personal observation.[2]

Dilating on the method of dissection, the text further adds,

> A dead body selected for this purpose should not be wanting in any of its parts, should not be of a person who has lived up to a hundred years (i.e. up to a very old age) or of one who died of any protracted disease or poison. The excrementa should be first removed from the entrails and the body should be left to decompose in the water of a solitary and still pool, and securely placed in a cage (so that it may not be eaten off by fish or drift away), after having covered it entirely with the outer sheaths of *munja* grass, *kusha* grass, hemp or with rope, etc. After seven days the body would be thoroughly decomposed, when the observer should slowly scrape off the decomposed skin etc. with a whisk made of grass-roots, hair, *kusha* blade or with a split bamboo, and carefully observe with his own eyes all the various different organs, internal and external, beginning with the skin as described before.[3]

The obvious difficulty involved in procuring such 'ideal' corpses must have restrained the teachers from handing them over to beginners for mutilation. This possibly explains the ancient surgeons' recommendation for a preparatory course in dissection with the help of dummies, fruits and vegetables before handling the actual corpse. The emphasis on direct observation as the supreme and irreplaceable source of knowledge was sufficient to annoy the upholders of orthodoxy, as this left no scope for the latter's advocacy of implicit faith in the scriptures. Surgery was becoming synonymous with rationality.

The acquisition of this precious fund of knowledge became the most crucial factor for the development of surgery in early India.

For the early Indian doctors, however, the acquisition of knowledge was not an end in itself; it was of significance only in so far as it ensured practical success. The *Charakasamhita* is explicit on this point: 'He is the best of physicians who can, in actual practice, cure people of diseases. Practical success depends on the right application of all the relevant measures. Thus it is practical success which makes one a first rate physician endowed with all the required medical qualifications.'[4] This attitude is markedly different from that of ancient Greece. Despite making meaningful advances in the field of clinical psychology and despite 'prodigies' accomplished by them in the observation of pathological symptoms, the actual therapeutic techniques used by the Greek doctors remained almost devoid of inspiring changes. The lack of congruence between knowledge and practice in the Greek tradition is a point noted by J.D. Bernal too: 'Unfortunately, in spite of their careful clinical studies, the school of Cos (i.e. the Hippocratic School) were also in no position to prescribe effective treatment. They excelled in prognosis and relied on the patient, if not given violent and unsuitable treatment, getting well through the curative power of Nature.'[5] Such criticisms of the Hippocratic doctors abound even in early literature— a Roman physician of the first century BC, Asclepiades, castigated the Hippocratic treatment as a 'mediation upon death'.[6] This assessment of the Greek medical profession remains unchanged throughout history. In 1836, a French doctor, M.S. Hondart, while talking about the Hippocratic doctors,

> violently attacked this medical doctrine on the ground that it neglected the physician's prime duty, which is to effect a cure. 'Diagnosis', he urges, 'is neglected in the cult of prognosis: no attempt is made to localize the seat of disease; the observations in the *Epidemics* are directed towards superficial symptoms without any attempt to trace them to their real cause. The writer is an interested but callous spectator who looks on unmoved while his patient dies.'[7]

The Ayurvedic tradition, unlike the Greek fascination for pure speculation characteristic of the Pythagorean school of philosophy, by laying emphasis on the aspect of actual practice, underlined the importance and necessity of the direct involvement of the doctor with every aspect of the science—from herb collection to the organization of theoretical knowledge. The element that injects vigour and vitality into Ayurvedic surgery in its formative phase is its crucial bond with manual work, or, as B. Farrington puts it, the head being enriched by the working hand. What is the meaning of the word surgery after all? It is but a simple modern rendering of the Greek word *cheirourgia*, which means manual labour. But this basic aspect of the surgical science was completely overwhelmed by the anti-manual labour prejudice of the slave-owning aristocracy of Greece, creating an unbridgeable gap between knowledge and practice. Vesalius documents this chasm,

> when the whole conduct of manual operations was entrusted to barbers, not only did doctors lose the true knowledge of the viscera but the practice of dissection soon died out, doubtless for the reason that the doctors did not attempt to operate, while those to whom the manual skill was assigned were too ignorant to read the writings of the teachers of anatomy. But it is utterly impossible that this class of men should preserve for us a difficult art which they have learnt only mechanically. And equally inevitably this deplorable dismemberment of the art of healing has introduced into our schools the detestable procedure now in vogue, that one man should carry out the dissection of the human body and another give the description of the parts. The latter is perched up aloft in a pulpit like a jackdaw and with a notable air of disdain he drones out information about facts which he has never approached at first hand but which he has committed to memory from the books of others, or of which he has a description before his eyes. The dissector, who is ignorant of languages, is unable to explain the dissection to the class and botches the demonstration which ought to follow the instructions of the physician, while the physician never applies his hand to the task but contemptuously steers the ship out of the manual, as the saying goes. Thus everything is wrongly taught, days are wasted in absurd questions, and in the confusion less is shown to the class than a butcher in his stall could teach a doctor.[8]

The creative phase of surgery in India did not suffer from such a constraint; therefore its superiority over the contemporary western tradition.

The entire corpus of surgical operations in the Indian tradition depends on the primacy accorded to the surgeon's hands, i.e. the attempts to translate into practice the concept of *jitahasta* or deft hands. Thus, the *Sushrutasamhita,* while introducing the discussion on the nature and types of surgical instruments, insists that their importance notwithstanding, the working hand of the surgeon is the most important of them all.

> The number of surgical instruments is one hundred and twenty-one—one hundred and one blunt and twenty sharp. But the hand itself is to be viewed as the most important of the instruments. Why is it so? Because all these instruments are ineffectual without the hand and only as subjected to the hand the instrument acquire their function.[9]

In the course of dilating upon the various aspects of these instruments, the text provides the following details:

> Surgical appliances may be divided into six different groups or types, such as the *svastika*, the *sandamsha*, the *tala*, the *nadi*, the *shalaka*, and the *upayantras* or the minor or accessory appliances. The *svastika* instruments (forceps), in their turn, are divided into twenty-four sub-classes; the *sandamsha* instruments (tongs) into two; the *talayantras* (picklock-like) into two; the *nadiyantras* (tubular) into twenty; and the *shalakas* into twenty-eight; while the *upayantras* admit of being divided into twenty-five different types. These instruments are all made of iron, which may be substituted for any other similar or suitable substance where iron would be unavailable. The mouths of these appliances are usually made to resemble the mouths of some particular animals in shape, or otherwise, according to the advice of old and experienced physicians (surgeons), or according to the directions as laid down in the *Shastras* (medical treatises of recognized authority), or according to the exigencies of the case, or after the shape and structure of other appliances used on similar occasions. Appliances should be made neither too large nor too small, and their mouths or edges should be made sharp and keen. They should be made with a special eye as to strength and steadiness, and they should be provided with convenient handles.[10]

How to get these instruments? 'It is imperative for the intelligent doctor to get his surgical instruments fashioned by the skilled and experienced blacksmith, using pure, strong and tempered iron.'[11] The active cooperation between surgeons and blacksmiths, a reflection on the former's positive attitude towards manual labour, is an indubitable fact of early Indian history.

A surgeon in early India was primarily concerned with the

management and healing of wounds. The *Sushrutasamhita* details sixty procedures for the same, ranging from the earliest manifestation of inflammation to its complete healing. The text is fully conversant with the concept of the pathogenesis of the disease, including wounds in six stages. The surgical procedure too admitted of a three-phase exercise:

Purva Karma	Pradhana Karma	Pashchata Karma
(i) Preparing the patient	i. Surgery	i. Bandaging
(ii) Preparing the operation theatre	ii. Eight surgical procedures	ii. Re-dressing
		iii. Cleaning the wound
(iii) Preparing the instruments		iv. Healing procedures
		v. Cosmetic restoration procedures

Besides providing detailed instructions regarding the pre-operative, operative and post-operative stages, the text cautions the surgeon against the dangers of postponing surgery as well as premature intervention.[12] Excision was prescribed for moles, tumours, piles and enlarged tonsils along with abscesses and other supportive lesions. Veins, hydroceles and ascites were punctured or tapped. Recourse was taken to scraping for chronic non-healing ulcers with hypertrophied lips and other skin lesions.[13] Operative extraction was practised to remove stones, loose teeth, impacted foreign bodies and dead foetuses. Detailed instructions regarding suturing underlines the level of surgical excellence attained by the early Indian doctors. Major operations, including abdominal interventions, paracentesis, carniotomy, cataract and lithotomy have been described in detail in the early Ayurvedic texts.[14]

The domain of 'traumatic orthopaedic surgery' also witnessed impressive advances during the period. Sushruta divides the bones of the body into five categories:

(i) *kapala* or flat bones,

(ii) *ruchaka* or small cubical bones,

(iii) *taruna* or cartilages,

(iv) *valaya* or thin curved bones without a medullary cavity, and

(v) *nalaka*, long bones with medullary cavity.

The following table may provide a better idea of this classificatory scheme:

Sushruta's terminology	Modern terminology	Details of bones included in the list
1. *Kapala*	Flat bones	Patella, hip, scapula, mandible, hard palate, temporal and other skull bones
2. *Ruchaka*	Small cubical bones	Teeth (carpels, etc.)
3. *Taruna*	Cartilages	Nose, ear, throat and eye-socket
4. *Valaya*	Thin curved bones	Ribs
5. *Nalaka*	Long bones	Femur, tebia, febula, humerus, etc.

Sushruta discusses the etiological factors and details the effect of trauma on bones. He classifies bone injuries into two groups: (i) *savranabhanga*, i.e. open or compound injury, and (ii) *avranabhanga*, i.e. simple or closed fracture. He also distinguishes between a fracture and a dislocation. The entire classificatory scheme is extremely interesting: six types of dislocation and twelve types of fracture. The methods of reduction and immobilization were known, and precautions were taken against infections. Besides taking recourse to splintage by healthy limb, a host of other techniques and rehabilitational exercises were adopted to treat limb injuries.

The developments in surgical practice notwithstanding, the ancient Indian doctors do not seem to have possessed a high degree of knowledge about anaesthesia. It is rather surprising to note that in the fairly advanced treatises on Ayurveda, there is no reference either to an anaesthetic or the science of anaesthesia, suggesting without doubt the absence of development in this area during that period. This situation becomes almost inexplicable if one keeps in mind the numerous indications pointing to the necessity felt by the contemporary surgeons, for an agent to produce insensibility to pain. Interestingly, wine was being used to produce this effect, a point made by both Charaka and Sushruta. The following provision of Charaka, though unconventional in nature, is illustrative of this practice: 'After extraction of a dead foetus before the full term of pregnancy, wine should be prescribed for her, for that will improve the condition of her uterus, make her happy and alleviate the pain of the operations.'[15] Sushruta more specifically provides that 'wine should be used before operation to produce insensibility to pain'. He further prescribes:

It is desirable that the patient should be fed before being operated upon. Those who are addicted to drink and those who cannot bear pain, should be made to drink some strong beverage. The patient who has been fed, does not faint, and he who is rendered intoxicated, does not feel the pain of the operations.[16]

That the early surgeons of India relied on prescribing the consumption of wine as an anaesthetic dose becomes all the more intriguing in the light of our information about the use of certain drugs by the contemporary Greeks and Romans to produce anaesthetic effects. Dioscorides refers to mandragora (Mandragora Atropa) as an internally applied anaesthetic, while Pliny, in his Natural History, informs us even about its external administration, a point corroborated by Galen, Araetaeus and Celsus as well. It is, however, to be noted that the Indian tradition talks about the inhalation of the fumes of burning Indian hemp as an anaesthetic in a period of antiquity that remains undated. It is, however, certain that the Indian doctors, by AD 927, were using drugs for this purpose. Ballala, in his Bhojaprabandha, alludes to a cranial operation performed on King Bhoja, in the course of which he was rendered insensible by a drug called sammohini. That by the tenth century AD the Indian doctors came to acquire a fairly good knowledge of anaesthesia, seems obvious.

What affected this highly developed system of indigenous medical science by the time the Europeans appeared on the scene? Besides the colonial imposition of the western system of medicine over the native medicinal structure, obviously to throttle the latter as a consequence of the colonial educational and cultural policies of dominance, Ayurveda came to be afflicted by the same crisis that had constrained the growth of medical science in the Graeco-Roman world, i.e. the anti-manual labour attitude of the social elite. As the varnashrama system got entrenched on Indian soil, a negative attitude developed towards manual labour. As early as the Manusmriti it was declared that the food offered by a surgeon was ritually as filthy as the food touched by a blacksmith.[17] The subsequent law-givers became more hostile towards the doctors. And this finally led to the separation of the hand from the head, more so due to the dominance of a feudal mentality, and the growth of a practical body of knowledge like surgery suffered.

Notes and References

[1] N.H. Keswani (ed.), *The Science of Medicine and Physiological Conceptions in Ancient and Medieval India*, New Delhi, 1974, p. 16.

[2] *Sushrutasamhita*, cited in D.P. Chattopadhyaya, *Science and Society in Ancient India*, Calcutta, 1977, p. 94.

[3] Ibid., p. 95.

[4] *Charakasamhita*, I.1.134–35.

[5] J.D. Bernal, *Science in History*, Vol. I, Harmondsworth, 1969, p. 190.

[6] W.H.S. Jones (ed.), *Hippocrates*, Vol. I, London, 1972, p. xviii n.

[7] Ibid., pp. xvii–xviii.

[8] Quoted in B. Farrington, *Head and Hand in Ancient Greece*, London, 1947, p. 347.

[9] *Sushrutasamhita*, I.7.1.

[10] Ibid., I.7.3–6.

[11] Ibid., I.18.19.

[12] Ibid., XVIII.10.

[13] Ibid., XXV, 3.10, 15; *Charakasamhita*, I.33, 34, 35.

[14] *Sushrutasamhita*, IV.2.39–48; 7.11–12; 7.14–22; 7.15–17; 7.17; *Ashtanga Samgraha*, VI.14.

[15] *Charakasamhita*, III.36–37.

[16] *Sushrutasamhita*, I.7.6.

[17] *Manusmriti*, IV.212–13.

Medieval Theories of Vision and the Introduction of Spectacles in India, c. 1200–1750

Iqbal Ghani Khan

The attempts to maintain one's natural ocular health and the trauma of a scholar gradually losing the ability to read or write are best reflected in the words of Petrarch (1304–74) who, in his *Letters to Posterity*, said: 'For a long time I had very keen sight which, contrary to my hopes, left me when I was sixty years of age, so that to my annoyance I had to seek the help of spectacles.' However, prior to the late thirteenth century (when evidence of the use of spectacles is first found), the prospect of losing one's eyesight would certainly have been quite a frightening prospect. Today, those of us fortunate enough to afford laser surgery and corrective lenses can hope to constantly push forward the day of our final break with the written word. After this there will be computers and software that will enable us to listen to the written word of our younger scholars from *e-books*; and then, if we are sharp enough, we shall dictate our responses, which will be read back to us for revision by our 'speaking PCs' before they are printed out for circulation. These latter inventions are the outcome of a technicalistic attitude that has come to dominate our mentality since some time in the sixteenth century, when inventions from China and Egypt combined with the efforts of the artisans of the Italian Renaissance to provide aids to a more durable life. However, prior to this, the earliest attempts at tackling the problem of failing vision were through sustaining one's health *per se* and securing the clarity of the eyes in particular.

The earliest studies in optics that are found among the Greeks had nothing to do with the behaviour of light; their concerns were centred around the problem of vision and of how the image is formed on the eye. For the pre-Aristotelians, vision was made possible by a ray of light being emitted from the eye. For the Atomists, the object sent forth a film of atoms that impinged an image on the eye, making the

26

object visible—this was one of the forms belonging to the genre referred to as the intromission theories. Plato settled for rays emanating from the object encountering another such entity leaving the eyes; where the two met, an image formed. These were, of course, very naive approaches and did not find favour with Aristotle, who replaced them with a theory based on his own construct governing natural laws. Basing himself on his four-element theory, he asserted in his *De Sensu et Sensibilibus*[1] that since all objects have a colour, it coloured the medium in-between, which in turn acted upon the eye and was, so to speak, seen. Furthermore, he added, the medium, in order to act upon the eye, must be continuous and illuminated. According to the earlier Greeks, the eye emitted a ray of light and the object was thus illumined.[2]

Light, according to Aristotle, was not an emission, as was the current belief, that propagates in time to the eye, but a state or quality that is acquired instantaneously by the medium from the luminous object. Whereas the later Graeco–Hellenistic physicists had a rather tortuous and largely misdirected debate amongst themselves on the causes underlying vision and on the elemental nature of light, the scientists in medieval Islam were in a position to select and reformat the more rational elements from within this vast treasury of Greek knowledge on light and vision, including, most notably, works written by the mathematician Euclid in the third century BC and treatises that the Egyptian astronomer Ptolemy produced four hundred years later. The former geometricized the study of light and brought it out of the realm of teleological argumentation that had plagued the Aristotelians. Ptolemy too sustained the mathematicization, but he remained committed to the axioms relating to the immutability of natural laws and therefore worked towards their reinforcement instead of demolishing them.

Yaqub Al Kindi, one of the first translators of ancient Greek texts in the ninth-century *Bait al Hikma* (House of Translation established in Baghdad by the Abbasides), was able to present a wealth of ideas on reflection, refraction, image projection through apertures, the rainbow, as well as on the anatomy and the working of the human eye. From the Greek texts that he was charged with translating into Arabic, he produced a new understanding, with a fair expression of his own critical comments, on the reflection of light as well as on the principles of visual perception. His ideas went on to establish the Renaissance laws of perspective and an entire new genre of art. Following the Quranic precept that since the Creator was one, his creation too could not be governed by separate laws, Al Kindi sought to reconcile the elements of the natural sciences with mathematics, and he opted for a definition of vision as that phenomenon which is generated by a luminous force that travels from the eye to the object in the form of a cone of radiation. Different angles subtended at the eye resulted in the changes in the perceived size of an object as it moved away or came closer.[3]

Two other scholars, Al Razi (ninth century) and Ibn Sina (eleventh century), also addressed the problems of light and vision in their texts, but the high point in Islamic science was the production of the *Kitab al Manazir*, or The Book of Optics, by Ibn al Haytham or Alhazen of the Latins, in the first two decades of the eleventh century. This tract was undoubtedly the single most original volume in medieval Islam that combined new ideas on light and vision with mathematical arguments on the behaviour of light along with experimental demonstration. Al Haytham studied the way light is refracted, or bent, by water, air, glass and mirrors. He came close to a theory of magnifying lenses. He examined the rainbow, aerial perspective and sunlight. He explained correctly why the diameters of the sun and the moon appear to increase as they approach the horizon (an optical illusion caused by their expected size in relation to familiar objects on the ground). He also demonstrated how refraction by the atmosphere causes the sun to remain visible when it is actually below the horizon. Furthermore, in order to study the solar eclipse, Al Haytham cut a small hole in a wall, allowing the semi-obscured solar image to be projected through it onto a flat surface. This early example of '*camera obscura*' optics anticipated modern photographic principles, just as his focussing by use of parabolically shaped burning mirrors pointed the way to the lenses of future telescopes and microscopes.[4]

Investigating the human eye, Ibn al Haytham studied its structure, analysed stereo vision, and formulated the hypothesis based on the Euclidean concept of the object sending out rays in all directions, some of which come through the pupils of the eyes and bring about an image of the objects. He added sophistication to this idea by adding that the rays from the perceived object, composing a 'form' representing an object's visible features, enters through the pupils (which act as lenses) and proceed to the brain, where the faculty of sense completes the process (see Figure 1). Therefore, in his model of

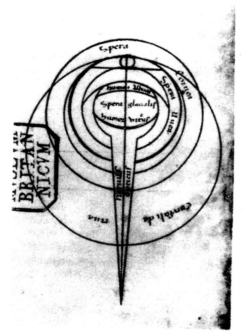

Figure 1: Diagram representing Ibn al-Haytham's
theory of vision. Ms illustration from a fourteenth-
century Latin version of his eleventh-century *Kitab
al-Manazir* (Book of Optics). Courtesy Howard
L. Turner, *Science in Medieval Islam* (New Delhi,
1999).

vision, the eye was involved as an optical system, in which psychology
too played an important part because pre-recorded images of the
object being viewed were also called into play by the psyche. This is
similar to the theories on vision that scientists today consider most
valid, and seems to have been influenced by the emphasis his famed
contemporary Avicenna was placing on psychology.[5] Al Haytham had
thus integrated Euclidean optics with the Aristotelian perception of
form and optics. It thus became a mathematical discipline, as did phy-
sics in general. Today, mathematics is the mutual language through
which the different sciences communicate.

Unfortunately Al Haytham's path-braking hypotheses, ideas
and, most importantly, methodology of repeated observations through
the earliest forms of instruments such as glass prisms and gratings,

were rather atypical of the ethos of scientific enterprise in medieval Islam, which depended to a large extent on the authority of established axioms whether of Greek or Ptolemaic origins. Al Haytham's ideas were therefore allowed to die for want of further studies and experiments. Three centuries later his work was taken up by the Iranian Kamaluddin al Farisi (*d.* AD 1318), whose *Tanqih al Manazir* added three more 'books' to Al Haytham's original seven, and widened the domain of optics irreversibly. While he revived the *Kitab al Manazir* as a master-text, Al Farisi also made some criticisms of Al Haytham's ideas and added sophistication to the experiments devised by his pre-

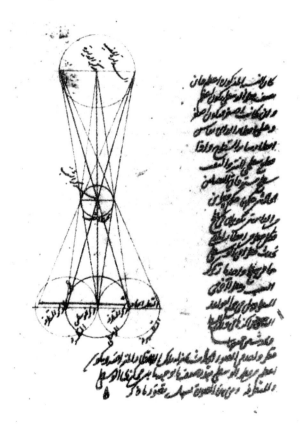

Figure 2: Diagram illustrating the principles of *camera obscura*. Ms. illustration from *A Résumé of Optics* by Kamaluddin al Farisi, Istanbul, fourteenth century. Courtesy Howard L. Turner, *Science in Medieval Islam* (New Delhi, 1999).

cursor—especially in the construction of the *camera obscura* (see Figure 2).[6]

Meanwhile, the absence of correspondence and continuity within the various centres of the sciences in Islam is tragically illustrated by the fact that when the celebrated twelfth-century Iranian astronomer Nasiruddin al Tusi wrote his *Tahrir al Manazir*, it was not a commentary on Al Haytham's ideas but on an Arabic recension of Euclid's *Optics* with the self-explanatory title of *Tahrir*, as in the case of Tusi's recension of the so-called *Kutub al Mutawassitat* or the Intermediate Books. The *Kitab al Manazir* of Al Haytham was probably not even available to Al Tusi. Since Al Tusi wrote in both Arabic as well as in his native tongue Farsi or Persian, the *manazira* debate was carried into Iran and treatises now began to be written not just on *manazira* (or the appearance of objects through air) but also on the subject of *maraya* to include indirect vision (i.e. appearance through another medium), such as in the case of reflected and refracted images. His student Qutbuddin al Shirazi (*d*. AD 1311), also a bilingual astrophysicist, wrote three volumes in Farsi on astronomy-related optics, and is said to have come into contact with Al Haytham's optics only in the 1280s.[7] This was followed by Al Amuli's *Nafais ul Funun* some time in the fourteenth century, and then by the work of an anonymous sixteenth-century writer belonging to Turkey with an Arabic title *Fi sabab i ru'yat al ashya. . .* (On the Cause of the Visibility of Objects. . .), which survives as part of a larger album of such MSS, entitled *Majmua fi 'ilm al Manazir*, in the Topkapi Palace Library in Istanbul.

After the establishment of the Delhi Sultanate, the flow of scientific ideas from the Arab–Iranian world was a regular feature of the ideological changes occurring across the subcontinent. Scholars in search of patronage, with their treatises and personal libraries in tow, who entered India throughout the medieval period, also constituted an 'invasion' of sorts. They were supported by Sultans like Firoz Shah Tughlaq (1351–88), who encouraged the translation of these treatises into Sanskrit and vice versa, so as to encourage a dialogue that Al Biruni had initiated in the eleventh century through his *Kitab al Hind*.[8] Medieval Indian ideas on optics and vision are found dispersed in Arabic and Persian manuscripts on astronomy, medicine, and in the encyclopaedias.[9] For all those involved in the debate between the *Mutakallimun,* the *Mu'tazilites* and the *Ishraqis,* light was an important issue, because what the orthodoxy were demanding was an end to speculation of the nature in which Ibn Sina and Al Biruni indulged. They had declared that all wisdom could only come through Revelation and must come from the Heavens into the purest hearts alone. The Mutazilites and the Ishraqis were trying to find a way out, and to continue their examination of the physical environment in which they defined Allah to be *Nur* or Divine Light. Unfortunately, in the absence of the institutionalization of experimental rigour initiated by Al Haytham, the debate degenerated into a metaphysical one.[10]

Al Haytham's influence on Latin optics seems to have been more extensive and translations of his works formed the basis of syllabi well into the seventeenth century. His *Kitab* was translated quite early and Risner published a Latin translation of it in 1572. However, what needs to be explored is the impact Al Haytham had on the original contributions to optics in the sixteenth and seventeenth centuries by men of the calibre of Galileo, Kepler and Descartes, since Al Haytham was definitely known to them and there are similarities in their approaches to the study of reflection and refraction, as well as in the explorations of both Al Haytham and Galileo into the roughness of the lunar surface.[11] There were obviously other arenas within which the debate on vision was in progress too—in the field of ophthalmology perhaps.

As soon as we turn our gaze towards the medical literature of the same century as the *Kitab al Manazir*, we find an exhaustive treatise entitled *Nurul 'Uyun* being written by one Abu Ruh Mohammad Bin Mansur al Jurjani, in 1087–88. This rare work on ophthalmology, in the form of questions and answers, has chapters on the diseases of the human eye visible to the naked eye, curable diseases of the eye, incurable diseases of the eye, measures to be taken during the early stages, surgical treatment, simple and compound medicines for treating the eyes and so on. It was possibly based on a treatise by Hunain ibn Ishaq —the first man to draw a detailed anatomical diagram of the human eye.[12] (See Figure 3.) Clearly the science of ophthalmology was developed not in order to understand the behaviour of light in the eye but to develop better eye health and thus to *prevent* eye disease. This attitude towards eye disease or weakening of eyesight prevented the development of optometry in Islam—despite the presence of one of the earliest glass industries at Alexandria since the Ptolemaic era.[13] Al Haytham had, like Ptolemy, utilized local skill for making glass prisms and hemispheres for verifying his laws on the refraction of light. However,

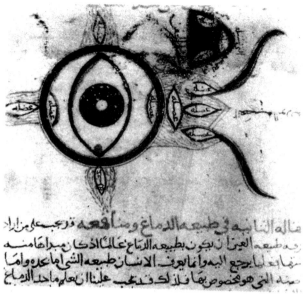

Figure 3: Diagram of the eye. Ms. illustration from *Kitab al-Ashr Maqalat fi'l 'Ayn* (Book of Ten Treatises on the Eye) by Hunayn ibn Ishaq, Egypt, thirteenth-century copy. Courtesy Howard L. Turner, *Science in Medieval Islam* (New Delhi, 1999).

it ought to be clarified here that the mirrors he used in his reflection experiments were made of steel, and it was only in the fourteenth century that sheet glass was made; it was then foiled into a reflective surface in about 1500.[14]

As for the earliest references to the use of spectacles, Joseph Needham dispelled the myth that China was the birthplace of this invention too. According to him, the earliest references to spectacles are found in Ming sources, namely, the *Chhi Hsiu Lei Kao* of Lang Ying (AD 1487–1566) and the *Fang Chou Tsa Yen* of Chang Ning (fl. AD 1452). From their accounts it is clear that spectacles were known in China, though not very common there, during the early years of the Ming dynasty, i.e. the fifteenth century. Even the first term for them, *ai-tai*, was clearly a corruption via transliteration of the Arabic *al uwainat* or the Persian *ainak*.[15]

As to the origins of spectacles in Europe, Needham admits that here too we are not on very firm ground, and this is evident also in Singer's conclusion that spectacles came into use at the end of the thirteenth century. They were reported first in Italy, beginning with convex lenses (*occhiali*) for presbyopia, and not developing concave lenses for myopia till as late as the mid-sixteenth century AD. From the more recent and exhaustive researches of Rosen it is now possible to date the first making of spectacles to shortly after 1286. The inventor was probably a layman of Pisa. The first appearance of spectacles in a picture is seen in a portrait dating to 1352 at Treviso. According to A.C. Crombie, the invention of spectacles was a singular achievement of the west, despite the fact that Islam had known of lenses, both in the eye and as experimental tools, for a much longer time. Crombie cites the *Opus Majus* of Roger Bacon (*c.* 1266–67) as containing the proposition that a convex lens in front of the eyes could cure the long-sighted. However the actual invention and use of spectacles was most probably done by the unknown artisan of Pisa in 1286, and the invention was made public by the friar Alessandro della Spina of Pisa, who saw them being made and thus constructed his own. The thriving glass industry at Burano in Venice has long been associated with the manufacture of spectacles. The earliest known occurrence of the term for spectacles is found in the supplementary regulations of the Venetian guild of crystal workers dating to 1300. In 1300 there is also reference to a *lapides ad legendum*, that seems to refer to a magnifying glass. The earliest absolutely certain medical reference is much later, when Guy de Chauliac in 1363 prescribed spectacles as a remedy for poor sight after salves and lotions had failed. By this time spectacles had in fact become fairly common, and this was the period during which Petrarch (1304–74) made the remark about finally having to take recourse to spectacles. However, all these early spectacles still seem to have been confined to convex lenses; it was only in the sixteenth century that concave lenses were fabricated and used by the short-sighted.[16] And here too they were preferably made of crystal, due to the ease with which the crystal could be polished into the required degree of convexity. No one knew about the behaviour of light through concave/convex crystals, so different lenses were tried on till the letters being read became clear, and they were then fitted into the frame. It is therefore clear that the earliest transmission to China must have taken place after *c.* 1300, and the process was facilitated by the intensification of trade relations with Europe, West Asia, and then with South Asia.

In fact, the Chinese references are just half a century earlier than the period to which P.K. Gode ascribes the earliest reference to the use of spectacles in India—i.e. in the *Vyasayogacharita*—wherein, in *c.* 1520, Vyasaraya is described as reading a book with the help of spectacles 'from which his great age could be inferred'.[17] The term *uplochangolak* is a 'very happy coinage' to describe 'spectacles' with convex eye-glasses. There is no word for 'spectacles' in Sanskrit, as spectacles as such were not known in India prior to the Portuguese contact. As regards the source of the *uplochangolaks* used by Vyasaraya, Gode suggests that they could have been presented to the pontiff by the Portuguese who, according to Somnath, were well known for their custom of 'strategic gift-giving' at the Vijayanagara court.[18]

In mid-sixteenth-century northern India, spectacles had become common enough to be used by painters. A painting shows one Mir Musawwir reading, and at the same time drawing attention to what is an entirely readable petition for assistance. The spectacles are set in a wooden frame and there are arms that go towards the ears, the nose clip seems to be made of wire (see Figure 4). That they were quite common by the close of the sixteenth century is evident from the fact that contemporary intellectuals were exchanging letters and verses that referred to the '*ainak*' in rather familiar terms. Thus, Faizi ends what

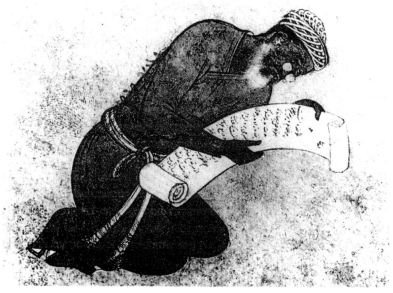

Figure 4: Portrait of Mir Musawwir (*c.* 1565–1570) shown using spectacles. Signed Mir Saiyid Ali. Collection: Musee Guimet, Paris.

35

was probably his last letter to Abdul Haq Muhaddis Dehlvi thus:

> Faizi you are old, watch where you step,
> And each step that you take let it be worthy of praise.
> From spectacles of glass nothing is revealed;
> Take a slice of your heart and place it on your pupils.

According to Badauni, Faizi had returned from his embassy to the Deccan in 1593 and was at Lahore, and this was perhaps the last letter from his pen before he died on 5 October 1595.[19]

The next reference to spectacles is found in Jamaluddin Inju's *Farhang-i Jahangiri* (1608–09), wherein 'the *chashmak* is a word that is said to have three meanings; the first being the "*ainak*". . . .'.[20]

The Jesuits were definitely important players in introducing this device into the subcontinent and we have evidence to the effect that Rudolfus, a Jesuit missionary at Akbar's court in 1580, used spectacles for reading.[21]

That spectacles continued to be imported from the west is clear from the next reference to them that occurs in the letter from President Kerridge at Surat to John Bangham at the Mughal court, 8 September 1625. He wrote: 'Mr Young (probably at the Mughal court) has stated that Asaf Khan (Nur Jahan's brother) desires some English spectacles; so a box containing two pairs is forwarded for him.'[22] There are many such references scattered throughout the English as well as Dutch factory records.

However, that it was all a hit-or-miss technique, and that vision had not till then been graded or quantified, is obvious from the fact that normally two pairs were sent to the recipients in the hope that at least one of them would work; the 'power' of the lenses were probably kept high to cover all deficiencies within a range. In fact the other reference to spectacles, which dates to *c.* 1706, highlights this very problem of matching the lenses to suit the eyesight. Abdul Jalil Bilgrami, a high-ranking officer, has just been posted to Bhakkar, and his son apparently thinks that he can squeeze a pair off his father and has probably asked his father to send him a pair. In the letter to his son at Bilgram, Abdul Jalil complains about the difficulty of finding a good pair for his son in Bhakkar; but as soon as he finds one, it shall be sent forthwith.[23] Nine years later the same Abdul Jalil is complaining about the loss of a good pair that he had obtained at Bhakkar. He reminds his son about the fine Europeans (*firangi*) pair with the wooden frames that he had left behind in Bilgram because he did not need them then. He gently reminds his son that he had given them to a friend and that now he must have them because they had suited his eyes well 'and up to the heaven I could see'. He adds that he was sending two pairs for his son that he had bought in Delhi, where there was no shortage of spectacles but none suited his own eyes. These exchanges not only establish the fact that the trial-and-error method was used in the matching of lenses. Qaisar uses this evidence to establish the presence of a thriving trade in spectacles by the advent of the eighteenth century. Furthermore, the low prices prevailing in the seventeenth century (approximately half a rupee each, landed cost, and retailing at one rupee and three-fourths each) also indicate a high turnover—probably due the vast army of copyists, calligraphers, painters, jewellers and metal engravers who constituted the market for spectacles.[24] Spectacles figured prominently in almost all the gifts of rarities to the emperor's courtiers and eunuchs on festivals even in the second decade of the eighteenth century.[25] It would seem, however, from Mir Abdul Jalil Bilgrami's letters, that by the early eighteenth century most of the spectacles were of Indian manufacture. Out of the four pairs mentioned by him, only one is described as *firangi* or European. It would be interesting to enquire if Indian spectacle-makers were using crystal besides glass, though Faizi in the verses we have quoted, speaks clearly of glass spectacles.

In the *Imperial Gazetteer of India*, the manufacture of spectacles from quartz crystals is referred to as follows: 'Vallan Vadikusetti, town in Tanjore Taluka, 7 miles from Tanjore. . . . The quartz crystals (pebbles) found here are made into spectacles of which the natives think highly.' This is really an indigenous manufacture in India current about 1886 when the *Imperial Gazetteer* was published.[26]

By the end of the reign of Aurangzeb's reign the Arabic *ainak* was being replaced by the more Persianized *chashma*. Tek Chand's *Bahar-i 'Ajam*, a dictionary completed in 1739, lists the numerous verses in which the word *chashma* and *chashmak* (the wink) occur. It also lists a number of optical instruments that were commonly known in India by then.[27]

However, the difficulty of sustaining temperatures high enough to melt silica (1723°C) made the Indian glass industry suffer the same fate as that met by those trying to make cast-iron—they both fell before cheap imports as well as due to bad furnace designs.[28]

Another reason for the failure was the disinterest on the part of the Mughal imperial elite to involve themselves in the production technology of even items that directly affected their lives.[29] This was also the case in Europe, where it took an artisan to invent the spectacles in 1300, and then another three hundred years for the combination of concave and convex lenses that we refer to as telescopes. The scholars were bound by the dictum that 'vision alone cannot be trusted'— fortunately for science, the artisans did not study at Aristotelian academies.

Notes and References

1 *Vide* Saleh Beshara Omar, *Ibn al Haytham's Optics: A Study of the Origins of Experimental Science*, Bibliotheca Islamica, Chicago, 1977, pp. 18–19.

2 The following ideas have been formulated after a survey of the translations of ancient Graeco–Arabic treatises embodied in recent works on optics such as Saleh Beshara Omar, *Ibn al Haytham's Optics*; Elaheh Khairandish, 'The Manazir Tradition through Persian Sources', in Gode, 'Some Notes on the Invention of Spectacles' in his *Studies in Indian Cultural History*, Vol. III, Pt 2, pp. 106–07.

3 Lindberg, *Al Kindi to Kepler*, Chicago, 1976, passim.

4 Howard L. Turner, *Science in Medieval Islam*, New Delhi, 1999, p. 196; see also the massive work by A.I. Sabra, *The Optics of Ibn Al Haytham*, 2 vols, London, 1989, passim. For a more accessible version see entry on Ibn al Haytham by Sabra in *Dictionary of Scientific Biography* (DSB), q.v. al-Haytham, Ibn.

5 Afnan, *Avicenna, His Life and Works*, London, 1958.

6 See details in Farisi's *Tanqih al Manazir*, Dairat ul Ma'arif ul Osmania, Hyderabad. See also Al Haytham's 'A Treatise on Moonlight' in the *Majmu'al Rasail*, Dairat al Ma'arif ul Osmania, Hyderabad.

7 Cf. A.I. Sabra, *The Optics of Ibn al Haytham*, Vol. 2, p. lxix, *vide* Kheirandish, *The Manazir Tradition*, p. 129.

8 *Alberuni's India*, translated by Edward Sachau, London, 1910.

9 Rahman, with Alvi et al., *Science and Technology in Medieval India: A Bibliography of Source Materials in Arabic, Sanskrit and Persian*, New Delhi, 1982.

10 See Mss in Arabic on the subject described in Imtiaz Ali Arshi, *A Catalogue of Arabic Mss in the Raza Library Rampur*, Vols I–VI.

11 Saleh Beshara Omar, *Ibn al Haytham's Optics*, pp. 151–52.

12 This rare work was believed lost until Max Meyerhof discovered it in 1926 and translated it into German. Ms No. Buhar 11/1, also at ASB PMC Society Collection No. 714, *vide* Rahman, Alvi, et al., *Science and Technology in Medieval India*, p. 11.

13 See details in S.D. Goitien, *Studies in Islamic History and Institutions*, Leiden, Brill, 1966. See also G.E.R. Lloyd, *Greek Science since Aristotle*, New York, 1989, chapter on Hellenistic Optics.

[14] See details of reflection instrument in Saleh Beshara Omar, *Ibn al Haytham's Optics,* p. 111. For the refraction experiment, see ibid., pp. 139–144. On the arrival of glass mirrors in India, see A.J. Qaisar, *Indian Response to European Technology and Culture,* New Delhi, 1982, pp. 72–74.

[15] Needham, *Science and Civilization in China,* Vol. IV, Pt 1, pp. 118–21.

[16] A.C. Crombie, *Medieval and Early Modern Science,* Vol. I, pp. 231–32.

[17] *Vyasayogi-Charita* of Somnath Kavi, edited by B. Venkoba Rao, Bangalore, 1926, p. xx. Rao refers to the word *uplochan-golak. Vide* P.K. Gode, 'Some Notes on the Invention of Spectacles', in his *Studies in Indian Cultural History,* Vol. III, Pt 2, pp. 106–07.

[18] Ibid.

[19] Badauni, *Muntakhab ut Tawarikh,* Vol. III, Bib. Ind., Calcutta, 1873–87, p. 117. Abul Fazl quotes the same verse when he refers to his brother's death in the *A'in-i Akbari,* edited by H. Blochmann, Vol. I, Bib. Ind., Calcutta, 1866–76, pp. 235–42. The verses being quoted are found on p. 241. These verses were again quoted in the late sixteenth-century source on geography, the *Haft Iqlim Amin Ahmad Razi,* Bib. Ind., Calcutta, 1918, 1927, 1939, Vol. II, p. 497.

[20] *Farhang-i Jahangiri,* Vol. I, Lucknow, 1876, p. 479.

[21] Cf. *The Commentary of Father Monserrate,* p. 193, vide, Qaisar, *Indian Response,* p. 75.

[22] W. Foster, *English Factories in India, 1624–29,* Oxford, 1906–27, p. 93.

[23] 'Abdu'l Jalil Husaini Wasiti Bilgrami, Letters to [his son,] Mir Sayyid Muhammad Bilgrami [1706–20], ed. and transl. anonymous, in *Oriental Miscellany,* Vol. I, pp. 138, 204–06. A.J. Qaisar, *Indian Response,* pp. 75–76; the letter does not indicate that spectacles were easily available at Bhakkar.

[24] Cf. Patna Diary, IOL, vide Qaisar, *Indian Response,* p. 75.

[25] As did prisms, kaleidoscopes, telescopes. See details in Wilson (ed.), *Early Annals of English Bengal,* II, 2, pp. 78–84.

[26] The term *durbin* also occurs in this dictionary and is described as the instrument by which distant objects can be seen clearly. It is used by navigators to assess the ocean and by contingents that are lost. The kaleidoscope is called the *ainak-i hazaar numa. Bahar—'Ajam,* Nawal Kishore, 1916, Vol. I, p. 315, and Vol. II, pp. 235, 466.

[27] On this question see I.G. Khan, 'Metallurgy in Medieval India: The case of the cast-iron cannon', *Proceedings of the Indian History Congress,* Chidambaram session, 1984.

[28] On the cultural failure as a reason for the decline of the Mughal empire, see Athar Ali, 'The Eighteenth Century: An Interpretation', in *IHR,* 1975, passim.

[29] *Science and Civilization.*

Physicians as Professionals in Medieval India

S. Ali Nadeem Rezavi

A study of Mughal society reveals the existence of a 'class' distinct from the landholding class and the peasantry, comprising physicians, architects, scholars, teachers, poets, painters, musicians and a large number of craftsmen, apart from merchants, who made their living by selling their professional skills.[1] Some recent studies have shown that this newly-arising intermediary professional group, by the seventeenth century, had started being recruited to influential bureaucratic positions.[2]

This paper attempts to analyse the role of the physicians as professionals and assess their position in the Mughal society as well as their relations with the imperial ruling class. Was their position just that of clients bound to their patrons in expectation of a respectable income, or did a general demand exist for their services among various sections of the society, against which they received a salary? Related to this is the status of these practitioners of medicine from the point of view of their clients and patients.

I

Commenting on the level of medical education in India, Fryer suggests that the field of medical science in India was 'open to all Pretenders, here being no Bars of Authority, or formal Graduation, Examination or Proof of their Proficiency; but every one ventures, and every one suffers; and those that are most skilled, have it by Tradition, or former Experience descending in their Families.'[3] Fryer further observed that the Indian physicians neither understood the pulse nor did they treat other ailments.[4] Careri goes still further when he says, 'In Physick they have but small skill, and cure several diseases by Fasting',[5] and Manucci is much harsher when he exclaims, 'From such doctors and such drugs *libera nos Domine!*'[6]

Although there were not many separate colleges exclusively dealing with the medical sciences, as in Alleppo, Egypt or Iran, their existence is testified in India as well. Monserrate pointedly mentions 'a very famous school of medicine' at Sirhind, 'from which doctors are sent out all over the empire'.[7] Abdul Baqi Nahawandi mentions the *madrasa* of Hakim Shams and Hakim Mu'in at Thatta, where they also gave lectures on medicine.[8] Similarly, Mir Abu Turab Gujarati, a contemporary of Akbar, had his own *maktab*, where he imparted education.[9] Abdul Hamid Lahori mentions a certain Hakim Mir Muhammad Hashim who used to impart instruction in his own school at Ahmadabad.[10] Hakim Alimuddin Wazir Khan is said to have built a *madrasa* at his native town Chiniot in the Punjab.[11]

One may assume that in these schools run by the *tabibs*, the curriculum included a study of texts on *tibb*. This impression is strengthened by Abul Fazl's statement in *Ain-i Akbari*, that Akbar had directed the inclusion of *tibb* with the other sciences in the school curriculum.[12] The well-known *Nizami* course included, besides other texts, the following well-known texts on *tibb*: *Sharh-i Asbab, Mu'jaz al-Qanun, Qanun* of Abu 'Ali Sina, *al-Nafisi* and *Hidayah-i Sa'ida*.[13]

Another form in which education in *tibb* may have been imparted was through *dawakhanas* (dispensaries) and *sharbatkhanas* (syrup houses /distilleries), often run through state munificence.[14]

The most important centres of medical education during the sixteenth and seventeenth centuries, however, were located in Iran, from where many physicians in India were recruited.[15] A sizeable number of physicians of the Mughal period are said to have attained their knowledge from various academies in Lahijan (Gilan), Mashhad, Isfahan and Shiraz.[16] Mir Muhammad Hashim, better known as Hakim Hashim, who later became tutor to Prince Aurangzeb and had also opened his own *madrasa* at Ahmadabad, remained in the holy cities for twelve years to acquire knowledge. In India he was a student of Hakim Ali Gilani.[17] Similarly, the famous Gilani brothers attained their education in Iran before migrating to India.

There exists evidence suggesting that sometimes Indian scholars too went to these institutions in Iran for training and education in *tibb*. One such person was Ahmad Thattavi who went to Iran from Sindh and studied in Shiraz under the guidance of Mulla Kamal-uddin Husain and Mulla Mirza Jan, two noted physicians of Shiraz; on completion of his studies he came back to India.[18] Muhammad Akbar Arzani, a noted physician under Aurangzeb and a native of Delhi, also went to Iran for further studies in *tibb*.[19]

A perusal of the Persian sources shows that medical education was tutor-oriented. Those desirous to learn would go to a reputed physician and get the education from him.[20] Thus Hakim Ali Gilani acquired his knowledge in the company of Hakimul Mulk Shamsuddin Gilani and Shah Fathullah Shirazi.[21]

II

In Mughal India, like other professions, the physician's profession also gained prominence. Historical sources reveal the important position held by physicians. Abul Fazl, Nizamuddin Ahmad and Lahori, while listing *ulema* (scholars) and poets, duly included the physicians of the period. Considerable interest appears to have been taken in patronizing them. In ethnic terms, the *tabibs* of Mughal India were a predominantly Irani group (see Table 1). This is borne out by the list of physicians mentioned in the Mughal chronicles as well as the observations of the European travellers.[22] But at Akbar's court the situation was slightly different in so far as there were also present a considerable number of Hindu *tabibs*, who are mentioned by Abul Fazl and Nizamuddin in their list of *Atibba*.[23] These 'Hindu' *tabibs* were probably brahmins by caste,[24] and experts of Ayurvedic rather than Unani *tibb*.

TABLE 1

Reign	Persians	Indians	Others	Total
Akbar	15	14	13	42
Jahangir	11	07	01	19
Shahjahan	10	08	05	24
Aurangzeb	04	?	01	?

We find that a sizeable number of *tabibs* joined Mughal service in various capacities and were sometimes also assigned *mansabs*. These were physicians who would be recruited directly to the service of the emperor; others would join the establishment of nobles.

Before a physician or a surgeon could join a service he had to pass certain tests, to the satisfaction of the employer. Extreme care was taken to select or appoint only the most accomplished and experienced physician.[25] Thus, at the time of Hakim Ali Gilani's employment, Akbar ordered several bottles containing the urine of sick and healthy persons, as also that of cattle and asses, to be brought before the Hakim for detection. The Hakim is reported to have diagnosed each one of them correctly and passed the test. From that time his reputation and influence increased and he became a close confidant (*muqarrab*) of Akbar.[26] Manucci recounts a similar incident that happened to him while in the retinue of Prince Shah Alam.[27]

From a stray remark of Manucci it appears that, as in the case of those in imperial service, there was a hierarchical division in the establishment of a prince. There used to be a chief physician under whose charge were placed a number of subordinate physicians and surgeons who were bound to obey his orders.[28] This chief physician was, in Mughal terminology, known as *saramad-i atibba* or *saramad-i hukama*.[29] This hierarchy is also discernible, at least in the imperial household, by the reference to the title of *Hakimul Mulk* (the chief of the physicians), which was quite independent of the *mansab* he was holding. Although the most visible of the state physicians and the holder of the highest *mansab* under Akbar was Hakim Abul Fath, the title (or office?) of *Hakimul Mulk* was held by Hakim Shamsuddin Gilani.[30] In 1627, on the accession of Shahjahan, the title was bestowed upon Hakim Abu'l Qasim, the son of Hakimul Mulk Shamsuddin Gilani.[31] In 1662 the recipient of this honour was Hakim Mir Muhammad Mahdi Ardistani,[32] followed by Hakim Sadiq Khan, who was awarded the title in the forty-ninth regnal year of Aurangzeb (1704–05).[33]

Mughal miniatures also confirm the hierarchical division amongst the physicians serving kings, princes and nobles. In three or four miniatures, a chief physician (*saramad-i atibba*) is depicted tending the patient along with his subordinate colleagues[34] (see Plate 1). The growing prosperity of the medical profession can be discerned through the depiction of the physician–bureaucrats. Muqarrub Khan (identifiable from an inscription, 'Shabih-i Muqarrub Khan'), in all his portraits, is shown wearing a white silken *dastar* with a golden design and standing amongst the nobles close to the emperor.[35] This attire is typical of a Mughal noble, with the exception that he is always wearing sober colours.[36] Unlike him, Masihuz Zaman is shown in a

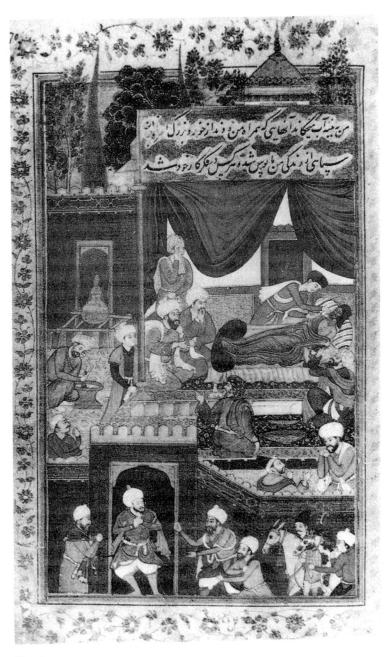

Plate 1

dress that was typical of the attire of the scholars and *ulema*.[37] Physicians who joined imperial service or that of a noble, but had not been assigned a *mansab*, were recruited on a daily (*yaumiya*) or annual (*saliyana*) salary.[38] Even after the grant of *mansab*, they received 'pocket-money' (*zar-i jeb*) to maintain a medicine box (*kharita*) comprising essential medicines.[39] From our sources it appears that the personal salary of a physician could vary between Rs 300 per month, i.e. Rs 3,600 per annum, and Rs 100,000 per annum.[40] According to Manucci, the salary of a blood-letter (surgeon) varied between Rs 2 per day and Rs 700.[41] Apart from remunerating a physician for his services through grant of *mansab* or cash allowances and salaries, they could also be given grants of bureaucratic offices or *madad-i ma'ash* grants.

Sometimes we find that the Mughal bureaucracy also included persons who were basically military or civil officers but had some knowledge of *tibb* which they used for treating people off and on. Such cases would include persons like Shaikh Faizi, Amanullah Khan Firuz Jang and Danishmand Khan. Khwaja Khawind, a noble under Humayun, is also said to have been a physician of some renown.[42]

Our sources also throw some light on the patron–client relationship between employer and employee. For example, Manucci observes that before being conducted into the royal *haram* or into the harem of a noble, the physician was covered from head to waist with a cloth and was accompanied by eunuchs.[43] Generally, a set of rooms, styled *bimarkhana*, was assigned for the ailing lady in the *haram*.[44] Manucci further informs us that in the case of a patient being of royal blood, prior permission had to be taken from the emperor in order to start the treatment.[45] Another piece of interesting information which hints at a patron–client relationship is provided by Manucci when he says that it was not the practice among the princes, and nobles to talk or have any sort of relations with the servants of other nobles or princes, for fear of treason. This applied to physicians particularly. When, in 1683, Diler Khan, an enemy of Prince Shah Alam, fell ill and with fair promises summoned Manucci to treat him, the prince strictly refused him permission to do so.[46]

There also exists evidence indicating the extent to which the ruler or nobles used to depend on the services offered to them by the physicians in their employment. This, for example, comes out very well from what we know about Jahangir's relationship with some of his physicians. On the one hand, he always had high expectations of their service and skilful treatment; at the same time he tended to denounce and denigrade them whenever they failed to come up to his expectations. He would, at the same time, criticize a *tabib* for not being able to give him relief from a disease and resent the *tabib* leaving his company on one pretext or the other.[47]

The dependence of the patron on his client is clearly brought out by a story narrated by Tavernier. In December 1665, when Tavernier passed through Allahabad, he was told that the chief of the Persian physicians in the governor's pay had tried to kill his wife by throwing her from the top of a terrace. The woman survived the fall. The governor dismissed the chief physician and the physician departed with his family. But soon after the governor fell ill and recalled the physician. On getting his message, the physician stabbed his wife, children and thirteen slave-girls, and returned to the governor at Allahabad. The governor said nothing to him and accepted him back in his service.[48] Similarly, Taqarrub Khan was retired and his son dismissed by Aurangzeb after the *hakim* had cured the imprisoned Shahjahan. But after some time when Aurangzeb himself fell ill, the *hakim* was restored to favour and the dismissal of his son was revoked.[49]

Further, it appears that a physician joining the service of the state or a noble was not bound to his patron. He could, like a true professional, change his employer as and when he willed. This becomes apparent by the way the author of *Ma'asir-i Rahimi* mentions approvingly that after joining the service of Khan-i Khanan, Hakim Muhammad Baqir remained attached to him throughout his life.[50] We also have the evidence of Hakim Muhammad Husain Gilani who, on migrating to India, initially joined the service of Mahabat Khan. After some time we find him in the service of Khana-i Zaman Bahadur. From there again he went to the court of Adil Shah at Bijapur, where he remained employed for a period of ten years. Later he joined the service of Khan-i Dauran.[51] A similar example is that of Hakim Momena Shirazi who, on coming to India, joined the service of Mahabat Khan.[52] In 1662 we find him employed with Bahadur Khan, the *subadar* of Allahabad.[53] In 1665 he joined the imperial service and became the chief physician treating an ailing Shahjahan.[54]

From the foregoing discussion it becomes apparent that the patronage extended to physicians after Akbar weakened under Jahangir but then rose again under Shahjahan, if we go by the number of physicians listed by various chroniclers (see Table 2). Secondly, the

TABLE 2

Reign	Those holding Mansabs	Others	Total
Akbar	8	34	42
Jahangir	7	12	19
Shahjahan	15	9	24
Aurangzeb	5	?	?
Total *mansab* holders:	35		

Iranian element remained dominant from the reign of Akbar to that of Shahjahan. Thirdly, those who joined service came after formal and proper training. Lastly, the recruitment and promotion of a physician was linked with his expertise in medical practice. It was more a demand-related relationship rather than a fixed relationship of the feudal type.

III

Darush-shifa or shifakhanas (hospitals) were also run by the government, which employed physicians for the purpose. According to *Bahar-i Ajam*, these places were buildings (*makan*) established by the rulers and nobles for the treatment of the poor and needy (*ghuraba wa masakin*).[55] The tradition of building hospitals in India appears to have been established much before the advent of the Mughals. For example, in 1442–43 orders were issued by Sultan Mahmud Shah Khalji of Malwa to establish a *darush-shifa* as well as a *darukhana* (dispensary or pharmacy) at Mandu, where those who had knowledge of the drugs (*adwiya shinas*) used in the systems of medicine followed by the Muslim physicians and Indians (*brahman-i hindi*) and 'accomplished physicians' were to be appointed, to look after the patients visiting the hospital.[56]

For the Mughal period, information about the establishment of state hospitals starts from the reign of Jahangir. In his twelve edicts of the first regnal year, Jahangir ordained the establishment of hospitals in all the great cities of the empire, where physicians were to be appointed for healing the sick. The expenses of these hospitals were to be met from the *khalisa sharifa*.[57] Sometimes, especially during Aurangzeb's reign, hospitals were also established in small places that were within the *altamgha* assignments of the biggar *mansabdars* and *umara*.[58]

It appears that in these hospitals, the state recruited a number of physicians and surgeons who were under the charge of a chief physician, who acted as the superintendent (*darogha*) of the hospital. To assist them in the general administration of the hospital, a number of clerks (*mutasaddis*) and a *kotwal* were also appointed.[59] From a reference to a *madrasa* being attached to a *shifakhana*, it appears that these hospitals sometimes served as medical colleges of sorts.[60] During the reign of Shahjahan, a government hospital was constructed at Delhi near Chowri Bazar, 'for the treatment of the travellers and the students (*talib-i 'ilman*) who cured the sick'.[61] A reference to a 'school of medicine' at Sirhind has already been given, from where, according to Fr Monserrate, 'doctors are sent out all over the empire'. Monserrate was probably referring to a medical college. Another government hospital that flourished was the *darush-shifa* of Ahmadabad, where Shahjahan appointed Hakim Mir Muhammad Hashim as the head.[62] This hospital was meant for treating the poor[63] and Unani as well as Ayurvedic (*tibb-i hindi*) physicians and surgeons were appointed here. We hear of two more government hospitals, the *darush-shifa* at Aurangabad and the *darush-shifa* at Surat.[64]

The physicians appointed in these hospitals were generally paid on a daily basis (*yaumiya*) from the treasury (*bait-ul mal*),[65] through the *mutasaddis* of *dar-uz zarb* (officials of the royal mint).[66] The superintendent and chief physicians (*darogha wa hakim-i darush-shifa*) of the government hospital at Aurangabad drew a salary, after usual deductions, of Rs 136 (i.e. Rs 6 per day).[67]

The physicians serving the government hospitals had to submit an attendance certificate (*tasdiq-i hazari*) before their salary was released. Sometimes, the *darogha-i darush-shifa* could be exempted from attendance.[68] To be appointed to the post of a physician, recommendations had to be made by the *bakhshi* or some other responsible person.[69] However, Aurangzeb did not like too much interference in the matter of appointment from ordinary people.[70]

Apart from government hospitals, hospitals could also be established by nobles. During Jahangir's reign, Saif Khan built a hospital complex at Jeetalpur comprising a mosque, a *madrasa* and a *shifakhana* which treated the poor.[71] During the same reign, Hakim Alimuddin Wazir Khan constructed a *madrasa* and a *darush-shifa* along with other buildings at his native town of Chiniot in the Punjab, and dedicated them to the residents of that town.[72] A certain Hakim Muhammad Rafi opened a *hawaij kadah* (clinic) for the treatment of the poor.[73]

Interestingly, Careri remarks that European soldiers were hesitant to be recruited into the Mughal army as they had 'no hospital for the wounded men'.[74] However, we have repeated information that the Mughal forces were always accompanied by physicians,[75] and it appears that the physicians thus employed in the retinue of the *mansabdars* enjoyed attractive perquisites. Many *tabibs* clamoured to be appointed to such positions.[76] But apparently these physicians, in spite of their perquisites, were an overworked and harassed lot.[77]

Another means of partronizing the profession of physicians in the Mughal empire was the system of rewarding expertise and service to the commonality through gifts and grants. Thus, when Nurjahan Begum was successfully treated by Hakim Ruhullah in 1618, the *hakim* was granted three villages in his native place as *madad-i ma'ash*, which were to be considered his *milkiyat* (private property).[78] The purpose of such *madad-i ma'ash* grants to the *tabibs* is clearly brought out by a number of Persian documents and chronicles. Hodivola has reproduced a number of documents relating to land and cash allowances granted to a family of Parsi physicians of Navsari, Gujarat, issued between 1517 and 1671.[79] According to these documents, these Parsi physicians received the *madad-i ma'ash* since they treated 'the poor and the diligent' of the locality.[80] A *parwana* quoted in *Muruqqat-i Hasan*, 1678, a compilation of letters written on behalf of Tarbiyat Khan, governor of Orissa, says that as a large number of ailing persons were being successfully treated by Hakim Muhammad Rafi, and as the people were greatly benefited by his medical knowledge, two *parganas* in *sarkar* Cuttack were given to him as *madad-i ma'ash*, from the income of which he was expected to meet the expenses of the *sharbat-khana* and the clinic (*hawaij kadah*) that he was running for the treatment of the poor.[81]

Importantly, this 'aid' was not confined to a particular religious or ethnic group of physicians. We have seen that apart from Muslim *tabibs* this grant was successively confirmed in favour of a family of Parsi physicians from the reign of Akbar to that of Aurangzeb.[82] A number of documents testify to similar *madad-i ma'ash* grants to Hindu physicians.[83]

IV

A general view which has found currency is that the physicians were completely dependent on royal patronage, or on the service of and endowments from the aristocracy. It is also sometimes held that the demand for the service was very limited.[84] This erroneous view seems to be based mainly on Tavernier's observation to the effect that: '... in all the countries we have just passed through, both in the Kingdom of Carnatic and the Kingdoms of Golkonda and Bijapur, there are hardly any physicians except those in the service of the Kings and Princes.'[85] But what the statement reveals is that Golconda and Bijapur were different in this respect from other areas. We have already noted in the preceding discussion that there were numerous physicians in Mughal India who ran their own clinics, imparted education and treated the poor. Apart from the evidence already cited, there are many more references to the private practitioners. Some of them however, were no more than quacks (*na-tabib*), a fact borne out by Badauni.[86] Manucci too, in one of his passages, refers to these unqualified *bazar* physicians. While giving an account of the caravan *sarais*, he mentions the 'endless cheating physicians' who pestered the travellers.[87]

These *bazar* physicians appear to have lived mainly on private practice. For instance, Badauni uses the term *mutatabib-Sirhindi*, that is, a private practitioner of Sirhind, when he mentions Shaikh Hasan, father of Shaikh Bhina, the surgeon.[88] Banarsi Das, in his *Ardha Katha-nak*, mentions a physician (*baidh*) of Jaunpur who treated him when he was young. He also mentions a *nai* (literally, barber), a term applied to local surgeons, who treated him for syphilis at Khairabad in 1602.[89] When his father fell ill in 1616, he was treated by yet another private practitioner at Banaras.[90] During Shahjahan's reign a physician called Hakim Basant had a flourishing practice at Lahore. Surat Singh mentions a 'specialist' of dog-bite at Kalanaur, to whom hapless patients would be carried.[91] During the reign of Aurangzeb, Hakim Muhammad Abdullah practised and taught at Agra.[92] Balkrishan Brahman, a petty official, in his letters written during the reign of Aurangzeb, mentions local medical practitioners like Balram Misr and Manka Tabib at Hissar Firoza. In one of his letters recommending Manka Tabib to a *mansabdar* for employment, he certified that 'a large number of people have benefited by associating with him'.[93] The presence of Hindu *bazar* physicians in the south is attested to by a number of European travellers.[94]

The practice of setting up private clinics in the *bazars* by physicians also finds place in the Mughal miniatures. A miniature attributed randomly to Abul Hasan and pertaining to the reign of Jahangir reminds us of Tavernier's descriptions (see Plate 2, next page). It depicts a physician sitting under a canopy (*shamiana*) on a platform and advising an old patient.[95] All around the physician (or is he just a druggist?) on the platform are displayed vials, bottles, jars, cups and bags containing a number of drugs, viz. *sufuf* (powder), *sharbats* (syrups) and *arq* (medicinal liquid extracts). A number of books are at hand, as is a small mortar and pestle to mix the medicines. On one of the bottles is inscribed '*sharbat-i diq*' (syrup for consumption). Every bottle and bag is labelled. Behind the physician stands a boy, who probably acted as his assistant.

Thus we see that not only was there considerable scope for private practice, in many cases physicians preferred establishing private clinics to government posts or accepting patronage from a noble. Yet, interestingly enough, we know on the testimony of Fryer that there was no dearth of physicians who coveted employment under a noble.[96] Presumably this was so because employment under a noble gave them a feeling of security and ensured a comparatively small but steady income.[97]

These medical practitioners tended to be very hostile to their European counterparts. Partly this might have been an outcome of the European physicians assuming superior airs vis-à-vis the Indian physicians. As Manucci tells us, the Europeans were often not agreeable to accept salaries on a par with those of Indian physicians.[98] However, Linschoten speaks very reverentially of the Indian physicians who, he says, had no scruples in treating the natives and Europeans alike.[99] Careri goes a step further and, in one of his very perceptive passages, suggests that persons suffering from particular kinds of diseases found in India respond more naturally to the treatment given by Indian physicians: 'Experience having shown', observes Careri, 'that European Medicines are of no use here.' He further says:

> . . . the physicians that go out of Portugal into those parts, must at first keep company with the Indian surgeons to be fit to practice, otherwise if they go about to cure those Distempers, so far different from ours after the European manner, they may chance to kill more than they cure.[100]

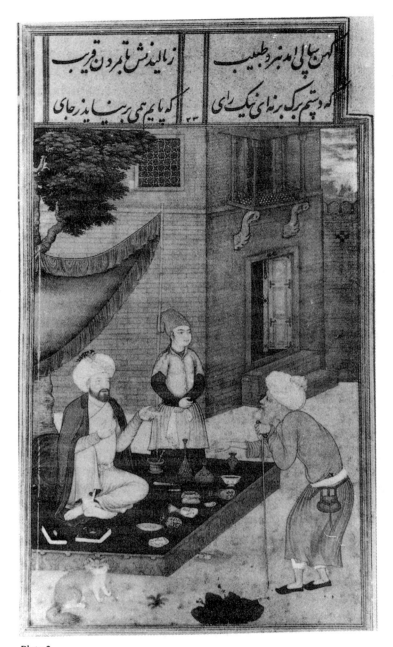

Plate 2

V

As far as the state of knowledge in the field of medicine during the Mughal period is concerned, many modern scholars, following the testimony of the European travellers of the seventeenth century, have expressed serious reservations. As a matter of fact, Manucci held a firm belief that these *tabibs* had no knowledge of medicine and were certainly not in a position to cure the stone, paralysis, epilepsy, dropsy, anaemia, malignant fevers or other difficult complaints.[101]

The available evidence, however, suggests that the medical profession in Mughal India had achieved a considerable degree of specialization within the frame work of Graeco–Arab medical science. The *hakims, tabibs* and *jarrahs* (surgeons) appear to have had amongst them ophthalmologists, specialized surgeons, pharmacologists, veterinarians, sexologists and anatomists. Manucci admits that the *tabibs* of the period were well-versed in the science of pharmacy. He says, 'In this country it is incumbent on a doctor to prepare medicines, ointments and distillation—infact all things that appertain to the apothecary's office. Many a times it is also necessary to instruct as to the fashion of preparing the patient's food.'[102]

Generally, the preparation of medicines was considered the responsibility of the physicians who prescribed them. The prescriptions, however, were generally kept a secret by the physician from each other, due to rivalry among them.[103] This was, perhaps, an important factor inhibiting the growth of pharmaceutical establishments. Generally, pharmaceutical preparations consisting of *sufuf* (powder), *mahlul* (suspension), *majun* and *jawarish* (electuaries), *sharbat* (syrups), *arq* (distilled medicinal water) and mixtures were prepared by the physicians themselves. Sometimes the physician possessed expertise in more than one field. For instance, during the reigns of Babur and Humayun, Hakim Yusum bin Muhammad Yusufi, who migrated to India along with Babur, was an expert in symptomatology, therapeutics, ophthalmology and general medicine. He was the author of at least twelve books. Two of his treatises dealing with symptomatology are preserved in the Maulana Azad Library, Aligarh.[104] His *Fawa'id-ul Akhyar* and *Ilajul Amraz* deal with hygiene and therapeutics.[105] He also compiled a short discourse on eye diseases and their cures.[106] Similary, Hakim Muhammad bin Yusuf ut Tabib al-Harawi, the personal physician of Babur, was, in addition to his other accomplishment as *tabib*, one of the most widely-read pathologists of his time.[107] Hakim Abdur

Razzaq, who was a contemporary of Humayun, wrote *Khulasat-ut Tashrih,* which deals with human anatomy.[108]

During Akbar's reign, much stress seems to have been laid on surgery. Shaikh Bhina, Mulla Qutbuddin Kuhhal (eye surgeon?), Hakim Biarjiu, Hakim Bhairon and Chandrasen were all reputed to be accomplished surgeons.[109] Hakim Shaikh Bhina wrote a book on medical prescriptions which is popularly known as *Mujarrabat-i Shaikh Bhina.*[110] Hakim 'Ainul Mulk 'Dawwani' Shirazi excelled himself in the field of opthalmology.[111] He was also an expert in the use of collyrium and pharmacology.[112] His treatise, *Fawaid ul Insan,* is a work on pharmacology in versified form.[113] Muhammad Hakim Gilani had expertise in sexology.[114] Hakim Ali Gilani, one of the most accomplished physicians of Akbar's reign, apart from his formula of *roghan-i deodar,* had also prepared *sharbat-i kaifnak,* which helped in removing exhaustion.[115] He also had considerable knowledge in fields like osteology (study of bone structures), myology (study of muscles), angiology, neurology and the digestive system.[116] Hakim Fathullah Shirazi translated the famous *Qanun* of Abu Ali Sina (Avicenna) into Persian for the benefit of the people.[117] Muhammad Qasim Ferishta, the famous author of *Tarikh-i Ferishta,* wrote *Dastur-i Atibba,* now popularly known as *Tibb-i Ferishta,* in order to create among the Muslims an interest in the Indian system of medicine.[118] During the same reign, Ma'sum Bhakhari, author of *Tarikh-i Sindh,* compiled a treatise on the treatment of diseases and drugs.[119] Similarly, in 1556 Shaikh Tahir authored *Fawaid-ul Fuad,* dealing with general medicine.[120]

During the reign of Jahangir, Muqarrab Khan and Hakim Ali Akbar were renowned surgeons.[121] Muqarrab Khan was also an expert bleeder and veterinarian.[122] Later his nephew Hakim Qasim also grew to become an expert bleeder.[123] Amanullah Firoz Jang Khanazad Khan, son of Mahabat Khan, famous noble under Jahangir and Shahjahan, had a sound understanding of medicine. His *Ganj-i Bad Awurd* is a good work on pharmacology. His second work, *Ummul Ilaj,* is a treatise on purgatives.[124]

Under Shahjahan as well, much work was done on pharmacology. Sheikh Muhammad Tahir, Hakim Ma'sum Shustari and Hakim Nuruddin Muhammad 'Ainul Mulk, grandson of Hakim Shamsuddin Ali Dawani 'Ainul Mulk (of Akbar's reign), have left behind books on pharmacology.[125] Hakim Ma'sum's *Qarabadin-i Ma'sum* deals with the preparation of drugs, electuaries, pulps, pastes, syrups, tablets, collyriums, enemas, gargles and ointments, as well as the effects of tea and coffee.[126] Hakim Nuruddin 'Ainul Mulk's *Alfaz-i Adwiyya* is an encyclopaedia of pharmacology,[127] while his *Ilajat-i Dara Shukohi* is a compendium of medical science basically instructing travellers on dietary precautions, anatomy, medicines etc.[128]

During the reign of Aurangzeb, Hakim Sanjak achieved much in the field of opthalmia.[129] Bernier says that Danishmand Khan was well-versed in anatomy.[130] He even had works of William Harvey on the circulation of blood, and Pecquet translated these into Persian for him.[131] Nurul Haq Sirhindi wrote *Ainul Hayat*, a rare work on plague.[132] Hakim Muhammad Akbar Arzani, a renowned physician of this reign, apart from translating a well-known commentary of the popular thirteenth-century pathological treatise by Najibuddin Samarqandi,[133] wrote a commentary on Chaghmini's *Qanuncha*.[134] Qazi Muhammad Arif wrote *Tibb-i Qazi Arif,* a general work on medicine containing prescriptions for diseases that are especially indigenous to India.[135]

It appears from the surviving manuscripts of works written on medicine and other sciences, now preserved in various repositories,[136] that in Mughal India a large number of books on medicine were either written or compiled, translated or commented upon (see Tables 3 and 4). Under the early Mughals (sixteenth to seventeenth centuries) and later Mughals (eighteenth century) the largest number of books written belonged to the field of medicine, as compared to astronomy

TABLE 3

Century	Medicine				Astronomy				Mathematics			
	Persian	Arabian	Sanskrit	Total	Persian	Arabian	Sanskrit	Total	Persian	Arabian	Sanskrit	Total
13th	4	33	31	68	11	21	8	40	5	30	2	37
14th	21	5	50	76	7	6	15	28	8	29	3	40
15th	18	1	36	55	25	32	47	104	8	22	4	34
16th	120	10	61	191	34	36	93	163	6	11	18	35
17th	102	12	122	126	39	30	190	259	23	25	14	62
18th	133	6	80	219	32	22	37	91	34	12	10	56

Source: A. Rahman et al., *Science and Technology in Medieval India: A Bibliography of Source Materials in Sanskrit, Arabic and Persian,* New Delhi, 1982.

TABLE 4: *Categories of Books on Medicine (Persian)*

Century	Total	General	Specia-lized	Antholo-gies/Com-pendiums	Diction-aries	Ency-clopaedias	Commen-taries	Trans-lations
13th	4	1	2	-	-	-	-	1
14th	21	5	11	1	1	-	1	3
15th	18	4	10	-	3	-	-	-
16th	120	15	93	5	1	-	-	6
17th	102	10	68	5	4	3	2	10
18th	133	10	98	8	1	3	3	10

Source: A. Rahman et al., *Science and Technology in Medieval India: A Bibliography of Source Materials in Sanskrit, Arabic and Persian*, New Delhi, 1982.

and mathematics, the other two popular fields of study. A sudden impetus to the collection and writing of books on medicine started in the sixteenth century, which continued down to the eighteenth century. This trend was confined generally to works in Persian and Sanskrit; books in Arabic, on the other hand, either decreased or remained stable numerically.

Table 4 shows the trend of specialized books on medicine developing during the sixteenth century. The seventeenth century saw some decline followed by a steep rise under the later Mughals. The trend of anthologies and compendia, as well as translations of previous works also developed from the sixteenth century onwards.

VI

An interesting question can be asked about the physicians of medieval India: were these *tabibs* dogmatic in their approach or were they open to change? Some idea in this respect can be had from the discussion that is reported to have taken place at Akbar's court in 1603, on the use of tobacco. In this year Asad Beg Qazwini brought to the court from Bijapur a small sample of tobacco and a smoking pipe for the emperor. When Akbar showed an inclination to smoke, he was sought to be dissuaded by Hakim Ali Gilani, who argued that as nothing was mentioned regarding tobacco in 'our medical books', it would be risky to use it without making further investigations.[137] While one may not disapprove in principle of the advice that Hakim Ali Gilani gave on that occasion, one cannot help noting the intrinsic cause of the *hakim*'s line of argument. For him nothing was permissible that was not sanctioned by the texts of *unani tibb* handed down by the great masters of earlier times. This obviously applied to the new ideas regarding medicine that were coming at this time from the west.

But then, did this not mean that the urge to improvize was absent among the Indian physicians? A stray reference by Manucci suggests that the surgeons, at least of the Deccan, improvized techniques that were a step forward towards the as yet unknown field of plastic surgery. He says that the native surgeons of Bijapur could fashion a crude nose for those who had this organ severed. They would cut the skin of the forehead above the eyebrows and make it fall down over the wounds on the nose. Then, giving it a twist, so that the live flesh might meet the other surface, and by healing applications, they fashioned for them a nose, though imperfect.[138] Manucci says he saw many persons with such noses.[139]

Thus we see that the physicians of Mughal India were members of a highly developed and skilled profession. It was only after proper training and schooling that they were allowed to become members of this profession. Although it cannot be denied that many of them were physicians by hereditary occupation,[140] a large number of them also became physicians due to training and interest. It further becomes apparent that these physicians could be classified into a number of categories. There were some who joined the service of the king or nobles, amongst them those who rose to high positions as *mansabdars*. Others joined service but were appointed to mediocre offices. From a number of Mughal miniatures, where physicians of these two groups are depicted, it is apparent that in spite of their affinity to the ruling classes, they were perceived to be different. Their attire resembles that of the religious classes. They are seen wearing heavy and circular *dastars* (headgear); the *jamas* they wore were shorter than those of the *mullas*, coming down only up to the knee, and had tight sleeves, quite unlike those of the religious classes. They are also frequently depicted wearing a shawl.

The third category of physicians receiving state patronage were those who, instead of being given *mansabs*, were awarded cash salaries. Then there were those who were only patronized through *in'ams* and grants. All these physicians were recruited and promoted on the basis of an assessment of their medical knowledge and experience. Further, they could leave their employers at will.

Largest in number were those who, for convenience sake, we may designate '*bazar* physicians'. These physicians had their own clinics and conducted private practice in conditions where the demand for their services was considerable. In general, physicians in Mughal India formed a distinct, non-theological professional class, held in high repute and able, as we have seen, to penetrate the ranks of the ruling classes. They thus formed a kind of primitive 'middle class' for their profession. The Mughal physicians, whether in government service or outside it, were much in demand and enjoyed a respected position in the society as well as at the court.

Notes and References

1 For this emerging class see, for example, Iqtidar Alam Khan, 'The Middle Classes in the Mughal Empire', Presidential Address, Medieval Indian Section, *Proceedings of the Indian History Congress*, 36th session, Aligarh, 1975 (revised version, 'The Professional Middle Classes', being published in J.S. Grewal (ed.), *Social History of Medieval India*, Vol. VIII). See also W.C. Smith, 'The Mughal Empire and the Middle Classes', *Islamic Culture*, Vol. XVII, No. 4, 1994; S. Ali Nadeem Rezavi, 'The Empire and Bureaucracy: The Case of the Mughal Empire', *Proceedings of the Indian History Congress*, Patiala, 1998.

2 A.J. Qaisar, 'Recruitment of Merchants in the Mughal Feudal Bureaucracy' (unpublished, mimeographed); S. Ali Nadeem Rezavi, 'The Mutasaddis of the Port of Surat in the Seventeenth-Century', *Proceedings of the Indian History Congress*, Burdwan, 1983, and 'An Aristocratic Physician of the Mughal Empire: Muqarrab Khan', *Medieval India 1*, edited by Irfan Habib, 1992, pp. 154–67. For a contrary view, see W.H. Moreland, *India at the Death of Akbar*, Delhi, 1962, pp. 73–77, 78.

3 John Fryer, *A New Account of East India and Persia in Eight Letters being Nine Years Travels Begun 1672 and Finished 1681*, Delhi, 1985, p. 114.

4 Ibid., pp. 114–15.

5 Careri, *Indian Travels of Thevenot and Careri*, edited by Surendranath Sen, New Delhi, 1949, p. 247.

6 Niccolao Manucci, *Storia Do Mogor*, translated with Introduction and Notes by William Irvine, Vol. III, Pt iii, Calcutta, 1966, p. 214.

7 *The Commentary of Father Monserrate, S.J (on his Journey to the Court of Akbar)*, translated by J.S. Hoyland, annotated by S.N. Banerjee, Calcutta, 1922, p. 103.

8 Abdul Baqi Nahawandi, *Ma'asir-i Rahimi*, edited by Hidayat Husain, Vol. II, Calcutta, 1931, p. 274.

9 Shah Nawaz Khan, *Ma'asir-ul Umara*, edited by Maulvi Abdur Rahim, Vol. III, Calcutta, 1888–90, pp. 280–81.

[10] Abdul Hamid Lahori, *Padshahnama,* edited by Kabiruddin Ahmad and Abdur Rahman, I, ii, Calcutta, 1867, p. 345.

[11] *Ma'asirul Umara,* III, p. 936.

[12] Abul Fazl, *Ain-i Akbari,* translated and edited by Blochman, Vol. I, Calcutta, 1927, p. 279.

[13] Cf. Abdul Jalil, 'The Evolution and Development of Graeco–Arab Medical Education', *Studies in History of Medicine,* Vol. II, No. 3, September 1978; see also Hakim Kausar Chandpuri, *Atibba-i 'Ahad-i Mughaliya,* Karachi, 1960.

[14] Ibid. For state aid to dispensaries, see, for example, Maulana Abul Hasan, *Muraqq'at-i Hasan,* MS., Rampur Raza Library (transcript of MS. in Department of History, Aligarh Muslim University), pp. 330–31.

[15] See for example *Ma'asir-i Rahimi,* III, p. 46. Hakim Jibrail, a famous physician, who later joined the service of Abdur Rahim Khan-i Khanan, while teaching at a *madrasa* known as *Darul Irshad* at Ardebil, heard people say that 'Iran was the *Maktab Khana* of Hindustan'.

[16] See *Ma'asir-i Rahimi,* III, pp. 44, 46, 51, 52, 745–55, etc. For example, Hakim Fathullah Shirazi attained his knowledge at the *madrasa* of Mir Ghiyasuddin Shirazi, the reknowned *hakim* of Shiraz, and Khwaja Jamaluddin Mahmud and Maulana Kamaluddin at Shiraz. *Ma'asir-ul Umara,* I, pp. 100–01. For other such examples, see Muhammad Sadiq, *Tabaqat-i Shahjahani,* MS., Department of History Library, Aligarh Muslim University, p. 466. Saqi Must'ad Khan, *Ma'asir-i Alamgiri,* III, Calcutta, 1870–73, pp. 17, 50, 45–46.

[17] Lahori, *Padshahnama,* I, ii, pp. 345–46.

[18] *Ma'asir-ul Umara,* III, p. 263.

[19] *Yadgar-i Bahaduri,* BM.MS.OR. 1652, f. 96, as cited in *Catalogue of the Persian Manuscripts in the British Museum,* Charles Rieu, Vol. II, 1881, p. 479.

[20] For details on medical education, see Abdul Jalil, 'Evolution and Development of Graeco–Arab Medical Education'; and A.H. Israili, 'Education of Unani Medicine during Mughal period', *SIHM,* Vol. IV, No. 3, September 1980.

[21] Badauni, *Muntakhab-ut Tawarikh,* edited by Molvi Ahmad Ali, Vol. III, Calcutta, 1869, p. 166. For other such examples see Khwaja Nizamuddin Ahmad, *Tabaqat-i Akbari,* edited by B. De, Vol. II, Calcutta, 1931, p. 483; *Ma'asir-i Rahimi,* III, pp. 51–52; Lahori, *Padshahnama,* I, p. 346.

[22] See, for example, in this regard, Manucci, *Storia Do Mogor,* II, iii, pp. 332–33, wherein the author says that the physicians in the Mughal court were basically Persians.

[23] *A'in-i Akbari,* I, pp. 542–44; *Tabaqat-i Akbari,* pp. 481–84.

[24] See, for example, the testimony of Fryer, *A New Account,* p. 115, also p. 27; also see Pyrard, *The Voyage of Francois Pyrard of Laval,* translated and edited by Albert Gray and H.C.P. Bell, Vol. I, Haklyut Society, London, n.d., p. 373.

25 Manucci, *Storia Do Mogor,* II, iii, p. 332.

26 *Ma'asir-ul Umara,* I, p. 569; Farid Bhakkari, *Zakhiratul Khawanin,* edited by Moinul Haque, Vol. I, Karachi, 1961–74, pp. 243–45.

27 Manucci, *Storia Do Mogor,* pp. 373–74.

28 Ibid., p. 215.

29 Khwaja Kamgar Husaini, *Ma'asir-i Jahangir,* edited by Azra Alavi, Centre of Advanced Study in History, Aligarh Muslim University, 1978, pp. 50–52; *Maasirul Umara,* I, p. 577; *Miratu'l Alam,* I, p. 332.

30 *A'in-i Akbari,* Vol. I, p. 542; *Tabaqat-i Shahjahani,* p. 465.

31 Amin Qazwini, MS.BM.OR. 173, Add. 20734 (transcript of MS., Raza Library, Rampur, in Department of History, Aligarh Muslim University), II, p. 281.

32 Muhammad Bakhtawar Khan, *Miratu'l Alam,* edited by Sajida Alavi, I, Lahore, 1979, p. 297.

33 Khafi Khan, *Muntakhabu'l Lubab,* edited by Kabiruddin Ahmad and W. Haig, Vol. II, Bib. Ind., Calcutta, 1905–25, p. 539.

34 See 'Babur stricken by illness in Samarqand', signed by Nama, *Baburnama,* BM.OR. 3714, f. 79(a), cf. *Miniatures of Baburnama,* Samarqand, 1969, p. l8; 'Doctors and Patient', signed by Mirza Ghulam, *Diwan-i Hasan Dehlavi,* Walters Art Gallery, W. 650, f. 127, cf. Amina Okada, *Imperial Mughal Painters, Indian Miniatures from 16th and 17th Centuries,* translated by Deke Dusinberre, Flammarion, Paris, 1992, pl. 120; 'One Physician Killing Another', signed by Miskina, *Khamsa-i Nizami,* BM.OR. 12208 (Dyson-Perrins Collection) f. 23(b), cf. Amina Okada, *Imperial Mughal Painters,* pl. 143. For details, see S. Ali Nadeem Rezavi, 'Depiction of Middle-Class Professions and Professionals in Mughal Miniatures', *Madhya Kalin Bharat,* 7, edited by Irfan Habib, New Delhi, 2000 (Hindi translation of the paper presented at the Indian History Congress, Aligarh session, 1994).

35 'Jahangir amongst his Courtiers', Victoria and Albert Museum, IM. 9–1925, cf. Ivan Stchoukine, *La Peinture Indienne a l'Epoque des Grands Moghols,* Paris, 1929, pl. XXVIII.

36 'Jahangir being offered food by Dervishes', *Jahangirnama,* Edward Binney 3rd collection, San Diego, cf. A.K. Das, *Splendour of Mughal Painting,* Bombay, 1986, pl. V; 'Jahangir holding his court in a garden', State Library, Rampur, cf. Percy Brown, *Indian Painting under the Mughals,* AD 1550 to AD 1750, Oxford, 1924, pl. xlix; 'Jahangir celebrates *Ab-pashi*', attributed to Govardhan, State Library, Rampur, No. 1/5, cf. P. Brown, ibid., frontispiece.

37 'Portrait of Hakim Sadra, Masihuz Zaman', signed by Mir Hashim, folio of an Album, BM. Add. 18801, No. 30, cf. P. Brown, ibid., pl. 65.

38 Discussing the salary of the state physicians, Manucci comments that 'those bearing the title of Khan—that is "noble", have a gross allowance of from twenty, thirty, fifty, one hundred to two thousand rupees a year'; Manucci, *Storia Do Mogor,* p. 332. See also Lahori, *Padshahnama,* II, p. 422; Muhammad Waris, *Badshahnama,* MS, IO Ethe 329 (transcript of MS., Raza

Library, Rampur, at Department of History, Aligarh Muslim University), II, p. 255.

39 Waris, II, p. 306.

40 For example see, Manucci, *Storia Do Mogor*, IV, pp. 205, 210. *Mirat ul Alam*, I, p. 332; Lahori, *Padshahnama*, II, pp. 8, 11–12, 184, 234, 301, 334, and also I, p. 177; Qazwini, MS.BM.OR. 173, Add. 20734, II, p. 277; *Ma'asirul Umara*, I, p. 589.

41 Manucci, *Storia Do Mogor*, IV, p. 205.

42 *Ma'asir-i Rahimi*, I, pp. 516, 585. *Science and Technology in Medieval India: A Bibliography of Source Materials in Sanskrit, Arabic and Persian*, edited by A. Rahman, M.A. Alvi et al., New Delhi, 1982, p. 21. Francois Bernier, *Travels in the Mogul Empire, 1656–68*, Constable, 1968, p. 4.

43 Manucci, *Storia Do Mogor*, II, iii, pp. 328–29, 332, 374–75; see also ibid., p. 195.

44 Ibid., II, iii, p. 319. In the royal harem, sometimes a woman having a sound knowledge of *tibb* could also be attached. Lahori (*Padshahnama*, II, i, p. 629) refers to sati-un Nisa Begum, the wife of Nasira, the brother of Hakim Rukna, who was attached to the household of Mumtaz Mahal.

45 Ibid., II, iii, pp. 193–94, 195.

46 Manucci, *Storia Do Mogor*, II, iii, pp. 383–84.

47 See in this regard Jahangir, *Tuzuk-i Jahangiri*, edited by Saiyid Ahmad Khan, Vol. II, Ghazipur, 1863, p. 334; also see ibid., II, p. 336.

48 Jean-Baptiste Tavernier, *Travels in India*, translated by V. Ball, Vol. I, New Delhi, 1977, p. 96.

49 *Ma'asir-ul Umara*, I, p. 493; *Ma'asir-i Alamgir*, p. 42.

50 *Ma'asir-i Rahimi*, III, p. 45.

51 *Zakhiratul Khawanin*, III, pp. 336–38.

52 Lahori, *Padshahnama*, I, ii, p. 349; *Ma'asir-i Jahangiri*, p. 345.

53 Manucci, *Storia Do Mogor*, II, p. 76.

54 *Miratu'l Alam*, I, p. 332.

55 Munshi Tek Chand 'Bahar', *Bahar-i Ajam*, 1739–40, litho. Nawal Kishore, Lucknow, 1336/1916, Vol. II, p. 166.

56 *Ma'asir-i Mahmud Shahi*, p. 64.

57 *Tuzuk-i Jahangiri*, I, p. 4.

58 Ali Muhammad Khan, *Mirat-i Ahmadi*, edited by Nawab Ali, Vol. I, Baroda, 1972–78, p. 376.

59 For a reference to the *mutasaddis* and *kotwal* in a government hospital, see Gopal Rai Surdaj, *Durrul Ulum*, MS., Bodleian Library, Oxford, Ms Walker 104, f. 45(b) (Rotograph in Department of History, Aligarh Muslim University).

60 *Mirat-i Ahmadi*, I, p. 209.

61 *Sairu'l Manazil*, p. 8. This *Danish Shifa* is probably the same which is referred to by Gopal Rai Surdaj (*Durul Ulum*, f. 45(b)).

62 Lahori, *Padshahnama*, I, ii, p. 345.

63 *Mirat-i Ahmadi* (supplement), pp. 186–87.

[64] For the hospital at Surat, see *Ruqqat-i Alamgiri*, Nizami Press, Kanpur, 1273 AH, Letter No. 125. See also *Surat Documents*, ff. 174(b), 175(a).

[65] *Mirat-i Ahmadi* (supplement), p. 187; *Selected Documents of Aurangzeb's Reign*, edited by Yusuf Husain, Hyderabad, 1958, pp. 122–23.

[66] *Surat Documents*, Blochet, Suppl. Pers. 482, ff. 174(a), 174(b).

[67] *Selected Documents of Aurangzeb's Reign*, pp. 122–23. The total salary was Rs 180 p.m. which, after the deduction of usual dues, came to Rs 136 p.m. For salaries and daily allowances in government hospitals at Surat and Ahmadabad see *Surat Documents*, ff. 174(a)–175(b), ff. 81(a)–82(b); *Waqa'i Ajmer wa Ranthambhar*, MS., Asafiya Library, Hyderabad (transcript in Department of History, Aligarh Muslim University) Vol. I, p. 9; *Mirat* (supplement), pp. 160–61, 186–87. Compare this with the salaries of local officials like *qanungo, muharrir, nawisanda*, etc., which ranged 'somewhere between Rs 10 to Rs 17 per month'. See S. Ali Nadeem Rezavi, 'The Empire and Bureaucracy'.

[68] *Selected Documents of Shahjahan's Reign*, edited by Y.H. Yahya, Hyderabad, 1950, pp. 211–12; *Daftar-i Diwani-o-Mal-o-Mulki-i Sarkar-i A'la*, Hyderabad (State Archives), 1939, p. 161.

[69] *Selected Documents of Aurangzeb's Reign*, pp. 120, 122–23.

[70] *Ruqqat-i Alamgir*, Letter No. 125.

[71] *Mirat-i Ahmadi*, I, p. 209

[72] *Ma'asirul Umara*, III, p. 936.

[73] *Muraqq'at-i Hasan*, Abul Hasan, MS., Riza Library, Rampur (Microfilm in Department of History, Aligarh Muslim University).

[74] *Indian Travels of Thevenot and Careri*, p. 218.

[75] See, for example, *Selected Documents of Aurangzeb's Reign*, p. 120; Manucci, *Storia Do Mogor*, II, pp. 95–96, 225, etc.; Bernier, *Travels in the Mogul Empire*, pp. 489, etc.

[76] Letter of Balkrishan Brahman, MS., Riell, 83, Add.16895 (Rotagraph in Department of History, Aligarh Muslim University), f. 31(b).

[77] See for example Manucci, *Storia Do Mogor*, III, iv, p. 459. These physicians were probably quite unskilled. See *Mirza Nama* of Mirza Kamran, cited in Iqtidar Alam Khan, 'The Middle Classes in the Mughal Empire', p. 19, n.68.

[78] *Tuzuk-i Jahangiri*, II, p. 253; *Nishan* of Maryam Zamani in *Edicts from the Mughal Haram*, pp. 50–52. See also *Tuzuk-i Jahangiri*, I, p. 91.

[79] Hodivala, *Studies in Parsi History*, Bombay, 1929, pp. 167–88. See also Irfan Habib, *The Agrarian System of Mughal India, 1556–1707*, 2nd edn, Oxford, 1999, p. 353. I am thankful to Professor Irfan Habib, for having brought this set of documents to my knowledge.

[80] Ibid. Of special interest in this regard is the public testimony explicitly mentioning this reason for the grant contained in a document of Aurangzeb's reign (Hodivala, *Studies in Parsi History*, pp. 185–86, 188); Irfan Habib, *Agrarian System*, p. 353.

[81] *Muraqqat-i Hasan*, pp. 330–31.

[82] *Parwana*, dated 1 Ramzan 1116AH/48th RY/28 December 1704, preserved

in National Archives, New Delhi, no. NAI, AD.2444; see also NAI, AD.2446 (dated 25 Ziqada 1127/3RY of Farukh Siyar/22 November 1715).

[83] See for example NAI, AD.2445 and NAI, AD.2447; *Some Firmans, Sanads and Parwanas (1578–1802 AD),* edited by K.K. Datta, Patna, 1962, pp. 30, 45, 68.

[84] Amongst others this view is strongly endorsed by Moreland, *India at the Death of Akbar,* Delhi, 1962, p. 79, and B.B. Misra, *The Indian Middle Classes,* London, 1961, p. 59.

[85] Tavernier, *Travels in India,* I, p. 240

[86] Badauni, *Muntakhab-ut Tawarikh,* III, pp. 163, 170, 315.

[87] Manucci, *Storia Do Mogor,* I, p. 115.

[88] Badauni, *Muntakhab-ut Tawarikh,* III, p. 169.

[89] Banarsi Das, *Ardha Kathanak,* translated and annotated by Mukund Lath, Jaipur, p. 14, text, verse 15 and pp. 31–32, text, verses 185–92.

[90] Ibid., p. 70, text, verse 488.

[91] Surat Singh, *Tazkira-i Pir Hassu Taili,* MS., Department of History, Aligarh Muslim University, ff. 48(b), 171(a), 125(b)–126(a).

[92] Abdul Hayy, *Nuzhat-ul Khawatir,* edited by Sharifuddin Ahmad, Vol. V, Hyderabad, 1962–79, p. 357. For another such example see Anonymous, *Iqbal Nama,* translated by S. Hasan Askari, Patna, 1883, p. 213.

[93] Letter of Balkrishan Brahman, MS., Riell, 83, Add.16895, ff. 125(a), 319(a)–31(b).

[94] See for example Francois Pyrard, *The Voyage of Francois Pyrard of Laval to the East Indies, the Maldives, the Moluccas and Brazil,* translated and edited by Albert Gray and H.C.P. Bell, Vol. I, Haklyut Society, London, n.d., p. 373; Manucci, *Storia Do Mogor,* III, iii, p. 129; J. Fryer, *A New Account of East India and Persia,* p. 27; Carre, *The Travels of the Abbe Carre in India and the Near East, 1672 to 1674,* Vol. I, translated by Lady Fawcet, edited by C. Fawcet and R. Burn, New Delhi, 1990, pp. 268–69.

[95] 'An old man consults a doctor', *Bustan-i Sa'adi,* Aboulala Soudavar Collection, f. 176r, cf. S.C. Welch, Annemarie Schimmel et al., *The Emperor's Album: Images of Mughal India,* New York, 1987, fig. 25.

[96] Fryer, *A New Account of East India and Persia,* p. 115.

[97] As a private practitioner, Manucci was offered Rs 4,000 by a patient (Manucci, *Storia Do Mogor,* III, iii, p. 132); in the service of Shah Alam he received Rs 300 p.m. (ibid., II, p. 215) apart from occasional gifts ranging from Rs 400 to Rs 200 for individual treatment of the members of the princes' *harem* (ibid., II, p. 331). The government physicians on the other hand had a salary of Rs 2 per day (i.e. Rs 60 p.m.). See *supra.*

[98] Manucci, time and again, laments over this hostility; see *Storia Do Mogor,* II, p. 381; IV, pp. 205–10.

[99] John Huighen Van Linschoten, *Voyages to East Indies,* Vol. I, Hakluyt Society, 1885, p. 230.

[100] Careri, *Indian Travels of Thevenot and Careri,* pp. 161–62. Compare this view regarding Indian surgeons with that of Tavernier (*Travels in India,* I,

p. 241) that the people of this country understand nothing about it. See also Manucci, *Storia Do Mogor*, II, pp. 89–90, regarding limitations of Muslim surgeons at Agra.

[101] Manucci, ibid., II, p. 333.

[102] Ibid., III, iii, p. 187.

[103] See for example, ibid, III, iii, p. 129.

[104] See *Dala'il ul Bul*, MS., Sir Sulaiman Collection, 493/14; Subhanullah Collection, 616/22; and *Dala'il un Nabz*, MS., Sir Sulaiman Collection, 492/12, Subhanullah, 616/22.

[105] MS., Maulana Azad Library, Aligarh, University Farsiyya Funun, No. 56.

[106] MS., Bodlein, Persian MSS. Catalogue, 3/76, 2757/3, cf. A. Rahman et al., *Bibliography of Source Materials*, pp. 266–69.

[107] *Bahrul Jawahir*, MS., Maulana Azad Libery, University Farsiya Funun, 4, pub. Calcutta, edited by Abdul Majid, 1830. Cf. A. Rahman et al., *Bibliography of Source Materials*, p. 113.

[108] MS., Bankipur Library, Patna, 11–40; 1013, cf. ibid., p. 4

[109] Badauni, *Muntakhab-ut Tawarikh*, III, pp. 169–70; *Tabaqat-i Akbari*, II, pp. 483–84.

[110] MS., Central State Library, Hyderabad, *Tibb*, 254; Asiatic Society of Bengal, Persian MSS Catalogue, Soc. 722, cf. A. Rahman et al., *Bibliography of Source Materials*, p. 41.

[111] Badanuni, *Muntakhab-ut Tawarikh*, III, p. 230

[112] Ibid., III, p. 164; *Tabaqat-i Akbari*, II, p. 481.

[113] MS., Salarjung, *Mashriqi Kitabkhana*, Hyderabad, cf. A. Rahman et al., *A Bibliography of Source Materials*, p. 16.

[114] Ibid., pp. 144–45.

[115] *Tuzuk-i Jahangiri*, I, p. 152.

[116] See R.L. Verma and V. Bijlani, 'Hakim Ali Gilani: Assessment of his Place in Greco-Medicine', *Studies in History of Medicine*, Vol. IV, No. 2, June 1980, pp. 98–99.

[117] *Tarjuma-i Kitab-ul Qanun*, MS., Riza Library, Rampur, No. 1272.

[118] *Tibb-i Ferishta*, MS., Maulana Azad Library, Subhanullah Collection, No. 616/17, ff. 1–7.

[119] *Mufradat-i Sahih*, MS., Maulana Azad Library, Subhanullah Collection, No. 616/37.

[120] Cf. A. Rahman et al., *A Bibliography of Source Materials*, p. 203.

[121] See *Tuzuk-i Jahangiri*, I, p. 347, II, pp. 344, 364; Lahori, *Padshahnama*, I, p. 350.

[122] *Tuzuk-i Jahangiri*, p. 347.

[123] Lahori, *Padshahnama*, II, pp. 350–51.

[124] Cf. A. Rahman et al., *Bibliography of Source Materials*, p. 21.

[125] Ibid., pp. 202,134,164.

[126] MS., Maulana Azad Library, Subhanullah Collection, No. 615/4.

[127] MS., Maulana Azad Library, Farsiya Funun (Suppl), *Tibb*, 9.

[128] MS., Maulana Azad Library, Subhanullah Collection, No. 610, 3/9.

[129] *Ma'asir-i Alamgiri*, p. 84.

[130] Bernier, *Travels in the Mogul Empire*, pp. 353–54.

[131] Ibid., pp. 324–25.

[132] Cf. A. Rahman et al., *Bibliography of Source Material*, p. 165.

[133] *Tibb-i Akbari*, MSS., Maulana Azad Library, Subhanullah Collection, Nos. 616/15, 616/6 cr.

[134] *Mufarrihul Qulub*, MSS., Maulana Azad Library, University Farsiya Funun, 58; Subhanullah Collection, 616/2; Sir Sulaiman Collection, 580/5.

[135] MS., Maulana Azad Library, Subhanullah Collection, 616/16.

[136] Tables 3 and 4 have been prepared on the basis of the information contained in A. Rahman et al., *Bibliography of Source Materials*.

[137] Asad Beg, *Ahwal-i Asad Beg Qazwini*, MS. BM. OR. 1996 (Rotograph in Department of History, Aligarh Muslim University), ff. 36–37.

[138] Manucci, *Storia Do Mogor*, II, p. 282

[139] Ibid.

[140] See in this regard the statement of Bernier, *Travels in the Mogul Empire*, p. 259.

A Sixteenth-Century Code
for Physicians

Shireen Moosvi

Once the treatment of disease separated itself from ritual and invocation of supernatural powers, the burden of responsibility of the physician was infinitely enlarged. It was, therefore, inevitable that there should develop in course of time a set of ethical norms for the profession. These are summarized today in what is called the Hippocratic oath (see Appendix). Administered in many universities and medical institutions, the broad terms of the oath are traced back to Hippocrates (*c.* 460–*c.* 377 BC). Jolly cites two ancient Indian medical texts, by Charaka (first century AD) and Sushruta (fifth century AD), for certain principles of conduct expected of a physician. He should attend wholly to the cure of the patient and not injure him in any way. He should not look at the patient's wife or property. He should not disclose events occurring at the home of the patient, and not utter a word even if he feels the patient's death is near. He should give his medicine gratis 'to a Brahman, spiritual teacher, [the] poor, friend, an ascetic and the like'. On the other hand, he should not treat 'hunters, fowlers, outcastes and sinners'.[1]

Admonitions that appear to have greater expectations from physicians are found in the Islamic or Graeco–Arab tradition, according to al-Ruhawi's *Adab al-Tabib*, written in the ninth century. The physician should avoid money-grabbing, slander and addiction to wines and drugs. He is to remain calm and patiently answer questions from the patient and members of his family. If the patient so wishes, he is not to object to a second opinion; and if that opinion differs from his, he should leave the decision to the patient himself.[2]

What I shall present in this paper is a statement on the ethics of the physician from the pen of a writer of a book of ethics, written in India in the last decade of the sixteenth century. Abdu'l Qadir Badauni was a theologian with a large amount of learning, having studied under Shaikh Mubarak, father of Akbar's famous minister Abu'l Fazl and a liberal scholar. Badauni himself was a man of narrow religious views, saddled with embarrassing employment as a translator of the *Mahabharata* in a project commissioned by Akbar. He is well-known for his history, the *Muntakhabu't Tawarikh*, which contains bitter and caustic criticism of his employer and sovereign.[3] His work on ethics, the *Nijatu'r Rashid*, formally composed in 1590–91,[4] is, however, very unlike his history, although the two works contain references to each other. It is, perhaps, the first major work on ethics written in India during the Mughal period.[5] It is significant in that while Badauni states the *shariat* position on many matters, he recognizes that ethics comprise a sphere broader than that of law, and that what the law permits may not be what ethics would condone, as in the matter of temporary marriages, divorce, slavery—and, surprisingly, cow-slaughter. And there are, of course, matters like the physician's conduct, on which the *Shariat* has nothing much to offer. Badauni is, therefore, very much on his own here.

I offer below a translation of what he has to say after discussing the habit of some juridical luminaries who give legal opinions without knowledge or study.

> And of this genre [of improper conduct] is the pursuit of medical practice without past experience. Just as legal opinion given without knowledge can ruin spiritual life, so medical treatment given without wisdom can destroy physical life. Any one who has not read the books of medicine with reputed physicians for a number of years, nor put them to use for long years of life, nor obtained knowledge of the properties of drugs, nor received authorization for medical practice from masters [in the profession], but simply wishes that by force of some intuition, he may treat people without having any experience and consider it the means of gaining proximity to rulers and kings, is not a physician, no expert master, but a blood-shedder like a crude executioner. It is incumbent on the rulers of Islam to suppress such a reputeless set [of persons].
>
> One of the conditions for the physician is this that he should be a proficient physician by knowledge, and in word and deed truthful, and compassionate towards all creatures. For him there should be no difference between friend and foe, acquaintance and

stranger. Nor should he be an idle-talker, favour-seeker, self-praiser, unjust, and indifferent. When he engages in treating a patient he should solicit success from the Almighty. He should not impose an insupportable burden on a patient who is destitute and needy and should not let his self-interest intrude. He should attend to the needy more than to the well-provided. So far as he can, he should himself provide medicine and diet to the destitute patients out of his own resources, obtaining [spiritual] recompense and gratitude in return. He should not abstain from instructing other people and should not fully rely on compounded drugs as such are all suspect.

He should not place entire confidence on his own opinion alone, and if he finds himself unable to treat an ailment, he should on his own consult a more knowledgeable physician, and should not at all consider it disgraceful to appear as a beginner, but rather make him [the senior physician] a collaborator with himself and not strive after contention. After exchanging opinions, whatever is found correct should be followed whether it means following someone else's opinion or his own.

If the disease happens to be incurable he should not terrify the patient and should not make him despair of life. Although [ultimately] no one can prevent death, yet the duty of the physician is that he should by artful devices lead the patient in this physical world of four elements from one year further to another. He should not be too much solicitous of praise by people, and of the wherewithal of splendour.

In seeking glory, there is no better deed than securing cures.

As far as possible he should personally attend upon the patient, and if he does not have the time he should depute his students and assistants, with full effort and effectual arrangement, to wait upon the sick.

These counsels are furnished out of sincerity. It is incumbent upon him [the physician] to investigate the human body. But in regard to counsels on matters that appertain to the practice of medicine, these are described in the books of godly physicians (*hukama-i-ilahi*). A recital of these does not fall within the province of the expounders of ethics. *And He is the curer of Disease, and is Himself free of Disease* (Quran).[6]

The entire section is of interest for several reasons. Except for one casual reference to God, where the physician is asked to seek his aid, and a formal Quranic quotation at the end, religion and ritual play no part in the 'code'. What the physician is called upon to do is to read books, and acquire knowledge and experience. Secondly, the patient's interests are given a primary place, and this is where Badauni scores over the present text of the Hippocratic oath (see Appendix for its text). The wealth and position of the patient should not determine the amount of attention he receives. By his insistence that the poor, the needy and the destitute must have primacy, Badauni shows an amount of humane compassion and a rejection of the demands of hierarchy that, in a writer of that age, is singular. Badauni is also practical in that, knowing the harm of a physician's individualism, he insists on a more cooperative approach. A second opinion is to be taken in a difficult case, not on the patient's request, but at the physician's own instance. He is enjoined to let reason and argument decide, not wilful insistence on his own opinion.

Badauni's exhortation to the physician to investigate the human body *(tan-i ausaf)* is particularly modern in approach, since anatomy was such a weak point in both the Tibb and Ayurveda.

Appendix
The Hippocratic Oath

'You do solemnly swear, each man by whatever he holds most sacred, that you will be loyal to the profession of medicine and just and generous to its members; that you will lead your life and practise your art in uprightness and honour; that into whatsoever house you shall enter, it shall be for the good of the sick to the utmost of your power, you holding yourselves far aloof from wrong, from corruption, from the tempting of others to vice; that you will exercise your art solely for the cure of your patients and will give no drug, perform no operation, for a criminal purpose, even if solicited, far less suggest it. That what-soever you shall see or hear of the lives of men which is not fitting to be spoken, you will keep inviolably secret. These things do you swear. Let each man bow the head in sign of acqueiscence. And now, if you will be true to this, your oath, may prosperity and good repute be ever yours; the opposite, if you shall prove yourself forsworn.'

I have taken this text from the *New Illustrated Columbia Encyclopedia*, X, New York, 1978/79, p. 3111.

Notes and References

1 Julius Jolly, *Indian Medicines*, translated by G.G. Kashikar, 2nd rev. edn, New Delhi, 1977, p. 27. A.B. Keith's dates for the two texts in their final form are much later: he places Charaka earlier than the ninth century, and Sushruta, earlier than the eleventh century. (A. Berriedale Keith, *A History of Sanskrit Literature*, Oxford, 1920, pp. 506–07.)

2 Cf. Howard J. Turner, *Science in Medieval Islam: An Illustrated Introduction*, Delhi, 1999, pp. 134–35.

3 *Muntakhabu't Tawarikh* (*c.* 1595–96), 3 vols, edited by Ali Ahmad and W.N. Lees, Bib. Ind., 1864–69. It is Vol. 2 that mainly deals with the history of Akbar's reign.

4 Badauni says in his preface and conclusion (pp. 2–3, 531) that the numerical value of the title *Nijatu'r Rashid* yields the date of the work, which implies AH 999/1590–91. But there are many indications that the work was completed, or went on being revised, until much later. The internal evidence strongly suggests that Badauni began writing the work in 999/1590–91, but did not finish it until 1598 or some time afterwards. Cf. Irfan Habib, 'Akbar and Social Inequities, a Study of the Evolution of his Ideas', *Proceedings of the Indian History Congress*, Warangal (53rd) session, 1992–93, Delhi, 1993, p. 308. There are two known extant MSS., viz., Asiatic Society of Bengal (Ivanow 1263), A.P. State Archives. S. Moinul Haq's edition (Lahore 1972) is solely based on the Asiatic Society MS. This edition is used here.

5 The characterization of Nur-ud-Din Qazi al-Khaqani's *Akhlaq-i-Jahangiri*, as 'the first major book on *Akhlaq* (ethics, including governance) produced under the Mughals in North India' (Muzaffar Alam and S. Subrahmanyam, *The Mughal State 1526–1750*, Delhi, 1998, p. 23) shows how little Badauni's work is known even among historians.

6 'Abdul Qadir Badauni, *Nijatu'r Rashid*, edited by Sayyid Muinul Haq (S. Moinul Haque), Lahore, 1972, pp. 168–69.

Inside and Outside the Systems

Change and Innovation in Medical and
Surgical Practice in Mughal India

Irfan Habib

Medical science, like any other branch of knowledge, has in its history tended to develop its own set of assumptions (or superstitions!) and accumulations of experience. Such of these as have remained confined to particular regions or cultures have tended to grow into 'classical' systems of which the Ayurveda and Yunani ('Graeco–Arab') systems are two obvious examples. It becomes important, therefore, to consider how much change these systems were capable of incorporating, and what areas (and so what changes within such areas) they tended to exclude altogether.

I present here, mainly from sources of the Mughal period and the eighteenth century, three cases to illustrate developments within and without the two major systems we have mentioned. The first is that of China root, a drug that was received immediately with what was perhaps undeserved credulity. The two others are smallpox inoculation and nasal surgery which, as undeservedly, remained unacknowledged in both the systems. I would not like to claim a heavier theoretical import than my evidence can bear. I therefore intend to lay out the information that I have been able to gather and wait hopefully for it to be supplemented and interpreted by much surer hands than mine.

Syphilis and China Root

When, in 1604, a Mughal officer, Asad Beg Qazwini, back at Agra from a mission to Bijapur, presented to Emperor Akbar a hookah well and truly made, along with a supply of tobacco, the emperor showed some inclination to try a smoke. But his favourite physician, Hakim 'Ali, put in the characteristic objection: 'In fact, this [tobacco] is an untried drug. None of the old medical authorities (*hukama'*) have

71

written about it. How can we suggest that His Majesty take such a thing whose real essence is unknown. It is not proper for His Majesty to take it.' It did not matter, said the *hakim*, if the Europeans had adopted it: 'It is not necessary for us to follow the Europeans and to adopt a thing not known to our sages, and without experiment.' To this, Asad Beg says, he gave the following spirited rejoinder, much approved by the emperor:

> It is a wonderful thing that all customs of the world have come about [at one time or another], and from the time of Adam to this day everything has come by and by. Whenever anything new appears among one people, it gets to be known all over the World, and all people adopt it. Scholars and physicians need to apply themselves to learn of its usefulness or ill-effect and to experiment (with it). May be, [of now] they just do not know its [tobbaco's] benefits. Thus China-root (*chob-i-Chini*) was not present in old times, and has appeared recently and is yet found beneficial in so many diseases.[1]

China root, then, was the drug which Asad Beg could see as the most recent intruder from outside of the classical systems. Unknown to them, it had quickly followed upon a disease that too was earlier unknown, and of which it was regarded as a cure. The disease was syphilis.

Archaeologists' examination of New and Old World skeletons has established that syphilis could have appeared any time in the New World between AD 400 and 1200, while no skeleton examined from the Old World before Columbus seems to have been affected by it.[2] This has confirmed what history has long accepted from literary sources: that syphilis appeared first within the Old World in Spain in 1493, having been brought there by the first sailors returning from the Americas. It then spread to Portugal, France and Italy. The Portuguese arrival in the Indian Ocean with Vasco Da Gama's voyage of 1498, hastened its spread in Asia. As reported by Pyrard of Laval, 1602–07, the people of the Maldives aptly called it 'farangui baescour' (*farangi basur*), i.e. European piles.[3] When the Portuguese ships reached China in 1513 and seized the island of Tunmen in Guangdong province, they gifted the disease to China. Li Shizhen, who completed his great compendium of *materia medica* in 1578, noted that syphilis, 'not mentioned in the ancient recipes', had arisen in Guangdong and then spread to all parts of China.[4]

It so happened that in China there existed a drug which had long been in use for diseases of the urino-genital system. It is mentioned as early as the sixth century AD, by Tao Hongjing in his commentaries on *materia medica*. This was the *Smilax China Linn*. (also called *Smilax Japonica*, A. Gray).[5] The Portuguese naturally termed it *raiz da China*, 'China root', since it was the tuberous root of the plant from which the drug was derived, to be used in the form of powder or of liquid after decoction.[6] When peeled and trimmed, the root looked like 'a piece of heavy, pinkish white wood',[7] so that the name *chob-i Chini* ('China wood') in Persian was also natural enough: this word was adopted not only in Hindustani, Bengali, Punjabi, Marathi and Gujarati, in the simple form of *chob-chini*, but also in Sanskrit (*chobachini*).[8] In his account of India, based on his sojourn in this country, 1583–88, Linschoten writes enthusiastically of China root, praising God for giving the Chinese this remedy which, ever 'since it became known in India, they would never use any other remedy'. He gives the date of its arrival in India as 1535.[9] Garcia da Orta, writing his 'Colloquies' in 1563 at Goa gives the same year (1535) as the one when a cure was first accomplished (presumably in India) through the use of China root.[10] The efficacy of the drug was acclaimed in Europe soon afterwards, and in 1546 Andreas Vesalius published a 'small but celebrated' monograph on it from Basle.[11]

As Asad Beg says, China root, though a novelty, won recognition in the established systems of medicine without much obstruction. In Ayurveda its incorporation is marked by its mention in Bhava Misra's *Bhavaprakasa*, which is assigned to the sixteenth century, a more precise date being apparently not available.[12]

About its reception in Yunani medicine there is some interesting material on which Elgood has already commented.[13] This mainly consists of three successive tracts on China root, the earliest of which, the *Risala-i Chob-i-Chini* of Nurullah 'Ata, was written in AH 944/AD 1537–38, or, as given in some MSS, AH 1954/AD 1547.[14] If the first date is correct, this tract would have precedence in time over the one by Vesalius. The author says that he had spent nearly twenty years in India, where he had heard of China root (*bikh-i Chini*, *bikh* meaning root), which the Portuguese (*mardum-i Firang*) were deliberately withholding from the Muslims. A European physician (an allegedly secret convert to Islam) called Aristotle ('Arasto') told him that it came from the extremity of the Inhabited World. But at last, he had obtained

73

a supply of the drug from Portuguese notables, and for twelve years now this was being taken from him by people to different parts and many had obtained cures thereby.[15] It can be seen that, depending on the two alternative dates of the work, China root must have come into the author's hands, presumably in India, in either 1525–26 or 1535, whereafter it reached Iran—so he seemingly claims—through his own agency.

To this 'Imaduddin Mahmud (fl. 1571–72) adds that, when introduced, China root was found efficacious 'in such ulcers and vapours of syphilis (*atishak*) as had become chronic and did not respond to laxatives or inunctions'. It was by experiment found to be useless for treating paralysis, and so was not administered to Jumla Begum, the widow of Shah Isma'il (reigned, 1501–24).[16] This passage not only stresses the specific disease with whose cure China root was associated, but tends to confirm that the drug was in use in Iran not long after Shah Isma'il's death in 1524.

Qazi bin Kashifuddin Yazdi, who wrote his *risala* on China root, coffee and tea in the reign of Shah 'Abbas I (1587–1629), refers curiously enough to tracts written on China root by 'European physicians', but he is certainly dating the drug's appearance in Iran too early when he says that its arrival in the early years of Shah Isma'il's reign, 1501–24, was one of the blessings on Iran conferred by that ruler's presence.[17]

Why China root came to be acclaimed with such enthusiasm in the educated worlds of medicine in China, India, Iran and Europe, and why so much credit was given to its curative powers everywhere for so long is now not easy to understand. As late as 1893 Watt records the reports from modern physicians and surgeons regarding 'good cures' of syphilis attained by its use, and of its use also in rheumatism, scrofula and even consumption, as well as of its functions as an 'alternative and nutrient tonic'.[18] And yet Watt noted not only its recent disuse in Europe, but also that 'no active principle' had been actually derived from it. China root and other liliaceous roots are now held to contain little of medicinal value beyond the saponins and sapotoxins they contain, and are at best mild nauseants.[19] It was only in the nineteenth century that its use was given up in western medicine in favour of protracted and specific treatments with arsenic, mercury and bismuth. Penicillin in the twentieth century, of course, supplanted everything else. One may perhaps, then, attribute the universal credit given to China root to little more than a desperate desire to get a remedy for a new and worrisome disease, for which the existing prescriptions held forth no means of cure. The readiness to accept a new drug was creditable for both the Ayurveda and Yunani doctors, but here, unfortunately, their credulity was as misplaced as Asad Beg's in tobacco.

Smallpox Inoculation

If syphilis came from the New World to assault the Old in the sixteenth century, the New World too, on its part, received a far more dreadful disease from its Spanish conquerors. Smallpox, brought by the Spaniards, decimated the Amerindian population on a scale that is hard to imagine today: some 95 per cent of the population of Central Mexico could have been wiped out, in the century after 1520, by smallpox, assisted by the different genocidal measures of the conquerors. In India, the disease (the *masurika* in its serious or fatal form) appears in medical literature probably as early as the seventh century, about the same time as it did in the west, and possibly a little after China.[20] By the seventeenth century it was certainly one of India's major scourges. How extensive its ravages were can be seen from a simple count. Out of twenty-five villagers, who had their descriptions recorded during 1653–1717, as parties or witnesses before *qazis*, in documents that survive in the Vrindaban collections, as many as ten bore the scars of smallpox.[21] If this sample is really representative, about 40 per cent of all the people must have become victims of the disease; and this, of course, covers only those who survived to bear its marks. The number of fatalities remains unknown.

Neither Ayurveda nor the Yunani system had any effective remedy for smallpox. It is perhaps of some credit to an Indian physician, Muhammad Akbar Arzani (*d.* 1722), that he attempted the relief of a patient (his own son) by pricking and draining out the vesicles with the aid of gold needles.[22] Where India has a significant place is not, however, in the history of the treatment of smallpox, but in that of techniques to prevent its visitation.

On variolation or inoculation against smallpox as practised in Bengal under the familiar name of *tika*, there are two early reports, one by R. Coult of 1731, and the other by J.Z. Holwell of 1767.[23] Francis Buchanan, in his famous surveys of eastern India, 1808–12, has also furnished much information on the practice and its practitioners.[24] These reports agree on the fact that inoculation consisted of introducing matter originally taken from the pus of smallpox pustules with a thick needle; but they agree on little else. Coult (1731) reports that the pus was taken from a patient when the pox came to maturity and was of a 'good' (presumably mild) kind. Holwell (1767) says it was taken from persons who got a mild attack of the disease from the inoculation itself, and was then kept in cotton within a rag for a year. Buchanan says it was only taken from the pustules of those who had caught the pox in 'a natural way', and kept in cotton for no more than three days.[25] According to Coult, several punctures were made with a needle, impregnated with the pus, the punctures (*tika*) being made on the upper arm or forehead. It could be supplemented with an oral administration of the pus in a 'bolus', repeating the operation of inoculation through punctures for two days. According to Holwell, the incisions were made usually on the outside of the arm by a barber's instrument for cutting nails, and the intrusion of variolous matter was then secured by placing it in a moistened cotton-wad put on the incisions for several hours. Buchanan's description is similar here to Holwell's; the incisions were made first, and then cotton impregnated with the collected matter was rubbed on them to introduce the infection. Holwell insists far more than Buchanan on a strict dietary regimen for the patient for a month both preceding and following the inoculation.

There is little agreement too in respect of who the inoculators were. Coult says they were brahmans, who spoke of an originator of the practice at Champa Nagar some 150 years earlier. Holwell says that they were brahmans who came on regular tours from Brindaban, Allahabad, Banaras, etc., and so having their headquarters outside Bengal, and that they had been pursuing the practice since 'time out of mind'. Buchanan says the inoculators were 'of both religions [i.e. Hindus and Muslims] and of all castes'; elsewhere he says they belonged to 'the same lowest dregs of the populace'.

What is clear through these variations in the accounts is that the inoculators expected to bring upon their patients a hopefully mild form of disease, which would thereafter prevent the virulent form of it attacking them. If an attack of fever and eruption did not follow the inoculation, the operation would be regarded as having failed (Coult). Once the expected fever broke out, however, the inoculator himself had no remedies to offer except spells and dietary prescriptions (Holwell, Buchanan).

Both Holwell and Buchanan rate the success rate quite highly. According to Holwell it was 'a miracle to hear that one in a million fails of receiving the infection' from the inoculation. And Buchanan tells us that when the fatal form of the disease struck in district Dinajpur, it could take only one out of a hundred of those inoculated. In district Bhagalpur too the operations used to be 'attended with the most complete success, very few indeed dying' during outbreaks of the disease. Buchanan notes, therefore, that vaccination (i.e. the inoculation of Jenner's vaccine) was 'of very little importance' in Bengal and Bihar, so much so that the vaccinator in Monghyr had to pay persons coming to him to be vaccinated.[26]

One may infer from the different descriptions of the practice in the three reports that it either underwent successive changes or there were different customs prevailing among different sets of practitioners. The tradition reported by Coult of an indigenous Bengali origin of the practice under brahmanical auspices may then possibly refer to one form of inoculation only; and Holwell's report of practitioners coming from up-country, to yet another. By Buchanan's time the practice was apparently much simplified and the inoculators were so numerous as to have shed all pretensions to being brahmans.

Yet, even as inoculation was spreading in Bengal and Bihar, many other parts of India do not seem to have heard of it. Buchanan did not come across it in his great tour of southern India in 1800–01. In fact, while in the vicinity of Coimbatore, where the epidemic was then raging, he found that inoculation was 'unknown to the natives'.[27] In 1837 Donald Butter, himself a physician, noted that 'various inoculation is not practised in Oud'h'.[28] Could it then be supposed that the tradition recorded by Coult in 1731 was right, and that the smallpox inoculation was developed independently in Bengal, had only spread thence to Bihar and neighbouring parts, and so had not yet reached other parts of India and entered the texts of either the Ayurvedic or the Yunani systems?

I would have argued on these lines, but for evidence that the practice of inoculation was in fact known in western India and further west. The *Gazetteer* of the Mewar Residency, originally published in 1908, tells us that the Bhils 'have inoculated from time immemorial under the name *kanai*, the operation being done with a needle and a grain of dust dipped into the pack of a smallpox case. The practice is, however, disappearing with the spread of vaccination.'[29] As anywhere else, one must take the reference to 'time immemorial' with some degree of scepticism; but certainly the report implies that the custom was not of very recent introduction.

There is, then, a report of the practice in the Las Bela district of eastern Baluchistan, adjoining Sind, from Charles Masson, the famous American traveller, communicated in April 1839 by J.W. Wonchester from Thatta (southern Sind):

> Inoculation is known in Lus, the virus being taken from a person labouring with small-pox and inserted on the wrist of healthy individuals (children), who, if the operation is successful, which is not often the case, are seized with small-pox, not limited to the hand and arm, but general; commonly mild, yet in some cases fatal.

In a note it is further stated that inoculation was also known in Kabul: 'there it is generally performed by the Syuds [cf. the brahman inoculators of Bengal!], who frequently make two or three trials before succeeding'.[30]

It is probable that if explorations of older records are further extended, more casual references to smallpox inoculation in these and other areas are likely to be discovered: Bengal and Bihar, therefore, did not stand alone.

It is certain too that the region of inoculation extended much farther west, not only to Afghanistan but up to Turkey, where, in 1717 (fourteen years before the practice is reported from India), the wife of the British ambassador, Lady Mary Wortley Montagu, in an oft-cited incident, protected her family by resorting to the local technique of producing mild infections through insertion of matter from smallpox pustules. On her return (1718), she introduced the practice in England; and this led ultimately to Jenner and true vaccination (1796). Clearly, then, the practice was prevalent in Turkey at least quite early in the eighteenth century. It could also have been current during the same century in Iraq.[31]

Such extensive distribution of the practice in the eighteenth century, with no previous record of it in medical literature,[32] shows, first, that it spread through a popular acceptance of the practice without any recognition by the higher medical profession; and, second, that the spread was relatively recent, since otherwise it would have received some mention in the texts. Needham has proposed that the ultimate source of the practice was China, where the practice of putting matter from smallpox pustules in the nostrils became widespread in the sixteenth century.[33] The obvious difficulty in accepting the suggestion is that the Chinese technique involved inoculation through inhalation, while in all other countries it was by skin-incision ('cutaneous scarification').[34] The Chinese surely have precedence over all others in discovering the principle behind inoculation, but the incision technique certainly represented an important advance over the nasal. Where this crucial step of introducing infected matter into the bloodstream was first taken, remains obscure. Yet, from wherever it originated, the rapid spread of the technique, as common people learnt of it from each other unassisted by 'intellectuals', fully deserves the status of a medical epic. Its illiterate practitioners were the harbingers of all immunization techniques that constitute such a major part of the achievements of modern medicine and biochemistry.

Nose-Cutting and Plastic Surgery

Medicine cannot possibly exclude surgery, or 'manual treatment of injuries or disorders of the body' (as defined in Fowler's *Concise Oxford Dictionary*), and yet in both Ayurveda and Yunani medicine, surgical operations, even in the treatment of wounds, occupy a rather limited space, and are seldom included among the duties of the physician. When, in 1528, young Mughal Princess Gulbadan's arm was accidentally pulled so hard by her Afghan step-mother that it got dislocated, it had to be set and bound up, not by a physician but by a bow-maker (*kamangar*).[35] Wounds were treated and blood-letting performed by persons called *jarrahs*, 'those who tend wounds (*jarahat*)'. A *jarrah* who rose to high status under Jahangir (1605–27) was Muqarrab Khan, who successively became governor of Gujarat, Bihar and Agra.[36] Still, it was a physician (Hakim Momina) who prescribed how much blood was to be sucked out when, in 1619, a blood-letting of Jahangir himself was undertaken by Muqarrab Khan and his nephew Qasim.[37] In ordinary life *jarrahs* were regarded as little more than glorified barbers (*hajjams*), as appears from the designation of 'the *hajjam's* glass' (*shisha-i hajjam*) given in two dictionaries (compiled at Delhi, *c.* 1740) to the glass (tube) that the blood-letter employed to suck out blood.[38] It is true, however, that professional *jarrahs* of any status did not in fact pursue the occupation of barbers.[39] In the Indian caste system the doctrine of pollution by touch could also have prevented the *vaidya* from undertaking surgical operations.[40]

The general separation of the two crafts of physician and surgeon probably explains why there is no indigenous textual evidence for India's remarkable participation in the history of plastic surgery. It is possible too that the performers of the feat were illiterate men who never wrote about what they were doing.

The first evidence for the practice of nose-restoration in India comes from a veteran seventeenth-century 'India hand', the Italian Nicolas Manucci, who wrote the following in 1686:

> At the commencement of the war [between Aurangzeb and Bijapur], when the men of Bijapur caught any unhappy persons belonging to the Moguls who had gone out to cut grass or collect straw or do some other service, they did not kill them but cut off their noses. Thus they came back into the camp all bleeding. The surgeons belonging to the country cut the skin of the forehead above the eyebrows, and made it fall down over the wounds on the nose. Then giving it a twist so that the live flesh might meet the other live surface, by healing applications they fashioned for them other imperfect noses. There is left above between the eyebrows, a small hole, caused by the twist given to the skin to bring the two live surfaces together. In a short time the wounds heal up, some obstacle being placed beneath to allow for respiration. I saw many persons with such noses, and they were not so disfigured as they would have been without any nose at all, but they bore between their eyebrows the mark of the incision.[41]

I have given this long quotation from Manucci because all subsequent observers of this practice have described it in practically identical terms, except that while Manucci had found the art practised in the Deccan, or at least in the Mughal army in the Deccan, these observers associate it unanimously with Kangra and the mountains around in what is now Himachal Pradesh.

Writing in 1852, Honigberger, a physician himself, recalled how while staying at Lahore, he saw an 'Akalee or Nahung' whose nose had been cut off by Ranjit Singh. But 'his nose had been so well restored in the mountains that we were all surprised and confessed it could not have been better done in Europe'. He noted that 'in the East' the turban served well to hide the scar on the forehead.[42]

G.T. Vigne, who visited Kangra in 1839, adds to Manucci's description of the operation by saying that 'opium, bang or wine' was used to make the patient senseless; that the skin cut from the forehead was sewn on the skin below and supported by a piece of cotton; and that an ointment containing blue vitriol was thereafter applied to the wound. The patients were drawn from as far as Iran, and local tradition traced back the practice to Emperor Akbar's reign (1556–1605).[43]

The famous archaeologist A. Cunningham has a long note on this operation in his report of 1872–73. He found the surgery still being practised in Kangra, the patients coming mainly from Kabul and Nepal which, after the fall of Sikh rule in the Punjab, were the only adjoining areas where nose-cutting was still in vogue. His description of the operation is the same as that of Manucci, Honigberger and Vigne, and he specifically denies that the skin used was taken from some other person. He cited the tradition reported by Vigne that the practice here seemingly dated from Akbar's time when Kangra was given in *jagir* to a surgeon of Akbar's court, who was proficient in it. The current story as heard by him was, however, that the practice was already established in Kangra when Akbar subjugated it.[44] The implicit suggestion in Vigne's earlier report that the practice was imported from the plains is perhaps more credible, especially in view of Manucci's account of 1686, which shows that the surgery was actually being performed in the Mughal army in the Deccan. But how it came to the 'surgeons' in the Mughal camp there remains a mystery.

Notes and References

[1] Asad Beg Qazwini, Memoirs (untitled), Br. Lib., Qr. 1996, f. 21a–b. The whole passage is reproduced in translation in Shireen Moosvi, *Episodes in the life of Akbar, Contemporary Records and Reminiscences*, New Delhi, 1994, pp. 106–08. My translation, though not substantially different, is independent.

[2] 'Origin of Syphilis', *Archaeology*, 50 (1), 1997, pp. 24–25. This report refers to Bruce-Rothschild's refutation of an alleged syphilis-affected foetus of the fourth century found at Costebelle, France.

[3] Francois Pyrard of Laval, *The Voyage of Francois Pyrard of Laval to the East Indies, the Maldives, Moluccas and Brazil*, translated (from the French edition of 1619) by Albert Gray and H.C.P. Bell, I, London, 1887, pp. 182–83. This traveller notes correctly that the word *Farangi*, derived from the

word Frank/French, was applied to Europeans in general, but it was more specifically applied to the Portuguese. Thus 'Portuguese piles' would be a better rendering of the Maldive name for the disease.

[4] Cf. Berthold Laufer, *Sino-Iranica, Chinese Contributions to the History of Civilization in Ancient Iran, with Special Reference to the History of Cultivated Plants and Products,* Chicago, 1919, p. 557. For Li Shizen's work and date, see Cai Jingfeng in Mao Yisheng (ed.), *Ancient China's Technology and Science,* Beijing, 1983, pp. 352–53.

[5] Joseph Needham, *Science and Civilization in China,* Vol. 6: *Biology and Biological Technology,* Part I: *Botany,* Cambridge, pp. 160–61. On Tao Hongjing (Thao Hung-Ching), see Cai Jingfeng, *in Ancient China's Technology and Science,* p. 353.

[6] George Watt, *A Dictionary of the Economic Products of India,* VI (3), Calcutta, 1893, pp. 253–54.

[7] Ibid., p. 254.

[8] Cf. ibid., p. 253, and Laufer, *Sino-Iranica,* p. 556. It is noteworthy that in other Indian languages too, as recorded by Watt, the foreign origin of the drug is implied: *Pirangi Chekka* in Telugu; *Paringay* in Tamil. It is *China-alla* in Sinhalese.

[9] John Huyghen van Linschoten, *The Voyage of John Huyghen van Linschoten to the East Indies,* from the old English translation of 1598, II, edited by P.A. Tiele, London, 1885, pp. 106–12.

[10] Laufer, *Sino-Iranica,* p. 556.

[11] Needham, *Science and Civilization,* Vol. 6, Pt. I, pp. 160–61.

[12] J. Jolly, *Indische Medicine,* p. 106, cited by Laufer, *Sino-Iranica,* p. 556. A.B. Kieth too, in his *History of Sanskrit Literature,* London, 1920, p. 511, does not have a more precise date to offer for the work.

[13] Cyril Elgood, *Safavid Medical Practice or the Practice of Medicine, Surgery and Gynaecology in Persia between 1500 AD and 1750 AD,* London, 1970, pp. 50–51.

[14] It is only in manuscripts where the work is attributed to 'Imaduddin Mahmud, that the year is altered to 945/1547 (C.A. Storey, *Persian Literature: A Bio-bibliographical Survey,* II, Part II, *Medicine,* London, 1971, p. 241). But this attribution is difficult to accept, and this makes the altered year also doubtful.

[15] Nurullah 'Ata, *Risala-i Chob-i Chini,* British Lib., Add. 19, 619, f. 263a–b.

[16] 'Imaduddin Mahmud, *Risala-i Chob-i Chini,* British Lib., Add. 19, 619, f. 248a.

[17] Qazi b. Kashifuddin Muhammad Yazdi, *Risala-i Chob-i Chini,* etc., British Lib., Add. 19, 169, f. 130a.

[18] Watt, *Dictionary of Economic Products of India,* VI, p. 254.

[19] Needham, *Science and Civilization in China,* VI (1), p. 160.

[20] For the history of smallpox in India, see Ralph W. Nicholas, 'The Goddess Sitala and Epidemic Smallpox in Bengal', *Journal of Asiatic Society,* XL (i), November 1981, pp. 25–26. For China, Europe and the Islamic world, see

Joseph Needham, *Clerks and Craftsmen in China and the West*, Cambridge, 1970, p. 375.

21 Irfan Habib, *Agrarian System of Mughal India, 1556–1707*, revised edn, New Delhi, 1999, p. 111*n*. For the Vrindaban documents see ibid., p. 473.

22 So he says in his *Mufarrihu'l Qulub*, as quoted by R.L. Verma, 'The Growth of Graeco-Arabian Medicine in Medieval India', *Indian Journal of History of Science*, V (2), pp. 359–60. The work has been printed; Verma cites a Delhi edition, n.d., p. 572. See Storey, *Persian Literature*, II (2)(E), pp. 219–20, 268–71, for the work and the author.

According to Holwell's account of 1767, this was a procedure followed by 'Eastern practitioners' generally. He says: 'in very critical cases, they will not trust the operation of opening the pustules to the nurses or relations, but engage in it themselves with amazing patience and solicitude' (J.Z. Holwell, 'An account of the manner of inoculating for the smallpox in the East Indies', in Dharampal [ed.], *Indian Science and Technology in the Eighteenth Century: Some Contemporary European Accounts*, Delhi, 1971, pp. 161–62.)

23 Published in Dharampal, ibid., pp. 141–42 (extract from Coult's report on 'the diseases of Bengal'), 143–63 (J.Z. Holwell's 'Account of the manner of inoculating &c.').

24 See, especially, his surveys edited by Montgomery Martin, *The History, Antiquities, Topography and Statistics of Eastern India, &c.*, II, London, 1838, pp. 690–91, for Dinajpur district (1808); Francis Buchanan, *An Account of the District of Purnea in 1809–10*, Patna, 1928, p. 187; and idem, *An Account of the District of Bhagalpur in 1810–11*, Patna, 1939, p. 173.

25 This would have been warmly approved by Jenner; see long extract from Edward Jenner, *An Inquiry into the Causes and Effects of the Variolae Vaccinae* (1798) in Arthur Rook (ed.), *The Origins and Growth of Biology*, Harmondsworth, 1964, pp. 344–45.

26 For references in this and the preceding paragraphs to Coult and Holwell, see f.n. 23, and for references to Buchanan, see f.n. 24.

27 Francis Buchanan, *A Journey from Madras through the Countries of Mysore, Canara and Malabar*, II, London, 1807, pp. 285–86.

28 Donald Butter, *Outlines of the Topography and Statistics of the Southern Districts of Ou'dh*, Calcutta, 1839, p. 169. He says that vaccination too was encountering much resistance.

29 E.D. Enskine, *Rajputana Gazetteers*, II–A and II–B, *The Mewar Residency*, rpt, Gurgaon, 1992, p. 87.

30 R. Hughes Thomas (ed.), *Selections from the Records of Bombay Government*, No. XVII, Series: *Memoirs on Shikarpoor, the Syeds of Roree and Bukkur, &c.*, Bombay, 1855, reprinted as *Memoirs on Sind*, with introduction by Mahmudul Hasan Siddiqui, I, Delhi, 1979, pp. 286–87. The interesting observation is also made that the inhabitants of Las Bela were aware that camel-pox ('Photo-Shutoor') was a preventive against smallpox but, in spite of this, they did not 'inoculate with its virus'.

[31] That is, if Muhammad Al-Chalabi (1776–1846) of Mosul in his tract on smallpox has not described 'vaccination', but the earlier practice of inoculation (see Sayyar K. Al-Jamil, 'Iraq', in Peter Bruke and Halil Inalcik (eds), *History of Humanity*, V, UNESCO, Paris/London, 1999, p. 237).

[32] Thus, C. Elgood in his *Safavid Medical Practice* fails to mention inoculation, presumably because it never entered the tracts and compendia of Yunani medicine that form his main sources.

[33] Joseph Needham, *Clerks and Craftsmen in China and the West*, pp. 375–76; and idem, *The Grand Titration: Science and Society in East and West*, London, 1969, pp. 58–59. These papers have now been reprinted in J. Needham, *Science and Civilization in China*, Vol. 6: *Medicine*, edited by Nathan Sivin, Cambridge, 2000. According to a review by C. Benedict in *American Historical Review*, Vol. 106 (3), 2001, pp. 929–30, the editor in his revisions confirms Chinese inoculation against smallpox from *c.* 1500 onwards, but doubts Needham's claim that it originated among Taoist practitioners as early as *c.* 1000.

[34] Cf. Nicholas, 'The Goddess Sitala and Epidemic Smallpox in Bengal', p. 27*n*.

[35] Gulbadan Begam, Memoirs [*Humayun Nama*], edited and translated by Annette S. Beveridge, London, 1902, text, p. 19 (trans., p. 13, has 'bonesetter' for *kamangar*, an obvious slip).

[36] See study by Syed Ali Nadeem Rezavi, 'An Aristocratic Surgeon of Medieval India', *Medieval India 1*, edited by Irfan Habib, New Delhi, 1992, pp. 154–67.

[37] Jahangir, *Tuzuk-i-Jahangiri*, edited by Sayyid Ahmad, Ghazipur and Aligarh, 1863–64, p. 347.

[38] Sirajuddin Ali Arzu, *Chiragh-i-Hidayat*, printed on margins of *Ghiyasu'l Lighat*, Kanpur, 1899, p. 604; Tek Chand Bahar, *Bahar-i-Ajam*, II, Lucknow, 1916, p. 186. These dictionaries give identical definitions, one obviously drawing from the other. Both say that in India only ox-horn (*shakh-i gau*) was used for the purpose.

[39] Cf. Donald Butter, *Outlines of . . . Southern Districts of Ou'dh*, pp. 174–76. He recorded his observations of the Awadh *jarrahs* in 1837, and contrasted them with 'the barber-surgeons of Europe'.

[40] Yet Butter, ibid., p. 174, noticed 'one vaid of considerable eminence who practices surgery also (amputations, &c.)'.

[41] Nicolao Manuchy [Manucci], *Storia do Mogor, 1656–1712*, translated by W. Irvine, II, London, 1907–08, p. 301.

[42] John Martin Honigberger, *Thirty-five Years in the East*, rpt, Calcutta, 1905, pp. 49–50. In Europe, he says, 'this operation is usually performed with the cuticle of the arm', which would involve a wholesale transplant of the skin.

[43] G.T. Vigne, *Travels in Kashmir, Ladak, Iskardu, &c*, 2nd edn, 1844, rpt, Karachi, 1987, pp. 140–41.

[44] Alexander Cunningham, *Archaeological Survey of India Reports*, V, Calcutta, 1862–84, pp. 168–69.

Smallpox and its Treatment in Pre-Modern India

Ishrat Alam

Before its control by vaccination, smallpox was a familiar and dreaded epidemic in India. It was responsible for a high rate of mortality and was a major source of blindness besides other disabilities. There has naturally been some interest in the history of the disease and of the fight against it, and this has produced some valuable studies.[1] There were two viruses of the genus *Orthopoxvirus* which used to cause smallpox amongst humans. One was known as variola minor poxvirus, which caused a mild form of the disease. It was also called alastrim and the fatality rate was low. It was possibly rare in India. The other was variola major poxvirus, in which the mortality was exceptionally high.[2] Ralph W. Nicholas has suggested that references to the pustular disease smallpox as *masurika* is found in Sanskrit texts dating back to over 2,000 years, showing that it was an ancient affliction in India. But his earliest references are actually from the medical treatises of Charaka and Sushruta, whose floruit period can be anywhere between fourth to sixth centuries BC and fourth century AD.[3] But even the *Charakasamhita*, passing through various hands, obtained its present final form through one Dridhabala who lived in the Gupta period or a little later, in the sixth century AD.[4] Similarly, the dating of the *Sushrutasamhita* has also been questioned and the possible date suggested is between second century AD to seventh century AD.[5] In subsequent centuries the presence of smallpox in India is well attested by frequent textual references.[6] In the medieval period the earliest reference we were able to trace dates back to the eleventh century. Alberuni (AD 1030) refers to smallpox. In a very brief but interesting passage he wrote:

> The Hindus who are the neighbours of those regions (of Lanka) believe that the smallpox is a wind blowing from the Island of Lanka

towards the continent to carry off souls. According to one report, some men warn people beforehand of the blowing of this wind, and can exactly tell at what times it will reach the different parts of the country.[7]

By Alberuni's time people had become familiar with both the viral strains. He writes, 'After the smallpox has broken out, they recognize from certain signs whether it is virulent or not.'[8] The familiarity with the disease and its devastating consequences also prompted attempts at medical control. Alberuni writes of both surgery and medicine: 'Against the virulent smallpox they use a method of treatment by which they destroy only one single limb of the body, but do not kill. They use as medicine cloves, which they give to the patient to drink, together with gold dust'.[9] This dreaded disease, in the absence of proper knowledge, also prompted use of ritual. Alberuni refers to the use of cloves as amulets. He writes, 'and besides, the males tie the cloves, which are similar to date kernels, to their necks'.[10] Alberuni's confident observation was that if those precautions were taken, 'perhaps nine people out of ten' had the chance to survive![11]

It is interesting to note the absence of any reference in Alberuni to the goddess Sitala. It seems that the worship of Sitala as the goddess of the disease started subsequently. This argument gains strength also from the fact that it was only in the late fifteenth and early sixteenth century that an appendix (*parisista*) on 'The Pathology of Sitala' was added to the text *Madhavanidanam* by Madhavakara (composed in the early eighth century).[12] By the twelfth century, in Dalhana's commentary on Sushruta, we find *Sitalika* as a popular designation for *masurika*. By the sixteenth century, the *Bhavaprakasa* written by Bhava Misra had an elaborate section on smallpox and appropriate therapy for different types of pustules.[13]

By the seventeenth century smallpox seems to have become still more widespread, and transformed from a disease into a calamity. In 1644 Antonio van Diemen reported that 600 slaves (male and female) had reached Batavia from Masulipatam, and 135 had died during the journey due to smallpox.[14] In the Mathura region, there are references to twenty-five villagers as witnesses in sale deeds. Their personal descriptions were recorded before the Qazis (1653–1717). Of them, as many as ten had suffered from smallpox because their faces had pock-marks.[15] In the Cambay documents too there are references to the incidence of smallpox. In a document dated 20 Rabi I, 1104, or 29 November 1692, there is a witness named Paswir, son of Rup Karan, who had smallpox marks on his face.[16] In another Cambay document, of 24 February 1716, the description of the face of a witness notes smallpox marks .[17] In 1718, the Dutch factors complained that 'due to the prevalence of smallpox one cannot get indigenous brick-layers to repair and restore the walls of Cochin (first)'.[18] On 21 October 1726, De Haan reported the prevalence of 'strong smallpox' in Malabar.[19] Similarly, it also affected the people of Punjab. In a sale deed of 1160/ 1748, both of two mortgagers, Gur Sahai and Karam Chand, have pock-marked faces.[20] Four years later, in 1752, another document from the same town has the description of a mortgager, Godaria, who bore pock-marks.[21] A careful scrutiny of these limited number of documents shows that from the middle of the seventeenth century the frequency and spread of the disease had increased considerably. The evidence of smallpox from Punjab assumes more significance in the light of its coinciding with the disease's occurrence in Bengal.[22]

It is in this context that the lengthy account about the goddess of smallpox in the Malabar region by a former Dutch reformed missionary to Ceylon should be analysed. This account was considered so important by its writer Philippus Baldaeus, that he wrote minute details of the disease.[23] The very title of the chapter on it is quite interesting. It reads, "Handling of the daughter of Ixora (i.e. Ishwara) and the Origin of Smallpox. Fear and Service of the Malabaris for this, robbing of their temple at Madiri by the King of Cochin, their arrival at Koilang'.[24] Philippus Baldaeus provides information about the representation of smallpox in religious belief and ritual.[25]

According to this Dutch account, there was a devil named Darida who, through his devotion to Brahma, got the blessing that he could not be killed by anyone.[26] Darida was overwhelmed by the powers given to him by Brahma and, with the thought of fighting Ishwara, reached Calaya, where Ishwara resided. Since Darida had the blessing that no man could kill him, Ishwara sent a lady called Sorga who cut off his head. Darida had his head restored by the blessing of Brahma. Then Ishwara sent five holy ladies, called Chamundiga by the Malabaris. They too chopped off Darida's head. But he reappeared the next day. Ishwara consulted Vishnu, and Patragali (identified as Bhadrakali) was born. Baldaeus describes the physical features and other paraphernalia of Patragali. We are told how goddess Patragali was infuriated and how she caused smallpox on the face of Ishwara. According to this version it was thus that smallpox was born. Though this text is not free from anthropomorphism, it still considers that the disease had some natural causes.[27] Baldaeus is here narrating the history of smallpox in India as being inter-related with the goddess of smallpox, although both are obviously quite different things. This reflects the common practice of seeking and then interpreting a relationship between disease and divinities. However it is clear from Baldaeus's account that the religious interpretation which the people of Malabar associated with the infectious disease did not exclude a naturalistic comprehension. Baldaeus refers to Greek and Jewish perceptions of the disease and compares them with the Indian perception.

> The diseases under which smallpox should be reckoned, were sent by God to punish the sin of the humans, but she has natural causes, she can originate from within or from outside, as air, food, drink, sleep, waking, rest and movement of the body, hunger, forcing and holding of excrement, fashions and times of the year . . . winds and venomous vapour of the air, as from the same scalding fever and pestilence.[28]

Baldaeus refers to the traditionally accumulated knowledge about the disease:

> Brahmins also know well, how, according to the size of the winds, each period of the year produces various diseases, so we found fault with in Ceylon island,[29] and specially in the kingdom of Jafnapatan, in the province of Pachirapalli, how there in the Winter severe fevers and swelling up of bodies are caused by the saline and nitreous water, [and] how the mortality prevails among their cattle, is not unknown to them, how the aching eyes especially in Malabar tease the people, occurring from a spoiled air, how very often the fish (created by a stench in the water) like mad and silly ones proceed to the beach, and die in thousands, as a few years ago happened in Amboina, and earlier in Ceylon, and other places, where more has happened.[30]

Baldaeus also describes the seasonal pattern of the epidemic's visitation. He writes:

> So sees one in spring that the Malabaris are attacked by smallpox, which without doubt originate from the heat and contaminated

blood, and from other vicious humidity and fruits, which the common people mostly partake, who also are attacked by smallpox, for this season is also considered deadly or remediable, after that dampness was found venomous, so that some poxes are cured lightly, while others die in 12 or 18 days.[31]

This passage suggests that during the spring season the transmission of the smallpox virus was greater, and shows a great resemblance with the seasonal pattern of its occurrence in Bengal.[32] It is now a known fact that the smallpox virus was more active and transmissible in dry weather conditions.[33] However, Baldaeus's account suggests that a season in which there was damp was more vulnerable to smallpox.[34]

As far as the medical treatment of the afflicted person was concerned, Baldaeus informs us that 'Some poxes were cured lightly, as against others that kill in 12 or 18 days (both) men and children, like the doctors and Comaras[35] abandon these in the country from their experience, or they are mortal or capable of cure.'[36] He adds:

The Pagans, thinking that Patragali sends this disease, leave the patient at once. This can be the reason why the image of a woman is [there] among the Pagans, there a child strikes the poor on the neck, as seeking help from this idol, being deserted by men. Because they judge the disease is infectious and sticking: they give the patient over to one of the Comaras, being the devotees of Patragali pagod. Believing that Patragali causes the smallpox, they do then many oblations and ceremonies for the sick; to please this idol, cut off the heads of one or two hens, whose blood falling on the earth, was licked up by dogs.[37]

Elsewhere too, he speaks about the worship and rituals associated with treatment of the disease.[38] Curiously enough, he speaks about *Basuri*[39] as the daughter of Ishwara. This was why

the Malabaris gave this name to the smallpox, which they also hold to be the ulcer and the dagger of Patragali, therefore, when they see a patient with smallpox, they will worship him, because they think that Patragali is in his middle; so they do also to dead-body, calling it Pandara [Bhandara?], that is a royal treasure, they know well also that God is good and does harm to none: but that Patragali, because she produces this evil, must be reconciled with offerings.[40]

Interestingly, an iconoclastic attitude was developing amongst the people. Philippus Baldaeus also refers to some kind of counter-ideology prevailing in Malabar about the disease. They had started rationalizing the cause of its eruption. The entire passage is so unique as to deserve quotation. People believe

> that also this disease is not caused by Patragali, because people have not sinned especially against her, it appears, because many *Brahmans* and devout *Comaras* die of this disease, though they are in friendship with this idol. Many have according to their own admission sinned greatly against Patragali and nevertheless do not die of this disease. Many dying of this disease, are known openly, they have certainly not sinned against Patragali.[41]

Despite such a sceptical attitude towards smallpox, Baldaeus does not refer to any medical treatment of the patient. However he refers to the diet that was prescribed. The patients were given *kanji*, that is, well-cooked rice.[42] But they were not forced to drink it.[43] They were also treated with bleeding, purgation and taking of cold food.[44]

The mortality rate was possibly pushed up because of a corrupt practice among the people of Malabar. Baldaeus reports: 'and some die well by infirmity, and are also killed by the Comaras, as they see that with their removal, their profits can come to them, because they inherit all the household goods.'[45]

The people in Malabar had a special temple for Patragali at Cranganore. It was also called the Temple of Pilgrimage 'because of the great influx of the people'. Since it had possibly acquired the status of a major shrine, popular religious fairs were held. Baldaeus writes about the day of the feast when thousands of Sanams(?) were sacrificed. It had become a very rich temple. The king of Cochin wished to take away part of this wealth. He stationed his people at strategic places near the rivers and roads in order to rob the travelling pilgrims.[46]

While fear of the disease led to a religious ritual invented to protect people from the wrath of the goddess on the one hand, it also encouraged a rational effort to discover the causes of the disease. In the eighteenth century they considered controlling it with the help of medical treatment. It has been suggested that the practice of variolation or smallpox inoculation may have had many independent sources of origin. It possibly developed independently in different parts of Eurasia and Africa.[47]

So far as variolation in India is concerned, all our information comes from the eighteenth century. As early as 10 February 1731, Robert Coult wrote to Dr Oliver Coult about it. According to Robert Coult's report, inoculation was known in Bengal for the previous 150 years. According to the 'Bhamanian' records it was first performed by Dununtary (Dhanavantari?), a physician of Champaner near Kasimbazar.[48] Therefore, by the time it was used for the first time they were familiar with the theory of infection. Baldaeus too spoke about contaminated blood.[49] This was an advance over the Ayurvedic explanation of the disease, which emphasizes the humours as being responsible for diseases. In this method of inoculation, Robert Coult wrote, a little of the pus of the infected person was taken and, with the help of a sharp needle, it was applied under the delloid muscle or forehead.[50]

Robert Coult referred to a second method also, i.e. through swallowing. He wrote, 'When they want the operation of the inoculated matter to be quick they give the patient a small bolus made of a little of the pus, and boiled rice, immediately after the operation which is repeated the two following days at noon.'[51] J.Z. Holwell (1767) made a detailed report about inoculation.[52] Holwell wrote that inoculation was practised by a special category of brahmins who were despatched from 'the different colleges of Bindooband (Vrindavan), Eleabas (Allahabad) and Banaras' to various provinces in small batches of three or four each.[53] Their common arrival time in Bengal was February.[54]

Subsequently there are many references to variolation in Bengal. Dr Edward Ives (1773), the Dutch commander Stevorinus who died of it (1770), and Cossigny (1799) wrote about it.[55] Dr Francis Buchanan (1808) saw variolation in Dinajpur district.[56] But he (1807) noted the absence of inoculation in southern India.[57] The death rate was as high as hundred per cent.[58] We find the process of inoculation continuing as late as the first decade of the twentieth century, as in Assam, along with vaccination.[59]

Notes and References

[1] Ralph W. Nicholas, 'The Goddess Sitala and Epidemic Smallpox in Bengal', *The Journal of Asian Studies*, Vol. XLI, No. 1, November 1981, pp. 21–44; David Arnold, *Imperial Medicine and Indigenous Societies*, Delhi, 1989, pp. 45–65; Dharampal, *Indian Science and Technology in the Eighteenth Century*, Delhi, 1971, pp. 141–63; Mridula Ramanna, 'Indian Response to Western Medicine: Vaccination in the City of Bombay in the Nineteenth

Century', in A.J. Qaiser and S.P. Verma (eds), *Art and Culture, Endeavours in Inter-pretation*, Delhi, 1996, pp. 67–78.

2 Ralph W. Nicholas, 'The Goddess Sitala', p. 24.

3 Debiprasad Chattopadhyaya, *Science and Society in Ancient India*, Calcutta, 1977, pp. 24–32.

4 Ibid., p. 32.

5 Ibid., pp. 38–44.

6 Ralph W. Nicholas, 'The Goddess Sitala', pp. 25–26.

7 Edward C. Sachau (transl.), *Alberuni's India*, Vol. I, London, 1910, p. 309.

8 Ibid.

9 Ibid.

10 Ibid.

11 Ibid.

12 Ralph W. Nicholas, 'The Goddess Sitala', p. 26. Madhava Kara has given an extensive and comprehensive chapter on *masurika*, or smallpox. Nicholas is of the opinion that by the seventh century, smallpox had become so widespread in India that it demanded careful attention from experts dealing with medicine. In the same century it was established in the countries around the Mediterranean.

13 Cf. ibid., p. 27.

14 Dr W. Ph. Coolhaas, *Generale Missiven Van Gouverneurs—Generaal en Raden aan Heren XVII der Verenigde Oostindische Compagnie, Deel II: 1639–1655*, Martinus Nijhoff, Gravenhage, 1964, p. 223.

15 Irfan Habib, *The Agrarian System of Mughal India*, 2nd rev. edn, Delhi, 1999, p. 111. The first edition did not have this information.

16 NAI, 2702/4. I am grateful to my friend and colleague, S. Ali Nadeem Rizvi, for giving me information from the Cambay Documents, preserved in the National Archives of India, New Delhi.

17 NAI, 2695/16.

18 *Generale Missiven, Deel VII: 1713–1725*, p. 374.

19 *Generale Missiven Deel VIII: 1725–1729*, p. 64.

20 J.S. Grewal, *In the By-Lanes of History, Some Persian Documents from a Punjab Town*, Shimla, 1975, pp. 175–176, 178.

21 Ibid., pp. 182, 184.

22 Cf. Nicholas, 'The Goddess Sitala', p. 33.

23 Philippus Baldaeus, *Nauwkeurige en Waarachtige Ontdekking en wederlegginge van Afgoderye der Oost-Indische Heydenen, Malabaren, Benjanen, Gentiven, Bramines*, Janssonius van Waasberge en Van Someren, Amsterdam, 1672, pp. 28–34.

24 Ibid., p. 28.

25 In some of the earlier literature on smallpox we find much information about the divine origin of smallpox. Compare accounts given by Nicholas, 'The Goddess Sitala', pp. 29–33.

26 Baldaeus, *Nauwkeurige en Waarachtige*, p. 28.

27 Ibid., p. 31.

28 Ibid. This important passage is deleted in the printed version by A.J. de

Jongh. It is possibly because of this and some other omission of passages that Ralph W. Nicholas could not have access to this information.

[29] Cf. Alberuni's account, and it appears that the eleventh-century perception of holding Ceylon responsible for smallpox continued.

[30] Baldaeus, *Nauwkeurige en Waarachtige*, p. 31.

[31] Ibid.

[32] Nicholas, 'The Goddess Sitala', pp. 38–39.

[33] David Arnold, *Imperial Medicine and Indigenous Societies*, p. 46.

[34] The dampness was because of the winter monsoon in India which causes rainfall in northwestern India and the Tamil NaduKerala coastal areas. It is to be noted that since the winter monsoon blows from land to oceans, it is by and large less humid than the summer monsoon, and the consequent rainfall is also smaller. Nevertheless it creates sufficient dampness.

[35] Comaras could be identified with the people called *Coramas*, who were low-caste illiterate people engaged in making baskets, and trading in salt and grain. See Francis Buchanan, *A Journey from Madras through the Countries of Mysore, Canara and Malabar*, I, London, 1807, pp. 249–50.

[36] Baldaeus, *Nauwkeurige en Waarachtige*, p. 32.

[37] Ibid.

[38] Ibid., pp. 32–33.

[39] The term '*basuri*' was possibly used for the Sanskrit equivalent, '*masuri*', which was the ancient term for smallpox. But *basuri* could be from the Arabic *basur*, 'piles, ulcers', etc.

[40] Baldaeus, *Nauwkeurige en Waarachtige*, p. 33.

[41] Ibid.

[42] Ibid., p. 32.

[43] Ibid.

[44] Ibid.

[45] Ibid.

[46] Ibid., p. 33.

[47] David Arnold, *Imperial Medicine and Indigenous Societies*, p. 49.

[48] Dharampal (ed.), *Indian Science and Technology in the Eighteenth Century: Some Contemporary European Accounts*, Delhi, 1971, p. 141.

[49] Baldaeus, *Nauwkeurige en Waarachtige*.

[50] Dharampal, *Indian Science and Technology in the Eighteenth Century*, p. 141.

[51] Ibid., pp. 141–42.

[52] Ibid., pp. 143–63.

[53] Ibid., p. 146.

[54] Ibid., p. 147.

[55] Cited by Ralph W. Nicholas, 'The Goddess Sitala', p. 28.

[56] Ibid.

[57] Francis Buchanan, *A Journey from Madras*, Vol. I, pp. 249–50, 262, 359; Vol. II, pp. 153, 285–86.

[58] Ibid., pp. 285–86.

[59] B.C. Allen, E.A. Gait et al., *Gazetteer of Bengal and Northern-East India*, rpt, Delhi, 1984, p. 121.

Of Therapeutics and Prophylactics

The Exegesis of an Eighteenth-Century Tract on Smallpox

Harish Naraindas

Introduction

In the current essay[1] I attempt an exegesis of a well-known text: a short essay addressed to the College of Physicians in London by J.Z. Holwell (1767). Titled, *An account of the manner of inoculating for the smallpox in the East Indies,* it offers a *theory* of smallpox in the eighteenth century. Late twentieth-century historiography, conditioned by a post-Pasteur view of the world, glosses over categories that are central to eighteenth-century conceptions of medicine and healing which, I shall currently show, are comparable and similar, if not altogether identical, in the east and the west.[2] In the specific case of smallpox, Holwell's text bears mute testimony to gloss and excision. Arnold's otherwise insightful essay on smallpox in India (1993), which quotes Holwell at length, is a prime example. But his essay is symptomatic of a larger disciplinary cleaving. Hence, while the paper is about variolation in eighteenth-century Bengal, it is also a methodological excursus about past and present and about the power of disciplinary boundaries to excise and occlude.

Contemporary accounts of smallpox in India carve out a unitary phenomenon and distribute them across different sites. One is caught in a bind between the interesting insights the studies offer and the simultaneous parcelling-out due to *disciplinary* interests. Anthropological accounts of smallpox are about *Sitala* and the language and structure of worship. Thorny issues about efficacy are skirted, or, if addressed, are seen as an accomplishment of faith (Wadley 1980; Egnor 1984). It results in *Sitala* studies, as we shall presently see, being caught in a vortex of culture, belief and ritual. Under the tutelage of the pervasive opposition of Hot and Cold, which ostensibly underlies all forms of healing in South Asia, *Sitala* is encapsulated as the 'Cool One' (Wadley 1980). That this 'Cool One' could actually mirror, through her worship, the practice of literally cooling the body as efficacious therapy, is not addressed. In the case of smallpox this took the form of external cooling (by cold bathing) and dietary restrictions that kept the body internally cool. This regimen is either amalgamated with worship and ritual or explicitly relegated, as in the following case: 'A series of dietary restrictions was also imposed, *and though these can have had little practical effect upon the operation's success,* they emphasized the importance and danger attached to variolation and the need to observe due care to prevent the disease from becoming contagious.' (Arnold 1993: 128; emphasis added.) While these recipes and regimen *may not* have had any *practical effect,* the dismissal precludes an exegesis in the rare instance that it is explicitly offered to us. Moreover, it is made to appear as an addendum to the practice of variolation, which is privileged.

Anthropology inspired by Indology, whose forte is textual exegesis, addresses the 'Ayurvedic' medical corpus *sui generis* (Zimmerman 1987). It is only rarely that it is addressed in a comparative context. In the instance it does, it shifts the time-frame and compares the Ayurvedic medical corpus to the Hippocratic/Galenic corpus (Zimmerman 1992). Although the choice of frames has interesting consequences,[3] it is an understandable comparison and we must be thankful to Zimmerman for the comparative casting. But we do not have a comparative rendering of an Indian and a European medical theory in the eighteenth century: the moment of its *contemporary* meeting; nor have the insights gleaned from textual exegesis been used to specifically address smallpox.

The exceptions, each in a different vein, are Nicholas (1981) and Marglin (1990). Nicholas alludes, in the beginning of an essay (1981), to the way in which the cultural anthropologist often sidesteps issues of actual historical correlation between epidemic and worship, and the notion of efficacy. In this and another essay (Nicholas and Sarkar 1976), he demonstrates two facets of the problem: of eighteenth-century Bengal as the site of an enormous outpouring of *Sitala* poetry, where Maratha 'raids' and the rise of British power led to a disruption of agrarian Bengal, resulting in an impoverished and malnourished peasantry who were ready for the picking.[4] Smallpox, symptomatic of the state of affairs, led to an exacerbation of *Sitala* worship. A worship that turned 'calamity to community', bringing to an end, even if momentarily, intra-community strife (Nicholas and Sarkar 1976). The worship, as performance, was also a didactic site that recast the historical into the mythical by using suffering as an occasion to instruct and edify transcendental truths (Nicholas and Sarkar 1976; Dimock 1976).

Nicholas also manages to trace a genealogy of the practice of inoculation in the medical corpus along with the occasional reference to it in eighteenth-century European sources. The eighteenth century now appears as the site of a *techné* and a poetics. But what escapes him is that the technique of inoculating for the smallpox was part of a theoretical enterprise.[5] One of the European sources that he cites (Holwell again!) is truncated and offered as a verification of the practice of inoculation. Apart from the misreading this occasions at moments, its consequences are momentous.

Marglin's essay addresses the problem squarely in so far as it treats *Sitala* worship as not merely ritual, performance, or faith, but *also* as *knowledge*. Marglin's study is a rare instance of seeing worship *as* knowledge and in the process breaking down the pervasive and tacit dualism that characterizes such studies. In an attempt to show the isomorphism between worship and healing, it shifts the locus to the grand festival at Puri, locates the ritual as part of a larger cosmos and draws out its metaphysics: healing as regeneration through disease and death.[6] In strategic terms, the shift transforms the healing to a valid cosmo-therapeutics that, unfortunately, seems wholly other. More importantly, the ritual at Puri is not a therapeutic site for an individual patient. The exigencies of practice may offer a different view of both its 'art' and theory: the act of 'opening of the pustules' captures this difference dramatically.

Quite in contrast is the well-known but under-interpreted (if not altogether misinterpreted) eighteenth-century tract by J.Z. Holwell, an 'improper' Scotsman primarily known for his writings on Hinduism (Marshall 1970). Holwell attempts to render the Indian understanding of smallpox in terms that are accessible to an eighteenth-century medical audience in England. Born of the exigencies of practice, it is not *anecdotal*. A practising surgeon in Bengal for close to two decades, and witness to four epidemics of smallpox, starting with one in 1744, Holwell sets out not merely to describe the practice of inoculating for the smallpox, as the title of the essay seems to suggest, but to record a *theory* and *practice* of its origin, cause and therapeutics.

Situating the Text

Holwell's essay recommends itself on many counts. It is probably the clearest extant text on the theory and practice of smallpox in eighteenth-century India recorded by a European.[7] It is neither a casual observation, nor a traveller's account. Written by an experienced practising medic in Bengal, it is not a rendering of the practice of variolation in India for the sake of record but an attempt to evaluate the eighteenth-century theory and therapeutics of smallpox as understood in India *and* Britain. Despite beginning with what seems to be a disclaimer, the text sets up an implicit dialogue in an attempt at a *confirmation and correction* of its practice in Britain (then less than half a century old and introduced into England from the east, which is here Turkey) and of British physicians in India.

Holwell's account is an oft-quoted piece. It is quoted to prove the antiquity of smallpox inoculation and the care with which it was practised in the eighteenth-century, in contrast to its subsequent decline and degeneration (James 1909). It is interesting that those who quote Holwell fail to notice, or comment on, the fact that his account is perfectly at ease with the 'Eastern' theory of smallpox as practised by their 'Professors of Physic', which he is attempting to describe *and interpret*. There is none of the anguish of translatability that comes from any felt notion of incommensurability. The motive that animates the text is to communicate to the College of Physicians the theory and practice of smallpox so as 'to introduce, into *regular and universal practice, the cool regimen and free admission of air*' that characterize its 'Eastern practice'. Interestingly enough, *Sitala* is virtually absent in his account. Except for the introductory invocation of her as the 'Gootee ka Tagooran (the Goddess of Spots)' and a passing reference later as the divinity to whom a thanksgiving is offered, what we have is a 'rational' account of a theory and therapeutics of smallpox that accords rather well with eighteenth-century notions of it in England, allowing for an easy and ready translatability on a presumed and demonstrable similarity in its understanding and practice.

This is at variance with the understanding of smallpox by the end of the century. With the advent of vaccination, variolation is reconstrued as dangerous, and its introduction in India in 1802 leads to a simultaneous conflation and reduction. Inoculation and the worship of *Sitala* are conflated and, more importantly, therapy in Holwell's text, of which inoculation is only a part, is reduced to the technique of inoculation and/or the worship of *Sitala*. As a synecdoche of *Sitala*, inoculation turns into a ritual craft.[8] The 'Professors of Physic' in Holwell's text reappear as *ticcadars,* whose prejudice and professional interest stand in the way of vaccination. The jettisoning of theory and the prescriptions that derive from it, which either vanish or are reduced and amalgamated with worship, leaves one with a triad of inoculation, worship and vaccination. Holwell's plea for the 'cool regimen and free admission of air'[9] is lost sight of. Instead, vaccination and inoculation are played off against each other with each trying to solicit *Sitala*. That roughly is the frame that sets the tenor for the nineteenth century and *also* for the historiography of smallpox in nineteenth-century India which, as I have said earlier, forms the thematic of my second essay (Naraindas 1998). By the late twentieth century, *Sitala* is replaced by a demon and the campaign against smallpox turns into an outright war against the disease, which I analyse in another essay (Naraindas 1997).

Holwell's essay has suffered a similar fate. Those who approach it have invariably done so from the present and impute a nascent present to the past: a bacterial theory of infection as in the case of Dharampal (1983) who, having resuscitated the text, does the disservice of placing it under technique. Others, by cue, have looked at the text as a confirmation of the sophisticated technique of inoculation present in the eighteenth century (Arnold 1993) and, in a retrospective act, read practices of attenuation where none exists (Nicholas 1981), and fail to find it where it may be found.

Unlike *Sitala* studies, or commentaries on Holwell, Holwell's text is an exception and does not suffer from these 'infirmities'. Largely due to historical context and also due to the author's idiosyncrasy, it approaches the business of smallpox in the eighteenth century neither through the end of worship,[10] nor primarily through the practice of inoculation as technique. It is a refreshingly pragmatic text about the theory that underlies it and is eager, on the basis of that theory, to borrow what it sees as the essence of its therapy: the 'cool *regimen* and free admission of air'. Both history and historiography have excised what is central to Holwell and the eighteenth century. The passage to the nineteenth century is effected not only by an *irruption* in the history of medicine or science, as we are often led to believe (Canguilhem 1988: 27–40), or by the *disruption* of the other, but also by an *excision and reordering of the self.*

Holwell's Janus Face

Marshall (1970) has pointed out that Holwell's more well-known writings on Hinduism were employed by 'non-Christians' in Europe as a weapon in the running battle against the clerics. He was far better received on the Continent than he was in England, where his idiosyncratic rendering of Hinduism often brought the worst out of his reviewers. Voltaire, however, was a great admirer, and probably took to his metempsychosis with alacrity. Marshall is silent on Holwell's short essay on smallpox and we are not in a position to say how he was received by the medics of his day. But we gather that he was in dialogue with contemporary medical opinion through an opening reference to a Dr Schultz. He says,

> the world has been already obliged with a performance of the kind which I have now undertaken, by a Dutch author a friend of Mr Chais; but as this is all I know of that work, it shall not discourage my proceeding with my own, the more specially as that performance is in a foreign language, and may not much benefit my country.

Under the sign of 'benefit', the eighteenth century was peppered with such accounts. Many of them were appreciative of various theories and techniques of the east, as is clear from Dharampal's collection (1983).[11]

Marshall's assessment of Holwell is, however, faintly disapproving. He seems embarrassed by what he probably sees as Holwell's peculiar rendering of Hinduism through a 'debased' Christianity. This is compounded by Holwell's penchant for a theory of metempsychosis, a plurality of heavens and hells, and his vegetarianism. Holwell, both through his writings and his biography, appears to be the antithesis of Jones who, on both counts, was a 'model Englishman'. Though deeply appreciative of Hinduism, he never for a moment thought it to be superior, with all the world's cosmologies derived from the original Hindu cosmology. Holwell, 'fortunately' for us, seems to portray the same skill when it comes to his rendering of smallpox in India: not just an 'empathetic' rendering of the principles behind the practice, but a rendering in terms that allows his audience to make sense of it. Consistent with his object, he swings in the opposite direction in the case of smallpox. It is merely tinged by religion and faith, and is in vigorous dialogue with practices present in his time. How are we to approach Holwell's text, especially in the light of Marshall's assessment of his other writings? We can easily show that the template Holwell uses is fashioned by mid-eighteenth-century medical theories in Britain. But for comparative purposes one needs to treat the text as *sui generis*: a corridor and passage between two worlds; and an independent voice and practice in India and Britain. We should not impute to the eighteenth century an imagined and irrecoverable gulf. The thematic and practices may have had much in common although the particulars may have had a different valence in each: much like the Greek and Christian problematization of pleasure whose resolutions were different (Foucault 1990, 1988); or the Galenic and Ayurvedic management of therapeutic violence whose practices and procedures seem identical and the principles comparable (Zimmerman 1992).

The line traversed between Holwell and Jones is marked by a turning away of the west from the east *and* the past.[12] The past/east no longer appears as a counter-model. Holwell bears witness to a moment: a moment before the Fall! And even if the Holwell of Hinduism is different from the Holwell on smallpox, the text on smallpox stands on its own: a Janus-faced text that allows a cross-over, and defines both itself and all that follows in its wake. In a future genealogy it could be an *origin* text: something more and other than a text that facilitated dialogue, let alone offering a 'debased' rendering.[13]

Holwell's Manoeuvre

Holwell begins his essay, after the initial reference to Dr Schultz, with a clever manoeuvre. He invokes *antiquity* to ground the narrative of a practice that probably still evoked a considerable amount of ambivalence in England. In a reference to someone who sounds like William Wagstaffe (Marglin 1990: 111), he concedes that though in several instances the art of medicine has been indebted to barbarism and ignorance, in the particular case of smallpox it was sanctioned by remotest antiquity, and with 'some variation' will 'illustrate the propriety of the present practice, and promote the obvious very laudable intention, with which that gentleman published his late essay on this interesting subject' (Holwell 1767: 196). Further on, this antiquity is given a name and a date: the *Aughtorrah Bade,* the scriptures of the Gentoos promulgated 3366 years ago (ibid.:198)[14] This is one of the few occasions when he invokes the 'Goddess of Spots' and claims that these scriptures institute a form of divine worship in the smallpox season for all the cutaneous eruptions (ibid.). In a parallel to his work on Hinduism, antiquity is invoked to claim that India was the original home from where the Egyptians derived their smallpox and measles (ibid.), the way they derived their cosmology (Marshall 1970). This rhetorical positioning is an attempt to sanctify all that follows, without ruffling the feathers of his intended audience. For once, the *original home* thesis, unlike later versions (the classic case being cholera from the 1830s, where India and the east are seen as the origin and locus of epidemics and disease), serves the opposite function. *Origin* and *antiquity* 'elevate' India and the intended narrative; and the contemporary practice in Britain is to be confirmed and measured in terms of the fare that Holwell is about to offer: its 'manner' in the 'original home'!

The Prelude: Of Season and Diet
Course and Vicissitude

Two of the concepts that animate and anchor the narrative are season and diet. The year had a particular rhythm marked by its seasons. Each season had winds, rain, heat, cold and moisture peculiar to itself. The year as a whole was marked by the nature, and the order of succession, of these elements. Smallpox, like other diseases, was endemic and seasonal. It came in the months of March, April and May: the middle of the 'hot season' that extended from the middle of February to about the middle of June, when the 'returning rains' brought it to a close. Every fifth, sixth or seventh year, the disease, otherwise 'benign' and 'unnoticed', turned epidemic.

As I have pointed out elsewhere (Naraindas 1996), Holwell is here addressing a question that was posed and re-posed in the eighteenth century, and well into the nineteenth. The question was: when did an endemic turn epidemic? Quite as in the mid-nineteenth-century answer to the advent of epidemics, here, too, it was 'the sudden vicissitudes in the weather', often unusual in its advent for the season, that produced an 'epidemic influence' (ibid.: 29).

This is borne out in one of the initial passages that frames the narrative, where he divides the year in Bengal into three seasons of four months each: rainy, cold and hot. The advent of disease was marked when the seasons and the weather ran foul of an intended *course*.

> From the middle of February to the middle of June is the hot, windy, dry season; during which no rain falls but what comes in storms of fierce winds and tremendous thunder and lightning, called North Westers, the quarter they always rise from; and the provinces, particularly Bengal, is more or less healthy, in proportion to the number of these storms; when in this season the air is frequently agitated and refreshed with these North Westers, accompanied with rain, (for they are often dry) and the inhabitants do not expose themselves to the intense sun and violent hot winds that blow in March, April and May, it is generally found to be the most healthy of the year; otherwise (as in the year 1744, when we had no rain from the twentieth of October to the twentieth of June) this season produces high inflammatory disorders of the liver, breast, pleura, and intestines, with dysenteries, and a deplorable species of the small-pox. (Holwell 1767: 199)

In a seeming paradox, the smallpox season of March, April and May—when the sun was intense, and violent, hot winds blew—is described as the 'most healthy of the year'. How are we to account for this paradox? It was the season when the air was 'frequently agitated and refreshed' by the 'North Westers'. These North Westers were usually accompanied by rain and the healthiness of the season seemed to depend, first, on the arrival of these North Westers and, second, on the amount of rain they brought along. In the fateful year of 1744, when there was no rain from the previous October to June of that year, it led to 'high inflammatory disorders' and 'a deplorable species of smallpox'.

Cooling and Ventilating

The first of the epidemics of smallpox that Holwell observed in 1744 was when the year and its seasons did not unfold according to plan. When the weather played truant the healthiest of seasons turned upon itself. The concepts that animate the notion of weather when it *is* true to its course are ventilating and cooling. If the North Westers did not keep their rendezvous, the natural ventilation they performed by *agitating* and *refreshing* failed. If the rains failed to appear, there was no natural cooling of the body of the earth. In what seemed an archaic and garbled narrative a moment ago, we meet the principles of cooling and ventilation. If we pause for a moment we realize that ventilation is also a cooling: *cooling by air*. We already have with us the single notion that animates Holwell's narrative: cooling! The cooling in two forms, by air and water (neither reducible to the other),[15] which we will confront when we get to the body of the fevered smallpox patient, is laid bare in a strict homology vis-à-vis the body of the earth and the natural elements. The healthiest of seasons was the hot season; it was dependent, however, on being periodically cooled—by air and water. When this fails to happen, when the rhythm and the course of the seasons goes awry, the earth burns, and 'produces high inflammatory disorders of the liver, breast, pleura, and intestines, with dysenteries, and a deplorable *species* of the small-pox' (Holwell 1767: 199; emphasis added).

The Theme of Diet and Intemperance

Apart from the vicissitudes in the weather, the year as a whole was divided into the delightful, healthy and unhealthy. But Holwell, in keeping with the oft-repeated eighteenth-century refrain, is extremely clear that intemperance in food and habit was as much the cause of disease. We should not be led into believing that the statements about diet and food were purely pious. Every item of food had a particular character. Each had a place in the seasonal cycle and the prescriptions depended on the context: the season, the disease and the patient. In an opening section he attempts to answer why the natives of the island of St Helena are singularly susceptible to the smallpox even when the disease has never taken root there. He pins it down to their diet. They were susceptible not because they migrated only as adults and hence lacked, as we would say, 'immunity'. Rather than the lack of exposure to the disease as children, it was due to their chief diet—a yam—that they consume from infancy. Its *acrid*,[16] unwholesome quality, which frequently subjects them to 'epidemic and dangerous dysenteries' and 'sometimes putrid sore throats', makes them susceptible to the pox.

> The blood thus charged, must necessarily constitute a most unlucky habit of body to combat with any acute inflammatory disease whatsoever, but more especially of the kind under consideration (so frequently attended with a high degree of putrefaction), always fatal

to these people, even in those seasons when the disease is mild and favourable to others. (Holwell 1767: 197)

Season and diet, course and rhythm, temperance and intemperance, ventilating and cooling: these are the terms that animate the text. Before Holwell arrives at the theory of smallpox in India, the narrative lays out the catalogue of categories and their principles of operation. Apart from season and diet and the principles that animate them, smallpox as a fever was among the 'inflammatory fevers' as opposed to the 'nervous fevers' (Smith 1981). This mid-eighteenth-century nosological schism structures his narrative: the narrative moves to smallpox via the *putrid nervous fever of Bengal*. The nosological schism was neither purely heuristic nor descriptive. It was embedded in theory: theories primarily motivated by therapeutics. And Holwell's essay constantly plays between the two poles of theory and therapeutics.

Of Smallpox
The Practice

Holwell's description of inoculating for the smallpox has been quoted often enough. I will not dwell on this at length except to say that inoculating for the pox was however part of a larger therapeutic *course*. The therapeutic course had a proscribed diet before, after and during the course of the disease; and a prescribed diet while it ran its course. The proscribed items were fish, milk and *ghee*, and the proscription commenced a month before the inoculators normally arrived and continued for a month from the day of inoculation.

The inoculation was not an arm-to-arm procedure but came from variolous matter of the previous year. It was preserved in a 'cotton pledget' and kept bound in a 'double callico rag' that was tied around the waist of the practitioner. The pledget was moistened with 'Ganges water' and applied to the intended area that had been previously given a dry friction for about 'eight to ten minutes' and then wounded by a series of 'slight touches, about the compass of a silver groat'. The pledget was placed upon the scarified area and tied with a bandage for about 'six hours'.

But the inoculation was merely the beginning of a set of prescribed techniques that were 'most religiously followed'. Let me quote Holwell at length here:

He extends the prohibition of fish, milk and ghee, for one month, from the day of inoculation; early on the morning succeeding the operation, four collons (an earthen pot containing about two gallons) of cold water are ordered to be thrown over the patient, from the head downwards, and to be repeated every morning and evening until the fever comes on, (which usually is about the close of the sixth day from the inoculation,) then to desist until the appearance of the eruptions, (which commonly happens at the close of the third complete day from the commencement of the fever,) and then to pursue the cold bathing as before, through the course of the disease, and until the scabs of the pustules drop off. They are ordered to open all the pustules with a fine sharp pointed thorn, as soon as they begin to change their colour, and whilst the matter continues in a fluid state. Confinement to the house is absolutely forbid, and the inoculated are ordered to be exposed to every air that blows; and the utmost indulgence they are allowed when the fever comes on, is to be laid on a mat at the door; but, in fact, the eruptive fever is generally so inconsiderable and trifling, as very seldom to require this indulgence. Their regimen is ordered to consist of all the refrigerating things the climate and season produces, as plantains, sugarcanes, water melons, rice, gruel made of white poppy-seeds, and cold water, or thin rice gruel for their ordinary drink. These instructions being given, and an injunction laid on the patients to make a thanks-giving *Poojah*, or offering, to the goddess on their recovery, the Operator takes his fee, which from the poor is a *pund of cowries*, equal to about a penny sterling, and goes on to another door. (Holwell 1767: 203)

There is nothing pell-mell about the narrative. It is a careful description of an assiduous practice, and captures the course and timing of a set of therapeutic techniques that merely begins with inoculation: abstinence; a cold-water douche that starts and stops; a cooling diet; ensuring the patient is not confined and enclosed but in an airy and well-ventilated space; and opening the pustules.

The Theory

The second half of Holwell's account, which is devoted to an analysis and explication of the 'principles on which the Bramins act', opens with an admission that he was both aware and already prejudiced toward 'the cool regimen and free admission of air in the treatment of this disease' (Holwell 1767: 204). His misgiving, if any, came from the fact that 'the Bramins carried *both* to a bold, rash and dangerous extreme'(ibid.).

The four themes that he addresses are the following. (1) The rationale for the interdicted articles of diet. (2) A theory of the origin and cause of the smallpox, which is the scaffolding on which the therapeutic practice is built. (3) The rationale for the cold bathing. (4) And the method and rationale for opening the pustules.

Abstinence: Of Preternatural Ferment and Inflammation

Fish and *ghee* were prohibited on the ground that while one was 'viscid' and 'inflammatory', the other was 'acrid': both fouled and blocked the free flow of passages. While the viscid nature of the fish was likely to 'obstruct the cutaneous glands and the excretory ducts', *ghee* ('*all* fat and oily substances') during the course of digestion acquired an 'acrimony' that was conveyed 'into the blood and juices'. Both, by their capacities to befoul and block the body's flow, were 'forbidden on the justest grounds' (Holwell 1767: 205).

In the case of milk, 'the basis (next to rice) of all the natives' food', the problem was that it was 'highly nutritious'. But the quality of its nutrition arose not only from its 'natural qualities' but also by its 'ready admission into' and 'quick assimilation' by the blood:

> it consequently is a warm heating diet, and must have a remote tendency to inflammation, whenever the blood is thrown into any preternatural ferment, and therefore, that milk is a food highly improper, at a season when the preternatural fermentation that produces the smallpox ought to be feared, and guarded against by every person who knows himself liable to the disease, or determined to prepare himself for receiving it, either from nature or art. (Holwell 1767: 205)

For this very reason, says Holwell, 'their women', and 'our European women' in India, abstain from it during their 'periodic visitation' or during the 'flow of the lochia', when it 'is avoided as so much poison' (ibid.).

What we have here is a body in ferment and flow. Anything that turned the natural ferment into a preternatural one ran the risk of inflaming the body's fluids or blocking its passages. Also present, sometimes at the margin and sometimes at the centre, was season. It was not that milk was improper *per se*: its impropriety was founded on the season 'when the preternatural fermentation that produces the small pox ought to be feared'; or during the *seasonal* flow of the blood which, presumably in an analogue, led to a preternatural ferment and hence was 'strictly forbid' (ibid.).

The important point to be noted is that the abstinence from certain articles of diet does not appear as an addendum to inoculation. Neither does it appear as a ruse to mark its danger and gravity and the possible spread of the contagion. We will see, when we get to examine the cause of smallpox, that it was presumed to rest two legs. The first was the notion of an 'immediate cause', which was stirred and brought into play by a preternatural ferment within the body. The other was a 'second or mediate cause' that triggered the first from the outside, either 'by nature or art'. A preternatural ferment led logically to inflammation, which worked itself out by eruption, ulceration and evacuation. Food that tended to either exacerbate inflammation, or led to a fouling of the passages and a blocking of the ducts, was dangerous. Hence the *practical effects* of violating the interdiction may have meant, *in terms of the theory*, that the operation of inoculation, instead of being unsuccessful, may turn too successful and result in a monstrosity. The disease, instead of being *true* to an intended course, a course designed and intended by 'art', may turn into something the therapeutic techniques may not be able to handle, thus ruining the patient and the reputation of the practitioner. But with the interdiction in place the practitioner probably had the confidence and the 'vanity' to 'ask the parents how many pocks they chuse their children should have': 'Vanity, we should think, urged a question on a matter seemingly so uncertain in the issue; but true it is, that they hardly ever exceed, or are deficient, in the number required.' (Holwell 1767: 201)

Origin and Cause: Immediate and Mediate

There were other reasons for the prohibition placed on these three articles of diet. Reasons that give us, through Holwell's interpretative grid, a theory of the origin and cause of smallpox. This theory rested, so to speak, on two causes, two media and mediation. It was a theory that had to account for many things. How did inoculation originate? Why was inoculation better than naturally contracting the disease? Why was a person not susceptible to a second attack? Why was there an interdiction on certain articles of diet? Why was the disease more prevalent at particular seasons?

The two causes were an '*immediate* (or instant)' cause and a '*mediate* (or second) *acting* cause'. The first 'exists in the mortal part of every human and *animal* form'. The second were '*imperceptible animalculae* floating in the atmosphere'. The second triggered the first by two media: food and blood. The animalculae were 'imprisoned' by the interdicted articles and conveyed via digestion and assimilation with the 'chyle', into the blood. If enough of these had been conveyed into the blood then it raised a '*peculiar* ferment which produces the small pox'. Once this peculiar ferment 'is raised in the blood, the *immediate (instant) cause* of the disease is totally expelled in the eruptions, or by other channels; and hence it is that the blood is not susceptible of a second fermentation of the same kind' (Holwell 1767: 207).

We must dwell on the notion of fermentation and the ferment. The immediate cause of smallpox present in all animal forms appears as both ferment and as triggered by fermentation. As Holwell says earlier, the animalculae received into the blood by digestion and assimilation 'excite a fermentation peculiar to the *immediate (or instant) cause,* which ends in an eruption on the skin. The animalculae do not directly *turn into* the ferment that erupted, nor do they automatically raise this 'peculiar ferment': 'though we all receive, with our aliment, a portion of them, yet it is not always sufficient in quantity to raise this *peculiar* ferment, and yet may be equal to setting the seeds of other diseases in motion; hence the reason why any epidemical disorder, seldom appears alone' (Holwell 1767: 207). Hence, if one was to come down with smallpox, enough of the animalculae had to be received by way of food, which threw the blood into a preternatural ferment and raised 'the peculiar (specific?) ferment' that would be 'thrown upon' the surface of the skin in the form of characteristic eruptions.

Once this *peculiar ferment* was raised the 'immediate or instant cause of this disease' was expelled. The body as brewery is the model at work. We have a principle, a thing and a result. The animalculae that triggered, depending on their charge and extent, turned an endemic into an epidemic. This in turn depended on season and course: 'driven by stated winds', or when there was no wind (the North Westers?) and hence 'generated on the spot by water and air in a state of stagnation (and consequently in a state of putrefaction favourable to their propagation)' (Holwell 1767: 208). The animalculae generated by the conjunction of these circumstances adhered to most things to a greater or lesser degree depending on the nature of their surface. They usually

> pass and repass in and out of the bodies of all animals in the act of respiration, without injury to themselves, or the bodies they pass through; that such is not the case with those that are taken in with the food, which, by mastication, and the digestive facilities of the stomach and intestines, are crushed and assimilated with the chyle, and conveyed into the blood. (Holwell 1767: 207)

The prohibited articles, given the nature of their surface, were particularly susceptible and the ban on them arose from a desire to keep them at bay.

We see once again that the interdiction on the three articles of food arises from a theory of the origin and contraction of smallpox: fish, milk and ghee not only ran the risk, by their viscid and inflammatory nature, of exacerbating the disease but were ideal and dangerous media for contracting it. The patient was usually not susceptible to a second attack as the 'internal and first cause' was expelled. While its occurrence was occasioned by the season, sudden vicissitudes in the weather turned an endemic into an epidemic by *charging* the air with the animalculae.

Having accounted for abstinence, its seasonal occurrence, and why one was not susceptible to a second attack, we are left with two allied questions: the origin and superiority of inoculation as opposed to naturally contracting the disease. Earlier commentators on Holwell's text have seen the practice of using the variolous matter from the preceding year as a principle of attenuation. I have no quarrel with such a view. But we arrive at this principle in Holwell's narrative by means and arguments that serve a different end. The structure of the argument does not privilege either the principle of attenuation or inoculation *per se*. We must be wary of retrospective imputations, not because they do not offer a (much-maligned) *precursor*. But an unproblematic rendering of animalculae as a precursor of bacterial infection, or preserved variolous matter as attenuation results in violating a *whole* and *excising* parts that no longer seem relevant to us. What it does, and what we have been at pains to show, is that instead of moving from theory to theory we move from empirically gleaned fragments in the past to theory today. All the tired categories by which we are imprisoned then rear their head. And we are back to the great theme of *light*, of the progressively unfolding light of the Enlightenment.

In Holwell's narrative we see the presence of the goddess in the notion of the immediate or instant cause that is present in all 'animal form'. It is the divinity presiding over the immediate cause, he says, that suggested the possibility of inoculation. The ferment triggered by a small portion of the variolous matter was better than naturally contracting the smallpox because: (a) it was similar to the immediate cause, and (b) since it '*had already passed* through a fermentation the effects must be moderate and benign' (Holwell 1767: 208). In opposition to this, the fermentation raised by the natural or mediate cause 'gives necessarily additional force and strength to the first efficient cause of the disease' (ibid.). It is this notion of a double cause, of a ferment raised by the one that raises the ferment *specific* to the pox, that holds together the rest of the theory. And it is a theory *of fermentation* that allows him to say why variolous matter from the preceding year is used. If it 'is effectually secured from the air, it undergoes at the return of the season an imperceptible *fermentation*', which gives 'fresh vigour to its action' (ibid.). It is the vigour imparted by the fermentation at the return of the season that 'constitute(s) its superiority over fresh matter'.

We must dwell on this for a moment. The superiority of the preceding year's vaccine arose from the fact that it was more vigorous than fresh variolous matter and, hence, more sure in its effect. While the variolous matter was preferred over naturally contracting it because it was more benign, the 'pickling' imparted to it just the right strength. But beyond the first year this capacity to re-ferment was lessened every year.

If we take away the theory of fermentation we are left to walk on one leg: the leg of inoculation. Season and diet, interdiction and temperance, course and rhythm, internal and external cause, and evacuating the pox by bathing and puncturing are jettisoned. Their possible insistence by a subject population is reduced to superstition and worship.

The Cold Douche

We have already alluded to the arguments for cold bathing put forward in eighteenth-century Europe and have pointed to the difference in the east of 'sluicing their patients over head and ears, morning and evening, with cold water, until the fever comes on' (Holwell 1767: 209).

The theory behind the cold bathing was once again accounted for in terms of fermentation and a circulatory pathology. The intense *shock* created by the sluice increased circulation, drove offensive matter to the extremities, and promoted the ferment of the smallpox. The fever was the first sign of the fact that the coction had begun. Once begun, the bathing ceased and the body was allowed to *ferment* without 'any additional commotion till the eruptions came on'.

The cold bathing and the opening of the pustules were to the eruptions what abstinence was to inoculation. If the interdiction against the three articles of diet were violated the practitioners refused to inoculate; and if cold bathing after inoculation was not attended to they refused to have anything further to do with the patient. Once the pustules appeared, it was the 'daily fresh impetus' provided by cold bathing that drove the ferment into the pustules.

> I have been myself an eyewitness to many instances of its marvellous effect, where the pustules have sunk, and the patient appeared in imminent danger, but was almost instantly restored by the application of three or four collons of cold water, which never fails to fill the pock, as it were by enchantment.

Opening the Pustules

If the plea for cold bathing by sluicing was a novelty in eighteenth-century Europe, the question of opening the pustules in the case of the smallpox was probably even more so. Holwell seems unable to find more than three people who thought similarly.

If abstinence prepared the ground and made the body ready for the reception of the ferment (and the goddess?), if inoculation introduced the ferment (the goddess?), if the cool diet housed it and controlled it (placated the goddess?), if the cold bathing fanned it and drove it into the pustule, opening the pustule was the last act in a performance where every patient was the actor (and the goddess). But this last act of a play in five acts had a crucial relationship to the life of the patient after the play. If the play was not to miscarry, if the actor was not to be left with 'inflammation and weakness of the eyes, biles, and other eruptions and disorders, which so commonly succeed the disease, however benign' (Holwell 1767: 212), then opening the pustules was mandatory. This last act toward which the others led *evacuated the pox*. The practitioners considered it so necessary that

> in very critical cases, they will not trust the operation of opening the pustules to the nurses or relations, but engage in it themselves . . . and when it has been zealously persevered in, I hardly ever knew it fail, of either entirely preventing, the *second fever*, or mitigating it in such sort, as to render it of no consequence. (Holwell 1767: 212)

If the fever was the first act of an excretory movement purificatory in intention, and opening the pustules the last act in allowing *nature* to accede to its own truth, then the *second fever* that interceded between the two was the sign of *nature* not having completed her work. The second fever becomes the occasion in Holwell's narrative of posing a question that is posed over and over again in European therapeutics: to bleed or not to bleed. The question was not whether one should *per se* bleed or not. Though that too was a question often posed, the issue was usually a 'for what and when' question.

'Eastern practitioners' advised against bleeding and cathartics on the ground 'that the first weakens the natural powers, and that the *latter* counteracts the regular course *of nature*, which in this disease invariably tends to throw out the offending cause *upon the* skin' (ibid.). Since nature had deigned that the pustules were the mode by which the ferment be thrown out of the body, nothing was to be done to subvert nature from its course. If the pock was to fill and the ferment rooted out, then any attempt to evacuate the body by other means was contra-indicated.

As we can see, both the technique[17] and the rationale for opening the pustule were dictated by theory: a theory in which inoculation was one act of a therapeutics that began with abstinence and ended by opening the pustules.

Of Therapeutics and Prophylactics

Where are we to situate Holwell's narrative in the eighteenth-century medical map? What are the concerns that animate him? By way of a quick recapitulation we can see that it is anchored by a fever nosology, a theory of proximate and ultimate, or internal and external causes, and therapeutics. But the motive of his essay, if one can say as much, is to introduce two of his pet concerns: the cool regimen and free admission of air. While the first of these concerns is backed by an elaborate practical description and the theoretical premise of cold bathing, his plea for ventilation is not similarly backed. The shorter and poorer descriptions by Coult, Deb and Wise, while they confirm the essentials of his description, make no mention of ventilation.[18]

One is not naive enough to assume that Holwell's theoretical explanation of the various practices he describes are a faithful rendering of native concepts. Their interest lies in the fact that they are not. But we should not jump to the conclusion either, that they were not backed by a theoretical edifice, or have no correspondence with native concepts. This is not the occasion to read against the grain and restore a possible misreading of native concepts that Holwell may have fallen prey to. While it is obvious that he was rhetorically positioning himself vis-à-vis his audience through his letter, what emerges through the exegesis is that the eighteenth century, both in the east and the west, did not privilege inoculation. The reasons for this lie in the fact that inoculation, which stands as the prototype for modern preventive public health, is not the only or even the main issue in the eighteenth century. Historical writing on smallpox works, as we have attempted to show, on this tacit premise and pays a heavy price for it.

The introduction of smallpox inoculation in Europe in the 1710s ushered in a new technique of prophylactics. The prophylactic measures before that were preventive in so far as they rested on the concept of distancing oneself from the disease: especially epidemics. Quarantine, segregation and internment were the three great themes that dominated the earlier approach. Smallpox inoculation certainly did not lead to the demise of these methods. But it ushered in something novel: of preventing it by giving oneself a little bit of it. In sites other than Europe one 'bought the pox'. It is not surprising that vaccination, based on this prototype, was to dominate the nineteenth century as a model of preventive public health. I think it is more than a coincidence that the history of vaccination and the history of state-organized public health are so closely allied to each other. But the eighteenth century was dominated by a model of therapeutics rather than prophylactics. If therapeutics, beginning with Linnaeus and Suvages, was to concern itself with nosological compendiums for didactic and pedagogical purposes, at the bedside, in the encounter between doctor and patient, it had to account for a temporal unfolding of the disease. We must bear in mind that inoculation was not vaccination. It produced smallpox, albeit a milder version of it. The disease had to be managed and prescribed for by the practitioner. Hence the need for a therapeutics that would understandably fit inoculation into a theoretical arsenal already in place for the management of smallpox. In the case of Bengal and Britain at least, that certainly seems to be the case.

This recasting of variolation versus vaccination as a movement from therapeutics to a prophylactic allows us to view the passage from the one to the other in a very different light. The nineteenth-century record of vaccination, especially in India, could then be read, as we have shown elsewhere (Naraindas 1998), rather differently.

Notes

[1] This is the first of a set of three essays on smallpox. The second of these essays has appeared as 'Care, welfare and treason: The advent of vaccination in the 19th century' (Naraindas 1998), where a small portion of the current argument has been reworked and at times reiterated, in so far as it impinges on the advent of vaccination in the nineteenth century. All three are part of a larger work (Naraindas 1997).

[2] I am aware of the pitfalls when I say east and west. Even India (or Bengal) may not stand in as a necessary substitute for the east, though it seemed to, for Holwell. Sumit Guha (2001) has drawn our attention to the fact that the practice of inoculation may not have been known in parts of western and northern India, while it was practised in many other parts of the east beyond eastern India (and one may add, in many other parts of the world, including rural England). While we may be called upon to revise this statement in due course, it indicates that contemporary boundaries and their labels may or may not be useful, and given the task in hand, may have no more than a heuristic value.

[3] An unintended effect of the frame of reference is that it freezes and *medievalizes* the corpus. In a familiar act, it empties tradition of either agency or innovation. In the light of a normative structure that textual exegesis creates, subsequent and contemporary practices appear as distortions and corruption. The tacit register of comparison is history, particularly a triumphalist history of science.

[4] Marglin offers evidence in support (1990: 117). Further evidence of the impact of British revenue policy on indigenous institutions (of specialists) is offered by Dharampal in his Pune lectures of 1986 (Dharampal 1987). Dharampal, in a perceptive introduction to his collection on 'science and technology' (1983), points out that inoculators in India, like other categories of specialists, 'were maintained on subventions from public revenues': subventions that were pervasive and made possible by the low tithe (which has been questioned by a number of scholars) imposed by pre-

British state structures (Dharampal 1987). The specialists appear in his text in a very different light. It rescues them from the ad nauseam back and forth in the literature: whether they were brahmins and high-status (as if there was no hierarchy within the brahmins), or low-caste and low-status. The issue of high and low probably betrays the particular valence that these possessed in England in the eighteenth and nineteenth centuries, that later-day history often unreflectingly takes over. Marglin, in part, and from the other side, attempts to break this when she uses Gomes' notion of 'circular hierarchy' to analyse the role of each caste in the healing of the goddess at Purl (Marglin 1990: 137).

5 At best he passes over it by alluding to it as 'humoral medicine'. This, as Marglin has pointed out, may create other problems: a dual explanation of the disease—theurgic and naturalistic—is offered (Marglin 1990: 116). It should not surprise us as it is precisely against such dualism that this essay struggles.

6 Dimock (1976) and Robinson (1976) have argued for a similar under-standing of the *Mangal Kavya* texts of Bengal, among which is the *Sitala Mangal.*

7 Arnold alludes to 'many accounts of variolation in eastern and northern India in the eighteenth and nineteenth centuries, most of them written by European doctors and surgeons' (1993: 126). The only account he quotes at length, like most others for the eighteenth century, is Holwell.

8 As Arnold says, variolation 'was seen more as a religious ceremony and a ritual invocation of *Sitala* than as a medical procedure as such' (Arnold 1993: 126). For a further elucidation of the problematic nature of this remark, see footnote 10 below.

9 Which, under the concept of ventilation, appears as an eighteenth-century innovation and is itself part of a larger tetrad of concepts: ventilation, lavation, drainage, interment (Riley 1987).

10 Holwell's 'rational' rather than 'religious' rendering is interpreted by Arnold as audience-induced (Arnold 1993: 128): the College of Physicians. This might be true. But the tacit premise of the remark (like the one in footnote 8) is that these (the words he uses are medical and religious) are necessarily opposed categories, and that the *truth* about smallpox in India is religious (see footnote 8 above). Holwell could then be seen as packaging it in a 'medical' garb to primarily reassure his audience about a practice only recently borrowed from the 'East'. In another perceptive but problem-atic passage he says, 'the greatest objection to vaccination was its raw secularity. There was no ritual or dietary preparation; no *Sitala* prayers or Ganges water; no appeal to the goddess of smallpox to guide the child safely through such a dangerous defile. Since there was "no preparation of the body or poojah", "no blessing could attend it" ' (Arnold 1993: 143).

While I readily agree that the problem with vaccination arises from the fact that it enjoined upon the person 'no preparation of the body or poojah' (which by authorial admission cannot possibly have any *practical effect*), what the statement does (what it is busy doing while telling the 'truth') is that it circumscribes 'a dietetics and a regimen' by religion and, having done so, relegates it to the margin and leaves it unaddressed. Or, to put it differently, the circumscription is explanation enough. Its opposite is vaccination in its 'raw secularity'. Apart from the reiteration of a tired trope (the conflation of India and religion), the conflation of dietetics, regimen, ritual and religion, in opposition to what is left unsaid, creates an eddy of meaning that is problematic. As the title of the essay suggests, smallpox in India is imprisoned by the iconic body of the goddess. There is no locus outside of that. And the only *response* to vaccination from the body politic is to oscillate between lament and protest.

11 Dharampal's collection offers a sample on 'science and technology' (Dharampal 1983). Coult's short note there, of 1731, on the inoculation of the smallpox performed in Bengal, is one of the earliest notices served to the west in English. It provides independent corroboration of some crucial features (like Wise [1860] and Deb [1831] in the nineteenth century) of Holwell's description.

12 This is precisely the argument that Latour too makes when he says that anthropology and history are flip-sides of each other: scientific truth irrupts into the present by annulling the past and the other. The past reappears in the contemporary west as commonsense which, like the other, is the past in the present and hence vestigial; and scientific truth constitutes itself as opposed to both commonsense and the past. It is not only Bachelard and Canguilhem who make this argument (Latour 1993: 92–93), but also Kuhn (1970). While I have attempted to elaborate the disciplinary effects of this dichotomy between 'Truth and Past/East' in a paper on 'Truth and Time' (Naraindas 2001), we can clearly see its effects throughout this essay in the way in which Howell's essay is truncated and mis-read, and how a unitary phenomenon like smallpox is parcelled out across disciplines.

13 Holwell on Hinduism is part of a long line of Janus-faced figures, starting with Fleming and Nobili in the sixteenth and seventeenth centuries, both of whom could be easily accused of rendering the Christian vision through a 'debased' Hinduism and, in the process, of debasing Christian doctrine. Nobili was indeed so charged from both sides (Cronin 1959). His fellow-Jesuits attempted an inquisition from which he was eventually exonerated. The brahmins of Madurai held a public examination where he was eloquently defended by his first brahmin disciple, at the end of which they found him a slot in their scheme of things. He was given a title called *tattuva bodhar*, 'teacher of reality' (Neil 1985), and allowed to ply his trade. I am not sure if *tattuva bodhar* means 'teacher of reality' but the upshot of it (the translation), if his chroniclers are to be believed, is interesting. It *confirms* Christian and Hindu doctrines in their respective (stereotypical) positions: the first, this-worldly and true, and the other, other-worldly and untrue. This is the sub-text in the dual sense of the term. A transcendental divinity, a one-and-only life, a real world and a day of judgment are opposed to metempsychosis and an illusory world, whose layers may be peeled by different doctrines. A depiction that reconfirms the 'misplaced' tolerance of

116

the one and 'righteous' evangelization *by* the other! The 'actual' historical record even as told by his hagiographers is fuzzy. One is struck by the fact that history often functions as hagiography. And the moment one sets out to write a history of *reason* it turns, willy-nilly, into its hagiography.

[14] For the implication of what dating, and this particular date, meant to his eighteenth-century audience, see Marshall's introduction (Marshall 1970).

[15] We must be careful not to reduce either to the other. Cooling by air and by water, apart from the fact that they cool, may perform the same function differently. That apart, ventilating also has a *mechanical* action upon the body. The same is true of water. Tobias Smollet, in *An essay on the external use of water* (1752), claimed: 'I can easily conceive how extraordinary cures may be performed by the *mechanical* [emphasis added] effects of simple Water upon the human body; and I fully believe that in the use of BATHING and PUMPING, that efficacy is often ascribed to the mineral particles, which properly belongs to the element itself, exclusive of any foreign substance' (Cayleff 1987: 20). Smollet's statement marks one trend, starting with John Floyer and John Smith before him, for the external effects of cold water. Not that it marks the demise of a 'mineral philosophy' of water: its transmutation and attempted appropriation by chemists from the late eighteenth century is recounted by Hamlin in his *The legitimization of English spas* (1990). We will see further on that cold bathing in the form of a douche that Holwell describes for the smallpox patient in India, is recommended for its *shock* and seems to derive primarily from its capacity to cool rather than act by pressure. The norm in England was bathing by immersion, and the 'circumambient pressure' that it created apart from cooling (Holwell 1767: 210). The douche by its suddenness cooled the body more dramatically.

[16] John Barker, in *An inquiry into the nature, cause, and cure of the present epidemic fever* (1742)), valorized the notion of the 'acrid' to the Acrid Stimulating Body, and made it responsible for all the nervous fevers. In an attempt to theorize about the cause of the inflammatory and nervous fevers, the 'circulatory pathology' then current was broken down into nerves and fluids, and causes into stimulation and obstruction. Fluids were obstructed and nerves were stimulated; the first gave rise to the inflammatory fevers and the latter to the nervous fevers: 'commonly, however, the two varieties of cause acted together or successively to "form a fever of *Mixt* or *Compound* kind, partly partaking of the Nature of the one, and partly of the other" ' (Smith 1981: 131).

[17] I have commented elsewhere on the theoretical necessity of the technique of opening the pustules with a fine sharp-pointed thorn (Naraindas 1998: 87).

[18] Constraints of length prevent me from situating and exploring how cold inaugurates a new sensibility in eighteenth-century Europe (see, for example, Vigarello 1988). As for ventilation, I have already alluded to its place as part of a tetrad of concepts in the eighteenth century (see footnote 9). I discuss both at some length elsewhere (Naraindas 1997).

117

References

Arnold, D. (1993). 'Smallpox: The Body of the Goddess', in D. Arnold, *Colonizing the Body: State medicine and epidemic disease in nineteenth-century India*, Delhi: Oxford University Press, pp. 116–58.

Bynum, W.F. (1981). 'Cullen and the study of fevers in Britain, 1760–1820', in W.F. Bynum and V. Nutton (eds), *Theories of fever from antiquity to the enlightenment, Medical History*, Supplement No. 1, pp. 135–48.

Bynum, W.F. and R. Porter (eds) (1987). *Medical fringe and medical orthodoxy 1750–1850*, London: Croom Helm.

Canguilhem, G. (1988). *Ideology and rationality in the history of the life sciences*, Cambridge, Massschussets: The MIT Press.

Cayleff, Susan E. (1987). *Wash and be healed. The water-cure movement and women's health*, Philadelphia: Temple University Press.

Deb, Radha K. (1831). 'Account of the tikadars', *Transactions of the Medical and Physical Society of Calcutta*, 5, pp. 416–18.

Dharampal (1983) (first edn 1971). 'Preface', in Dharampal (ed.), *Indian Science and Technology in the Eighteenth Century: Some Contemporary British Accounts*, Delhi: Impex India, pp. 17–58.

Dharampal (1987). *Some aspects of earlier Indian society and polity and their relevance to the present*, Pune: A New Quest Pamphlet.

Dimock, E.C. (1976). 'A theology of the repulsive: Some reflections on Sitala and other Mangals', in M. Davis (ed.), *Bengal studies in literature, society and history*, Michigan: Asian Studies Centre.

Egnor, M.E. (1984). 'The changed mother, or what the smallpox Goddess did when there was no more smallpox', *Contributions to Asian Studies*, 18.

Foucault, M. (1988). *The Care of the Self, The History of Sexuality*, Volume 3, New York: Vintage Books.

Foucault, M. (1990). *The Use of Pleasure, The History of Sexuality*, Volume 2, New York: Vintage Books.

Guha, Sumit (2001). *Health and Population in South Asia: From earliest times to the present*, Delhi: Permanent Black.

Hamlin, C. (1990). 'Chemistry, medicine, and the legitimazation of English spas, 1740–1840', in Roy Porter (ed.), *The medical history of waters and spas, Medical History*, Supplement no. 10, pp. 67–81.

Holwell, J.Z. (1767). 'An account of the manner of inoculating for the Smallpox in the East Indies', in Dharampal (ed.), *Indian Science and Technology in the Eighteenth Century*, pp. 195–218.

Holwell, J.Z. (1970). 'The religious tenets of the Gentoos, Excerpted from J.Z. Holwell, 1767, Interesting Historical events relative to the province of Bengal and the empire of Indostan', in P.J. Marshall (ed.), *The British Discovery of Hinduism in the Eighteenth Century*, Cambridge: Cambridge University Press, pp. 45–106.

James, S.P. (1909). *Smallpox and vaccination in British India*, Calcutta: Thacker, Spink and Co.

118

Kuhn, T. (1970). *The structure of scientific revolutions*, second edn, enlarged, Chicago: The University of Chicago Press.

Latour, B. (1993). *We have never been modern* (translated by Catherine Porter), New York: Harvester Wheatsheaf.

Marglin, F.A. (1990). 'Smallpox in two systems of knowledge', in F.A. Marglin and S.A. Marglin (eds), *Dominating knowledge. Development, culture, and resistance*, Oxford: Clarendon Press, pp. 102–44.

Marshall, P.J. (1970). 'Introduction', in P.J. Marshall (ed.), *The British discovery of Hinduism in the eighteenth century*, Cambridge: Cambridge University Press, pp. 1–45.

Naraindas, H. (1996). 'Poisons, putrescence, and the weather: A genealogy of the advent of tropical medicine', *Contributions to Indian Sociology* (n.s.), 30, 1, pp. 1–35.

———— (1997). 'Knowledge, Institution, and Environment: Aspects of the culture of science and medicine', Ph.D. Thesis, Department of Sociology, University of Delhi, Delhi.

———— (1998). 'Care, welfare and treason: The advent of vaccination in the 19th century', *Contributions to Indian Sociology* (n.s.), 32, 1, pp. 67–96.

———— (2001). 'Truth and Time', paper presented at the workshop on 'Theory and Method: Disciplinary practices and intellectual genealogies', Department of Sociology, University of Delhi, 27–28 March 2001.

Nicholas, Ralph W. (1981). 'The Goddess Sitala and epidemic smallpox in Bengal', *Journal of Asian Studies*, 41, 1, pp. 21–44.

Nicholas, Ralph W. and Aditi N. Sarkar (1976). 'The fever demom and the census commissioner: *Sitala* mythology in eighteenth and nineteenth century Bengal', in M. Davis (ed.), *Bengal studies in literature, society and history*, Michigan: Asian Studies Centre.

Riley, J.C. (1987). *The eighteenth-century campaign to avoid disease*, New York: St. Martin's Press.

Robinson, S.P. (1976). 'Death and revivification in the *Dharma Mangal*', in M. Davis (ed.), *Bengal studies in literature, society and history*.

Smith, D.C. (1981). 'Medical science, medical practise, and the emerging concept of typhus in mid-eighteenth-century Britain', in W.F. Bynum and V. Nutton (eds), *Theories of fever from antiquity to the enlightenment, Medical History*, Supplement No. 1, pp. 121–34.

Vigarello, G. (1988). *Concepts of cleanliness: changing attitudes in France since the Middle Ages* (translated by Jean Birrell), Cambridge: Cambridge University Press; Paris: Maison des sciences de l'homme.

Wadley, Susan S. (1980). 'Sitala: The Cool One', *Asian Folklore Studies*, 39, 1, pp. 33–62.

Wise, T.A. (1867). *Review of Hindoo Medicine*, 2 volumes. London: Churchill.

Zimmerman, F. (1987). *The jungle and the aroma of meats: An ecological theme in Hindu medicine*. Berkeley: University of California Press.

———— (1992). 'Gentle purge: The flower power of Ayurveda', in C. Leslie and A. Young (eds), *Paths to Asian medical knowledge*, Berkeley: University of California Press, pp. 209–23.

Modern India

Environmental Factors Contributing to Malaria in Colonial Bengal

Ihtesham Kazi

Writing about the predicament of people especially caused by diseases is not an accepted norm in the historiography of Bengal. But many other disciplines, like anthropology, economics and sociology, take a lead in this respect. They concentrate mostly on recent times, work within a confined locale and with a narrow data-base, and hence have limited scope. But a historian can give a wider dimension to and a greater perspective about disease. Moreover, the stigma in South Asia that the historian's trade is the politics of the past, and at best as a narrator of society's solvent people, is not tenable any longer. Historians in advanced countries are working on all aspects of human endeavour, from women's issues to workmen's compensation, from the history of species to space exploration. Yet, most historians in Bangladesh are doing what W.W. Hunter justly said a century ago: 'Eloquent and elaborate narratives have indeed been written of British ascendancy in the East; but such narratives are records of English Government, or biographies of English Governors of India, not histories of Indian people. The silent millions who bear our yoke found no analyst.'[1] He did not forget to narrate the condition of countryfolk, and lament about their sufferings from painful diseases. His words still hold good to some extent, in a different time and context. Things have not changed much since the days of Hunter. The Britishers have gone, but they have been replaced by more jealously-guarding bureaucratic Bengalis. Any research effort on human suffering is very much constrained because of limited access to materials. My effort to fill that gap and to probe into the history of malaria, more so about the environmental causes of malaria, will certainly be inadequate.

Although literature on malaria in India may be traced back to antiquity, as it was one of the oldest of diseases, its endemic and

123

epidemic prevalence in Bengal does not have a long history. From the middle of the nineteenth century malarial fever, originating from a small area in western Bengal, gradually spread its virulence to the whole of Bengal. People called it *natun jwar*, new fever; it was officially designated as 'Burdwan Fever'. It was said that the epidemic was killing 'numbers without number'.[2] Bengal as a political and administrative unit during British rule in India, comprised roughly the present-day state of West Bengal in India and the sovereign nation of Bangladesh. Today mosquito-vector-borne diseases like malaria and dengue are emerging again in this region, with devastating effects. The factors contributing to malaria at present may be similar to those in the past. The resurgence of floods last year (AD 2000) both in West Bengal and the western part of Bangladesh had many ramifications due to past neglect of and present indifference to environment. The flood in itself is disastrous to people, and the aftermath of it is bound to bring vector-borne diseases, malaria being one of many. This paper is only a tip of the iceberg in locating the environmental causes of malaria, one among many other factors contributing to malaria in colonial Bengal.

Some of the best work on tracing the cause of man-made malaria in Bengal was done by Bentley[3] and Ira Klein. Shireen Moosvi refers to dying rivers in Mughal Bengal in *Man and Nature in the Mughal Era* (Symposia Papers: 5). An elaborate study of malaria in the Punjab was done by Christophers. All of these hardly discuss in depth, the environmental causes of malaria. Ira Klein[4] studied mortality due to malaria but not the environmental causes of malaria in Bengal. In a recent article in a popular journal, *Desh* (December 2000), Kallyan Rydra talks about the devastating effects of the Farrakha barrage in West Bengal. Because of the barrage, the Ganga river (the Ganges) is changing course, resulting in a minimal supply of water from the same source to Bangladesh, creating large-scale economic and health problems. Environmental concerns are very real today, and for in-depth understanding of these detailed historical study is important.

The British colonialists seldom noted the ecological disturbances due to the expansion of communication through roads and railways, and at the same time neglected waterways such as canals and rivers which, for centuries, had served the need of transportation. While engineering works increased the facilities for travel, in many cases they were responsible for the great increase in the prevalence of malaria by creating conditions of mosquito-breeding. Engineers and contractors, in the course of construction of roads, railways, irrigation projects or in the lay-out of new townships, created burrow pits, quarry pits and badly-designed culverts. In the construction of large engineering works, they naturally tried to complete projects as cheaply as possible. They often paid no heed to, or did not realize the disastrous consequences to the health of the people. By their careless operations they created conditions for the progress of diseases and displacement. Communication networks also spread diseases; malaria is aptly called a disease of development. Commenting on the harmful effects of man-made malaria, Cartwright remarked: 'Roads meant easier and faster travel and new diseases are able to pass more swiftly along such roads, striking down unprotected populations in mass pandemics.'[5] Bengal was one of the few regions where the development and spread of malaria were, to a great extent, due both to the neglected and disturbed environment.

Environmental Change through Natural Causes

Let us first look at the neglect of environment. The rivers of Bengal were once an important highway for trade. They were enormous and served both the purposes of communication and a drainage system, with so many tributaries. Travelling in the eighteenth century, William Hodges was surprised to see the vastness of these rivers and compared them to oceans. He said, 'The rivers I have seen in Europe, even the Rhine, appear as rivulets in comparison with these enormous waters.'[6] But a century later some of those rivers had taken a different turn either for natural reasons or due to human interference.

An examination of the topographical map of Bengal and its river system would show that a large portion of the province comprised of deltas. Western Bengal contained the deltas of the Kasai, the Damodar, the Ajoy and Mor rivers, and part of the deltas of the Ganges, which were very much silted up. North Bengal, north of the Padma was wholly alluvial land. The general level of this region was very low and suffered from obstructed drainage. Central Bengal, or parts south of the Padma, between the Bhagirathi river on the west and the Madhumati on the east, was formerly the Ganges delta. East Bengal, the country east of the Madhumati, including the present deltas of the Ganga and the Brahmaputra which was in the process of land formation, remained healthier than the other regions. This was so in the late nineteenth century. Today, the Brahmaputra is a dying river.

The problem of siltation and the death of rivers were the result of human agency as well as changes in the courses of rivers. S.C. Majumdar, a health official in the Bengal government, believed that human interference caused rivers to become swamps, causing havens for the mosquito and malaria.[7] In Murshidabad, where the Bhagirathi was degenerating, malaria fever was a great scourge. The whole of the centre and east of Rajshahi were characterized by O'Malley as a swampy water-logged depression in which fever was rife. He explained the situation by saying:

> The drainage system in short, disjointed, and the bills which should get an influx of fresh water annually are left to stagnate. These bills are mostly shallow and their number is large. . . . The great Challan Bill has now largely silted up—all of which help to corroborate Dr Bentley's theory about the cause of malaria.[8]

Today, most of Chalan Bill (a huge marshy land) is dry, and a recent road-link through it caused it to gasp for its last breath. A similar correlation existed in the districts of Burdwan, Malda, Nadia, Jessore and Rangpur, between disrupted irrigation and drainage, and the increase of malarial fever. Opposite to this effect was the flooding of the countryside with spill water from the rivers, which had the effect of flushing that kept the mosquitoes out of breeding centres. It was said that 'a village situated on a live river is ordinarily much more healthy than one lying upon the banks of a dead river'.[9] Hence, the increase of malaria in the delta tracts of Bengal is directly attributable to the silting of the rivers and the obstructed condition of the drainage system.

Man-Made Environmental Change

There was reason to believe that many of the changes that occurred in the deltas of rivers and channels in western and northern Bengal were man-made. Improvement of communications almost invariably meant the construction of roads and railways which, in the delta areas, entailed a multiplication of embankments. The construction of embankments against floods and for irrigation led in the first place to a great amount of excavations and resulting burrow pits. Irreparable damage was done owing to the restrictions of free river flow, as a direct consequence of the construction of thousands of miles of embankments. These embankments were designed either for controlling the rivers or for constructing railways or roads. Whatever the object, the effects were the same, preventing the natural drainage systems. These combined to bring about widespread water-logging, agricultural decline and consequently breeding-grounds of mosquitoes.

The chief exponent of the theory that the outbreak of epidemic malaria had a direct causal relation with the construction of embankments was Raja Digambar Mitter, the Indian member of the first committee appointed by the government in 1863, to go into the causes of the epidemic of fever. Among the instances mentioned by the Raja was the construction of extensive embankments in the villages around Halishsahar to Kancharapara.[10] The people in these villages suffered from a severe type of fever, which broke out exactly in the order of the months and years in which the railway embankments progressed and passed along their eastern borders. His ideas were hardly accepted at the time, not even by sanitarians. But in 1873, reporting on the epidemic fever in Burdwan and Birbhum, Dr C.J. Jackson, Sanitary Commissioner of Bengal, was of the opinion that the spread of the disease exhibited a remarkable and persistent association with the lines of communication. He said:

> The main causes to which . . . the natural drainage of the country has been interfered with many ways of the late years; amongst these may be mentioned the many embanked roads that have been thrown up during the last sixteen years. These roads must materially interfere with the drainage of a country.[11]

In 1877, a committee was especially appointed to investigate certain localities where it was alleged that the drainage had been obstructed. Between 1878 to 1880, the need for efficient drainage was urged by the local authorities to the government, with no positive response. The subject was especially discussed by the Nadia Fever Commission of 1882, but after a protracted local enquiry the conclusion was that the outbreak of fever could not be attributed to local obstruction to drainage. In 1900 Captain Rogers noted that the places at 24-Parganas with the highest spleen rates lay for the most part to the east of the railways. Finally, a Drainage Committee was appointed by the Government of Bengal in 1906, to inquire into the causes of malarial fever in Bengal, and the possibility of undertaking some remedial measures.[12]

The investigation was confined to the Presidency Division because it was the most malaria-prone area at the time. Moreover, this division comprised the area in which 'the factor of defective drainage was most apparent'.[13] The committee observed that a live river bestows a more healthy living situation than a dead one.[14] The obstruction of drainage due to the construction of embankments or decaying of rivers was only one among other and possibly more dangerous sources of malaria.

Similar unhealthy results followed due to the embanking of the rivers for the purpose of flood protection. The earliest known example is that of an outstanding break of fever following the embanking of the river Nabaganga in 1858. An outbreak was reported in Krishnanagar *thana* in Hooghly district in 1873 as a result of embankment.[15] In 1893 Murshidabad district suffered the same fate because of embankments. Villages on the east bank of the Bhagirathi were examined by health officials, and the result was surprising. The mean spleen index of twenty-six villages outside the embankment was 27.0 per cent, whereas twenty-nine villages inside gave a mean spleen index of 60.0 per cent, a sufficient reason for malarial fever.[16] Changes of this kind were reported in the embankments in Birbhum, the Sara Bridge and the Sara-Sirajganj railway embankments. From the middle of the nineteenth century, embankments were spread out in the western part of Bengal through construction of railway roadbeds and for irrigation purposes. These embankments added to the siltation of rivers and canals, and created more breeding places for mosquitoes.

Another factor was that there was serious apathy on the part of the government in maintaining the embankments. While the large works were to be done by the government, the zamindars were to construct and maintain all the others. But no machinery was evolved to enforce this. Acts were passed in 1851 and 1873 redefining the powers of different authorities, but the cumbersome process of approval of plans became counter-productive; rather, it 'helped to keep the status quo of negligence'.[17]

Construction of Railways

The building of railways started in the middle of the nineteenth century. In fact, the first opening of Calcutta to Ranaghat via railway was started in 1862, and by 1872 there were no less than 900 miles of railway.[18] It is an interesting coincidence that in the very year the railway was built there were reports of fever epidemics in Burdwan. The change in situation was recorded in the following way:

> Before 1862 the district was noted for its healthiness, and the town of Burdwan particularly was regarded as a sanitarium. . . . But in 1862 the terrible epidemic fever . . . crossed the border of Burdwan. Thence it spread gradually but steadily over the district, following the main lines of communication, until it was fairly established in all the eastern thanas.[19]

The development of the railway was the beginning of malaria epidemics. The epidemic malarial fever of Burdwan was attributed to the obstruction of the natural drainage system because of railway embankments. It was rightly said by K.C. Ghosh, 'Railways are a most prolific source of Anopheline breeding places and malaria of virulent type.'[20] Similarly, an outbreak of malaria in Malda district was blamed on the extension of the railway. An outbreak of malaria took place in Murshidabad district coinciding with the construction of a new line there.[21] The sanitary report alluded to an epidemic of malaria which broke out when the railway was constructed between Dhaka and Mymensingh.[22] In later days Bentley thought that the areas of greatest railway construction in Bengal in the 1920s were the most intensely malarial ones.[23] 'More railway, more malaria', became a common saying in Bengal.

If government is based on the motto of maximum profit for minimum cost, the result is always disastrous for the people. This was quite evident in the letter of Lord Lawrence to Charles Wood, the Secretary of State for India, at Whitehall, with reference to the railway schemes. In his words: 'Our main object should be to complete the railways . . . which are the great arteries . . . but I doubt if most of them will pay our present financial difficulties. . . . We are at our wits' end for revenue: any increase of taxation is sure to produce discontent.'[24]

The main purpose behind the construction of railways, embankments and roads was to enhance the revenue of the state, not the well-being of the people. The widespread prevalence of malaria or other vector-borne diseases was due to serious environmental disturbances created because of the government's greedy policy of exploitation. Through its effects, the whole population of Bengal suffered, the majority of whom were farmers and labourers.

In the process of so-called development, malaria was only one of many devastating diseases. The number of deaths in Bengal from malaria was an economic factor of serious importance. It was estimated that in each year one million people died of malaria. If this was the death figure then the suffering and productivity loss would have been ten times more. Thus, the economic and human loss was colossal. The deaths due to malaria had a personal level of pain, but the records were collected in a blanket fashion. Moreover, during the colonial period the underlying causes of calamities were recorded with a view to blame the subject people rather than the sovereign. There was an imperialist argument that diseases are inherently linked to racial inferiority. This argument was based on Social Darwinism,[25] which says that weakest of races will die out in the natural selection process. When imperialism was at its high peak, any argument was rendered sensible in a distorted prism. The causes of diseases lay squarely with administrative, environmental and nutritional factors. The natural causes of decadence of the environment, along with man-made measures, brought untold suffering to the people. Unfortunately, that suffering is unabated today, and unluckily, we no longer have foreigners to kick about for our miseries. If it is rightly said that the knowledge of history is more than anticipated experience, then our knowledge of the history of environmental degradation could bring some foresight to the future.

Notes and References

[1] William W. Hunter, *Annals of Rural Bengal*, Calcutta, 1897, p. 6.

[2] Bholanauth Chunder, *Raja Digambar Mitra, His Life and Career*, Calcutta, 1983, p. 103.

[3] Charles Bentley, 'Some Problems Presented by Malaria in Bengal', *Indian Medical Record*, November 1913, pp. 154–62; *Report on Malaria in Bengal*, Calcutta, 1916; *Relations between Obstructed Rivers and Malaria in Bengal*, Calcutta, 1922.

[4] Ira Klein, 'Malaria and Mortality in Bengal, 1840–1921', *The Indian Economic and Social History Review*, Vol. IX, No. 2, June 1972.

[5] Frederick Cartwright and Michael Biddiss, *Disease and History*, New York, 1972, p. 3.

[6] William Hodges, *Travelling in India, during Years 1780, 1781, 1782, 1783*, London, 1893, pp. 33–43.

[7] S.C. Majumdar, *Rivers of Bengal Delta*, Calcutta, 1943, p. 93.

[8] *Bengal District Gazetteer*, XXXIII, 'Rajshahi', Calcutta, 1916, p. 70.

[9] *Report of the Drainage Committee, Bengal*, Calcutta, 1907, p. 32.

[10] Charles A. Bentley, *Malaria and Agriculture in Bengal: How to Reduce*

Malaria in Bengal by Irrigation, Calcutta, 1925, p. 35.

[11] *Report of the Sanitary Commissioner for Bengal for the Year 1874*, Calcutta, 1874, p. 90.

[12] *Report of the Drainage Committee, Bengal*, Calcutta, 1907.

[13] Ibid., p. 2.

[14] Ibid., p. 30.

[15] 'East India (Railways), Administration Report on the Railways in India, for the Year, 1911', *House of Commons Sessional Papers*, Feb. 1913–March 1913, Vol. 62, London, 1912.

[16] J.C. Peterson, *Bengal District Gazetteers, Burdwan*, Calcutta, 1910, p. 78.

[17] K.C. Ghose, 'Railway and Malaria', *The Indian Medical Gazette*, Vol. LXII, March 1928, p. 169.

[18] A.B. Fry, *Second Report on Malaria in Bengal*, Calcutta, 1914, p. 36.

[19] *Report of the Sanitary Commissioner for Bengal for the Year 1884*, Calcutta, 1885, p. 73.

[20] C.A. Bentley, 'Some Economic Aspect of Bengal Malaria', *The Indian Medical Gazette Advertiser*, Calcutta, Sept. 1922, pp. 324–26.

[21] *Report of the Sanitary Commissioner for Bengal for the Year 1873*, Calcutta, 1874, p. 90.

[22] Stewart and Proctor, *Final Reports on the Districts of Jessore, Nadia and Murshidabad*, Calcutta, 1970, pp. xiii–xiv.

[23] *A Review of the Legislation in Bengal Relating to the Irrigation, Drainage and Flood Embankments*, Calcutta, 1911, p. 6.

[24] Quoted from Sir George Dunbar, *A History of India: From Earliest to Nineteen Thirty-nine*, London, 1949, p. 539.

[25] Gertrude Mimmelfarb, *Darwin and Darwinian Revolution*, London, 1959, pp. 347–51. Ronald Ross, W.H.S. Jones and Ellett, *A Neglected Factor in the History of Greece and Rome*, Cambridge, 1907, pp. 2–3. Charles Bentley, *Report on Malaria in Bengal*, Calcutta, 1916, p. 60.

Malaria in Nineteenth-Century Bombay

Simkie Sarkar

Bombay seems to have suffered from the plague of mosquitoes for many years. Aungier writes of 'the vermin created in the wells and tanks', and Ovington mentions that 'The prodigious growth of vermin and the venomous creatures at the time of the monsoon do abundantly demonstrate the malignant corruption of the air. I cannot without horror mention to what pitch all vicious enormities were grown in this place.'[1] One of the chief reasons was, doubtless, the gradual silting-up of the creek which divided Bombay into a group of islets. At high tide the sea swept through the beaches, overflowed the major portion of the island, and laid a pestilential deposit highly productive of malaria.[2] Lady West, in her diary written between 1825–28, repeatedly complains of being tormented by mosquitoes, which appear to have been numerous in the Fort in her day.[3]

The Epidemic

A malaria epidemic broke out in Colaba about 1838–41. This outbreak seems to have occurred in association with the construction of the Colaba Causeway, which involved the reclamation of a large area of low-lying land previously covered by the sea. There appears to have been an outbreak of fever in Bombay during the period of extraordinary commercial activity between 1861–66, which followed the inflation of cotton prices as a result of the American War. A large number of reclamation schemes were started in different parts of the island at this time, and they were probably responsible for an increase of malaria.[4] During the four years from 1863 to 1866, fever deaths averaged 12,577 a year and in 1865 the recorded fever mortality reached a maximum of 18,767.

132

Ten years later, the proposal to construct Princes' Dock resulted in considerable alarm, as it was feared that it would affect the health of the city. Between 1903 and 1907, there was an increase in malaria at Malabar Hill in the neighbourhood of the waterworks with the enlarging of the filtering plant and reservoir, and similar works at Mazagaon also increased the incidence of malaria there.

The construction of Alexandra Dock and Hughes Dry Dock caused a considerable increase of malaria in the adjoining areas. Work on these docks commenced in 1904. In 1908, the disease broke out with increased severity and as a result there was an exodus of coolies and labourers employed in the neighbourhood of the docks.[5] The 1908 outbreak caused a considerable outcry and it was stated by many people at the time, that the dockworks were entirely responsible for the presence of malaria in Bombay.

It is not difficult to map the area influenced by direct diffusion of infection from the new dockworks. The most southerly berths in Victoria Dock are used by the P&O Company, and during the epidemic in the summer of 1908, the crews of many of the P&O vessels lying there, contracted malaria. On boat after boat, from 80 to 100 cases of the disease occurred among the crew during the homeward voyage.[6] During the Spleen Census of 1909, it was found that high blocks of houses separating two narrow streets in the middle of Chakala showed a high spleen rate, reaching 20 per cent, among residents on the side facing the harbour; but among residents in the tenements facing away from the harbour, the spleen rate was only about 3 per cent.

Guards, porters and sweepers belonging to the G.I.P. Railway were attacked and, at one time of the epidemic, as many as ten of the local trains had to be cancelled. St George's Hospital, which is situated so that it overlooks the new dockworks, became the most malarious place in the city; members of the nursing staff were frequently prostrated with malaria and few of the patients who entered the hospital escaped contracting the disease.[7]

Passing westward from Frere Road into North Fort, malaria becomes more intense again, but investigation has shown that this is due to the existence of hundreds of open wells and permanent foci of malarial infection in the Fort itself. A similar centre of infection due to entirely local cases is to be found in the Dhobi Talao section, situated on the west side of the island.[8] A medical man born and brought up in the Fort volunteered the information that he well remembers

133

possessing an enlarged spleen as a boy and being treated for it, and some Europeans residing near Elphinstone Circle repeatedly suffered from malaria so severely that they had to leave the neighbourhood.[9]

There is no reason to suppose that the labourers brought much infection with them, as the examination of newly-arrived coolies living on the works has usually shown them to be free both of enlarged spleens and parasites in their blood; but those resident a few months show a considerable amount of infection.[10]

In 1910, the headman of a gang volunteered the statement that of 300 working coolies who came with him from their district (Marwar), 100 had died and another 100 had deserted their work during the preceding eighteen months. He ascribed the occurrence of fever and enlargement of the spleen among his men to the water they drank at the docks, and stated that in his own village the people did not suffer in this way.[11]

The *Indian Spectator* of 20 November 1908 stated that the outbreak of malaria has already caused serious loss of life and affected the business of the city. The belief has spread that certain parts of the city have become practically uninhabitable in consequence of the outbreak.[12]

The Disease

We all know the old theories about malaria—the Italian derivation of the word illustrates them:

> '*mala aria*', bad air; air tainted by injurious emanations from animal or vegetable matter; noxious inhalations of marshy districts; in other words *miasma*. Those were beliefs of old days and it was not until 1880 that Lavaran, a French army surgeon, discovered the malaria parasite and his views were not accepted until 1894 when Sir Patrick Manson suggested that the malaria parasite probably had some kind of mosquito as an intermediate host which was necessary for its development and it was only in 1897 that Major Ross made the brilliant discovery that solved the problem of the etiology of malaria that earned for him the admiration of scientists and the world at large.[13]

Malaria is produced by a parasite which is carried from a sick man to a healthy man by certain kinds of mosquitoes. An attack begins with shivering, then fever and headache if the temperature is very high, then profuse perspiration and the fever goes down. There may be second attack a few days later or after a few months or even a few years. A malarial fever attack lowers the patient's vitality. Successive attacks of malarial fever, particularly in children, produce enlargement of the spleen.[14] The disease is spread from man to man by the mosquito. When a mosquito bites a person who has malaria, it sucks in the germs of malaria fever with that person's blood. These germs undergo some changes in the body of the mosquito and finally come to the mouth of the insect. In the process of biting another person, it injects the germs into his blood. This is how malarial fever is spread. There are two main varieties of mosquitoes, viz.

1. Those that convey the germs of malaria (Anopheles).
2. Those that do not convey the germs of malaria (Culex and Stegomyia).

Anopheles breed only in clean water. Culex breed anywhere, preferably in dirty water. Another fact, which is often not realized, is that weeds or grass growing in stagnant pools favour the breeding of Anopheles since they provide a foothold for the mosquito to deposit her eggs. The malaria-carrying female mosquito bites only at night.[15]

Agent of Transmission

In November 1908, Captain W. Glen Liston, I.M.S., published the important announcement that *Nyssorhynchus stephensi* was the species of Anopheles responsible for the transmission of malaria in the Frere Road area. Captain Liston found only two species of Anopheles present: *Nyssorhynchus stephensi* and *Myzomyia rossi*. It was confirmed that while the former is an active agent in the propagation of malaria, the other common Anopheles, *Myzomyia rossi*, plays no part in the spread of the disease.[16] Moreover, a survey of the city south of Grant Road, has shown that *Myzomyia rossi* is widespread everywhere, often in great numbers where there is little malaria—an observation that supports the conclusion that it bears no relation to the disease. On the other hand, *Nyssorhynchus stephensi* may be found with varying frequency in every section of the city and appears to be the only important carrier of malaria present in the south of the island. Another potential carrier of malaria, *Nyssorhynchus jamesi,* exists at Malabar Hill and at Bhandarwada, and has also been found breeding in Gowalia Tank. It has been found only in association with *Nyssorhynchus stephensi*.

During the monsoon, a hundred vehicles, including Victorias, Shigrams and Broughams, were examined in the different stables in the city. It was found that mosquitoes were invariably present in these vehicles unless they had been recently disturbed.[17] Among factors which tend to limit the number and restrict the distribution of *Nissorhynchus stephensi* in Bombay, one of the most interesting and important is the existence of another mosquito belonging to the culicine group. This mosquito, *Culex concolor*, appears to exert a directly antagonistic influence upon other mosquitoes, the Anopheles in particular, because its larvae are specially adapted for preying upon those of other mosquitoes. It is frequently found breeding in collections of water haunted by *Nissorhynchus stephensi*, and destroys large numbers of them. Four large larvae of *Culex concolor* were placed in a bowl containing a number of larvae of *Nissorhynchus stephensi* of different sizes. These, they immediately began to seize and devour, and in the course of two hours, they had destroyed over fifty. In Bombay, and possibly in other places, *Culex concolor* plays a definite role in reducing the number of *Nissorhynchus stephensi*, and is possibly one of the factors that assists in producing fluctuations in malaria from year to year.[18]

Certain species of fish may serve to keep a breeding place free of mosquitoes, or to clear one which has become infected, but can only do so when conditions are favourable. A small fish, known locally as 'Piku', belonging to the class of top-swimming minnows, is very useful, but it must be present in sufficient numbers and its efforts must not be hampered by floating weed, leaves or rubbish. This fish was introduced experimentally into fifteen wells, which contained large numbers of larvae of *Nissorhynchus stephensi*. All but two wells were rapidly cleared of mosquito larvae and in the latter they had been reduced in number but a few escaped because of leaves, flowers and floating matter. The rootless duckweed *Wolffia arhiza* is inimical to mosquito larvae, provided it is present in large amounts. Several waterweeds, among which may be mentioned 'Azolla' and 'Lemna' have been supposed to prevent the breeding of mosquitoes.[19]

Malaria Prevention

The appointment of a committee by the Corporation in September 1901 to consider certain matters regarding the presence of

Anopheles mosquitoes and the measures that may be taken to reduce or suppress them, appears to have been the first occasion on which the adoption of specific measures against malaria, on the lines laid down by Ross, received consideration in Bombay. At that time it was assumed that malaria was responsible for a very large amount of sickness and considerable mortality in the city. Mosquito gangs consisting of a sub-inspector and four men was formed. Three wards, A, B, and C, meant three sub-inspectors and twelve men and the total wages amounted to Rs 260 per month. These gangs found Anopheles larvae chiefly in fountains, drinking troughs, tubs and buckets, open cisterns and certain drains. The Executive Health Officer records that the holes in the ground were filled where possible; open drains were cleared; drinking troughs, tubs and buckets were emptied once a week; fish were placed in fountains, and other breeding places were treated with a mixture of tar and kerosene.[20]

In 1907, the Corporation sanctioned the expenditure of a considerable sum of money for the repair of Bandarwada Hill Reservoir at Mazagaon, which had been subject to severe leakage for some time. The leak gave rise to springs and streamlets near the base of the hill and these became the breeding places of Anopheles mosquitoes, the presence of which caused the spread of malaria among the residents in the neighbourhood. During the same year, complaints were received regarding the prevalence of malaria at Frere Road and Chowpati, and as a result a certain amount of preventive work appears to have been done in both areas.[21]

In 1905, the Municipal Corporation of Bombay passed a resolution that a comprehensive and searching inquiry should be instituted with regard to the cause and spread of malaria and the measures necessary for its prevention. The action taken as a result of this resolution led to the appointment of a special committee, which sat for two years and published a report in 1908.[22] In 1907, malaria became prevalent in certain parts of the city and culminated in an epidemic in 1908. The alarm occasioned by this epidemic emphasized the need for a detailed investigation into the conditions relative to the disease, and as a result it was decided to conduct a special inquiry. The Executive Health Officer, on being asked to report on the matter, stated that all stagnant pools in the New Dock Compound were being frequently treated with Pesterine (crude petroleum) by the Municipality as in 1907, and he recommended that the Port Trust should be asked to take up the question also.[23]

Therefore the Municipal Commissioners addressed the Port Trust and as a result the Agent of the New Dock Contractors undertook to drain off or fill in as many pools on the high ground as possible, and treat the remaining ones with Pesterine, and also to cut down the grass. On 17 September 1908, an assistant sanitary inspector and four men were deputed for special mosquito destruction work in Ward A, and a sub-inspector and four men for similar duties in Wards B, C and D respectively. In spite of these measures, a severe outbreak of malaria occurred in the last quarter of 1908, the disease being especially prevalent in Frere Road, near the Docks.[24]

Early in 1909, Captain A.G. McKendrick (I.M.S.) was appointed to conduct the investigation of the epidemic of 1908, and a committee was formed consisting of representatives of the Municipal Corporation of Bombay, the Bombay Port Trust, the G.I.P. Railway Company and the B.B.C.&I. Railway Company, for the purpose of carrying out any measures that may appear necessary for the immediate mitigation of malaria.[25] As a result of the Spleen Census undertaken by Captain McKendrick, it was possible to map the areas most severely affected by malaria. A house-to-house census was undertaken in different sections of the city and a very large number of children were examined.[26] Children coming forward or brought by their parents were rewarded with a pice. Usually, in the course of an hour it was possible to collect 50 or 60 blood films, specimens being taken from everyone in the crowd who appeared willing. In this way, a large number of blood films from different localities were obtained and examined.[27]

There are three varieties of malarial fever:

1. Benign Tertian
2. Malignant Tertian
3. Quartan.

The terms are based on the periodicity of fever: in the first two, the fever comes on every third day but sometimes, especially in the case of Malignant Tertian, it may recur every day. This is due to the person being infected by more than one mosquito. Quartan fever comes back every fourth day. The parasites of all three varieties are distinguishable from each other.[28] During the examination of the blood films, all three forms of the malaria parasite were enountered. Benign Tertian appears to have been the most widely distributed, encountered in every part of the city. Malignant Tertian was more confined to the areas where malaria is severe and not nearly so common north of Mumbadevi Tank. Quartan infection occurred in groups and was fairly widely distributed and not nearly so rare as has sometimes been supposed.[29]

Prevention of mosquito breeding is the most important item in a campaign against mosquitoes. Measures for individual protection resolve themselves into: (1) Avoidance of being bitten by mosquitoes; (2) Regular use of Quinine. As regards the first, there has to be (a) the use of mosquito nets, (b) the use of *punkhas* and electric fans, (c) the use of mosquito repellents. As for the use of Quinine as a curative, when a man is attacked by fever, he should take a purgative and go to bed. He should start taking Quinine directly once the purgative has begun to act and take twenty-four grains of quinine per day in the form of a mixture.

The preventive measures to be adopted by a local body are:

1. Free distribution of Quinine
2. Prevention of mosquito breeding
3. Destruction of mosquitoes.

Kundis or garden cisterns should be emptied regularly once a week and all the water brushed out. Wherever water cannot be drained, it should be treated with larvaecide once a week. A mixture of one part crude oil and three parts kerosene oil with a little castor oil forms a most effective larvaecide. This mixture should be spread on the surface of the water by using a spray pump. Paris Green can also be used to destroy the larvae of the Anopheles mosquito. Paris Green contains arsenic and kills the larvae.[30]

Another useful method is fumigation. For fumigation, the best disinfectants are the following: (1) Sulphur—2 lbs to 1000 cubic feet for three hours; (2) Pyrethrum—3 lbs to 1000 cubic feet for three hours. Pyrocide is a solution prepared by mixing Pyrocide –20 with kerosene oil in the proportion of one part to nineteen parts oil. One-third part of the solution is sufficient for spraying 1000 cubic feet per day. Every year brings the necessity of eradicating malaria from a locality more forcibly before the public mind.

Malaria is essentially an economic disease, sapping the vigour and physique of the community and though its prevalence draws less attention than more 'sensational' diseases like plague and cholera, it does more damage by lowering vitality and thereby preparing the ground for other diseases like tuberculosis, etc. Apart from the suffering it causes among human beings, malaria is a disease which seriously interferes with the commerce and industry of a place. In India itself, it has been officially calculated to cause a mean annual death rate of five per 1000. This is more than the mortality from plague or cholera and dysentery put together. Malaria not only raises the death rate but lowers the birth rate, and is a common cause of miscarriage.[31] The small attempts to limit the spread of malaria have only served to mitigate the disease to a slight extent, and though it has been checked a little in some areas, unless more radical measures are adopted and carried through to successful termination, the city will remain as liable to epidemic outbreaks of malaria in the future.[32]

Cost of Malaria to Bombay

It is always difficult to estimate the cost of a disease to a community, even when there are exact figures to go upon, because there are so many different factors to take into account. Malarious fever was the disease for which most patients applied for treatment.[33] In India, the number of malaria cases attending hospitals is no criterion of the total number of sick; and in a city like Bombay, where there are probably not less than 700 qualified men, a host of unqualified practitioners and many hundreds of chemists and druggists of all sorts, only a portion of the total sick among the population attend hospitals and dispensaries. There are many people among the working classes who do not think of seeking treatment until after they have suffered from repeated attacks of fever. The total number of cases of all kinds receiving treatment is between 3,00,000 and 4,00,000, giving an admission rate for sickness among the whole population of nearly 400 per 1000 per annum. During the years 1901–03, the diagnosis of fever cases based upon a careful examination of the blood, conducted by an expert, showed that 75 per cent were due to Malaria.[34]

As about 60 per cent of the population of Bombay are workers, we may estimate that about 2,25,000 cases of malaria would occur among them and would result, on an average, in the loss of about a week of work in each case. Taking the average earnings of workers at

Rs 20 a month, this would mean a loss of about Rs 5 per case either in wages to the worker or in terms of loss of work to the employer, and the total loss would be equivalent to Rs 11,25,000. If we estimate a loss of Re 1 on every case of malaria occurring among non-workers, this would amount to another Rs 1,60,000, making up a grand total.[35]

In 1908, Police Hospital expenditures exceeded Rs 15,000, of which 25 per cent may be put down as the proportional cost of treating cases of fever, which form over half the total admissions. Broadly speaking, we may state that fever caused a loss of about Rs 7,500 or £500 per annum to the police establishment of the city, of which Rs 5,625 or £375 was due to malaria.[36]

As regards workers, Rs 10,50,000 may be assumed to have been lost on account of malaria. This estimate takes no account of the 3,89,000 dependants in the city supported by the actual workers, sickness among whom causes considerable loss to the latter. An estimate of Rs 12,00,000 or Rs 13,00,000 as the cost of malaria to the city is very low and much less than the real amount. This figure does not include loss of rent to landlords caused by abandonment of houses in malarious localities, loss to tenants who are forced to incur considerable expenses for medical attendance, or loss to a business organization, a portion of whose staff falls sick from time to time.[37]

If all these losses are totalled up, it would be found that the sum of Re 0.25 to Re 0.125 per head of the population, which has been taken as the estimate, represents only half or one-third of the amount paid away without return each year by the citizens of Bombay because of the existence of an easily preventable disease in their city. Because malaria is endemic in Bombay, it is necessary that measures for the prevention of the disease should be adopted.[38]

The *Bombay Samachar* of 25 November 1908 stated that the Government of Bombay is to be congratulated for stepping in at the right moment and expressing their readiness to appoint a special officer to investigate the causes and devise ways and means for the prevention of malaria in Bombay city. Considering the gravity of the situation created by the malaria epidemic and the benefits that would be derived from the labours of the proposed committee, we trust that these bodies will not grudge the payment they have been asked to make.

The *Parsi* of 29 November 1908 stated that although the Municipal Commissioner's statement that the malarial fever is quite a common disease in India does not in any way reconcile us with the epidemic in Bombay, it is a fact that the government, at least, is bound to recognize and act upon it, if any regular system of combating the disease is to come into vogue.

Though the government at that time spoke of investigating into all aspects of the malaria epidemic, obviously subsequent governments and corporations have been generally apathetic to the issue of its prevention. It is surprising that today too, the same attitude and picture of the past prevails, and mortality rates of malaria have caused concern about the general neglect of public health in Bombay city.

Notes and References

[1] *Gazetteer, Bombay City and Island,* Vol. III, p. 163.

[2] Ibid., p. 163.

[3] *Medical Files: Report on the causes of malaria in Bombay and measures necessary for its control,* p. 61.

[4] Ibid., p. 54.

[5] Ibid., p. 55.

[6] Ibid.

[7] Ibid., p. 56.

[8] Ibid.

[9] Ibid., p. 57.

[10] Ibid.

[11] Ibid.

[12] *Native Newspapers,* 1908, p. 168.

[13] *Report of the Imperial Malaria Conference at Simla* (October 1909), p. 2.

[14] *Bombay Government Manual of Public Health,* p. 199.

[15] Ibid., p. 202.

[16] *Report on Malaria in the Southern Part of Bombay Island,* p. 12.

[17] Ibid., pp. 13–14.

[18] Ibid., pp. 14–15.

[19] Ibid., p. 15.

[20] *Report on the Causes of Malaria in Bombay,* p. 89.

[21] Ibid., p. 89.

[22] *Report on Malaria in the Southern Part of Bombay Island with suggestions and measures for prevention,* p. 1.

[23] *Report on the Causes of Malaria in Bombay and measures for control,* p. 91.

[24] Ibid.

[25] Ibid., p. 92.

[26] *Report on Malaria in the Southern Part of Bombay Island,* p. 4.

[27] Ibid., p. 10.

[28] *Manual of Public Health,* p. 200.

[29] *Report on Malaria in the Southern Part of Bombay Island,* p. 11.

[30] *Manual of Public Health,* pp. 203–06.

[31] Ibid., p. 200.
[32] *Report on the Causes of Malaria in Bombay*, p. 58.
[33] *Bombay Administrative Report*, 1880–81, p. 402.
[34] *Report on the Causes of Malaria in Bombay*, p. 59.
[35] Ibid.
[36] Ibid., p. 60.
[37] Ibid.
[38] Ibid., p. 147.

'Clouds of Cholera'[1] and Clouds around Cholera, 1817–70

Dhrub Kumar Singh

Without a snapping of the umbilical cord and subscribing to the mother–child relationship, 'cholera' serves the analogy of the umbilical cord between the metropole Britain and the colony named India. 'Cholera emerged in epidemic form in India in 1817, and after an initial false start, arrived in Britain in 1831.'[2]

Taking into account all that happened in the political realm after the acquisition of Diwani, the East India Company in fact remained the surrogate mother, and it was only after the 1840s that the real mother increasingly took charge. But before this happened, both the mother and the child had become infected by what was later identified as 'comma bacillus' or 'vibrio cholerae'. Thus there came into being two very different 'cholera-stressed societies', one claiming to be the redeemer, protector and civilizer of the 'other'.

Examining this claim of the metropole during the whole of the nineteenth century from a statistical standpoint, Watt's synoptic and sarcastic comment is indicative of the different epidemiological paths that the two 'cholera-stressed' societies were to follow.

Britain lost an estimated 130,000 of its resident subject people to five cholera epidemics, each of which, after 1848, claimed fewer and fewer lives. During the same century and first quarter of the next, India lost in excess of 25 million of its people to the same disease. Even more striking was the fact that while England's cholera rates moved steadily downwards, those of nineteenth-century India dramatically increased. In 1900, the most disastrous of the year for which statistics had been kept, cholera claimed the lives of upward of 800,000 people, 163,889 in the single province of Bombay. These

144

vastly different totals of cholera death, relatively small in Britain and absolutely enormous in India[3]

reveal the indifference of the 'mother'; the 'recalcitrant' child appears forlorn and abandoned.

The Beginning

Cholera, 'as a highly political disease', 'seemed to threaten the slender basis of British power in India and to stand at the critical point of intersection between colonial state and indigenous society'.[4] The virulence of and far-reaching devastation caused by cholera, the impact on the colonial economy and military, the unrest that it created among local people, unsettled political debates. It necessitated state intervention and fuelled debates on Hindu religious rites and practices which were seen as antithetical to medical well-being and hygiene. It also indicated the limitation of state intervention. Debates around cholera also provided the space that illustrated how the local and colonial power structures converged and contested. In contrast to the cheap, simple, and to some extent successful, smallpox vaccination, which became emblematic of the colonial state's 'self-declared benevolence and humanity towards the people of India',[5] cholera as an unsettling and incomprehensible disease mocked at medicine's effort to understand it. Cholera leaped across all the preventive hurdles, and therefore cholera as an entry-point to social history is capable of unfolding the crudeness of the benevolence of the *Raj* epitomized in the mother–child relationship. The disease named cholera, commonly known today as *haija* in Hindi (from the Arabic word *hachaizia*), was called by various names such as *morysey, mirtirissa, vizucega, mordeyin* and *mordechien* in the different regions and different languages of India.[6] As per a historical note written on cholera in India in 1911 by P. Hehir, '*mordechien*' was in all probability derived from the French name '*mort de chein*', literally meaning a dog's death[7]—a clear indication of its virulence as reflected in the mounting mortality rate all along the nineteenth century, but more particularly when the census outgrew its infancy after 1870.

It is generally understood that cholera had been known to Europeans in India for several centuries. But contending this view way back in 1854, John Snow opined that 'The existence of Asiatic cholera cannot be distinctly traced back further than the year 1769. Previous to that time the greater part of India was unknown to European medical men; and this is probably the reason why the history of cholera does not extend to a more remote period.'[8] Citing the report on the cholera epidemic authored by one Mr Scot, Snow makes us aware that cholera was prevalent at Madras in the year 1769 and that 'it carried off many thousands of persons in the peninsula of India from that time to 1790'.[9] Subsequently it almost disappeared or was not recorded. But it soon reappeared in June 1814, 'when it hit with great severity the first bat. 9th reg. N.I on its march from Jaulnah to Trichirapally; while another battalion, which accompanied it, did not suffer, although it had been exposed to exactly the same circumstances.'[10]

As the disease is almost absent in the recordings of military commanders who, by professional compulsion, had to take notice of the health of their men, it can be safely assumed that cholera incidence was relatively infrequent and it did not in any sense dominate medical discussion. But things changed suddenly in 1817, when a cholera epidemic ravaged Bengal and by 1831 'the cholera began to spread to an extent not before known and in course of seven years it reached eastward, to China and the Philippines islands; southwards, to the Mauritius and Bourbon; and to the north-west as far as Persia and Turkey'.[11] Europe was just a step ahead.

Reporting on the virulent and mysterious nature of the epidemic from Jessore town, a hundred miles to the north of Calcutta, in August 1817, Dr Tytler, the civil surgeon of the town wrote: 'An epidemic has broken out in the bazaar, the disorder commencing with pain and uneasiness in different parts of the body is succeeded by giddiness of the head, sickness, vomiting, gripping in the belly and frequent stools.'[12] Within a month this bodily disorder was to spread spatially, increasingly implicating newer victims—cholera crossed 100 miles and spread to Calcutta, and in the following six months engulfed the whole of Bengal from Sylhet to Cuttack. In the next twelve months, the disease spread along the Coromandel and Malabar to the west, reaching Madras by September–October 1818.[13] Reporting from Madras, the then secretary to the Madras Medical Board explained that 'this disease is characterized by suddenness of its attack'[14] and that in 'this severe epidemic death has hitherto been observed to ensue from 10 to 24 hours from the commencement of the attack'.[15] From Madras it was conveyed by ships to Ceylon and thence to Mauritius. By 1819 it had appeared in Bangkok and shortly afterwards in Singapore and Malacca, and by 1821 it had reached China.[16] Travelling almost the whole of the country, the cholera epidemic between 1817–21 wrought terrible devastation in India in general and Bengal in particular. This 'baffling disease', an 'inscrutable malady' which knew no logical 'line of progression', was a little more favourable to Bengal and lasted there till 1823. Maintaining its elusiveness, it disappeared from there in the years 1823–25; it returned again in 1826 with much greater virulence and ferocity, taking almost the whole of India under its sway. In 1827 it visited Hardwar, the NWFP, the Bombay Presidency, Sind and the Punjab. Slowly cholera began to race through Khiva and Herat via Kabul by 1829.[17] When the first pandemic ended, in 1823, it had stopped short of Europe. But the second pandemic, which started in 1826, brought it to the doors of Europe. A complacent Europe, which had suffered no lethal epidemic since its last visit by the bubonic plague almost two centuries earlier, was caught unawares. The 'Asiatic cholera' emerging from a distant corner of the British empire warranted attention. In John Snow's words, 'its approach towards our own country (England) after it entered Europe, was watched with much more anxiety than its progress in other directions'.[18] Now that Britain in particular and Europe in general were feeling the stress of cholera, medical discourse began to be focused on this new disease both in the metropole and in the colony.

After 1817, deltaic Bengal was regarded as the nucleus, the endemic centre; Calcutta, which had grown far beyond expectations, even in the early nineteenth century, was a 'dirty, teeming warren'. As colonialism entrenched itself, and as the public works department became a permanent, independent arm of the colonial state, India saw itself laced with new roads, railway tracks, canals and busy ports. In the wake of the increasing trade and annexation exercises by the troops, there was constant movement of merchants, troops, administrators and religious pilgrims. The context of a pan-Indian colonial government in fact enhanced the possibility of pilgrimage and 'the rising tide of pilgrims crested in the age of colonialism'.[19] Colonial intervention changed the 'disease ecology' of India. If developments fostered in the wake of colonialism helped in the epidemicization of cholera in India, the rise of maritime trade, the increasing frequency of pilgrimage to Mecca and the slave trade helped in the pandemicization of cholera, and Britain did not remain untouched.

Contagion Contested

In England the ravages of cholera were disastrously felt during all the four principal invasions of 1831, 1848, 1853 and 1866. The disease seemed a product of 'colonial backwardness', carried back to Britain. In all these four epidemics, cholera assaulted not only 'bodies but Englishmen's pride in race, class and nation'. Its symptoms became a humiliating fate for Victorian gentlefolk. They saw that cholera afflicted them less than it did the poor, ill-fed, ill-housed, dirty and drunk. To chronically moralizing Victorian minds, the lower classes' weak resistance to disease proved their physical and moral inferiority.[20] 'The significance of invading cholera lay mainly in its capacity to open up fissures within society, particularly between the rich and the poor, or between the host society and immigrant communities.'[21] The cholera epidemic humbled the medical and civil establishments. The baffled administration fell back upon the earlier wisdom of 'quarantine'. Nations had tried to prevent the import of exotic diseases by this method. Way back in the fourteenth century, Venetians had invented 'quarantine'—a method of isolating arriving ships for thirty to forty days. In 1403, Venice enacted that travellers from the Levant must be isolated in a detention hospital for the same period—*quranta giorni*, from which the word quarantine is derived.[22] As it happened then with regard to plague, so it happened with regard to cholera: the 'quarantine' proved abortive. Cholera leapt over quarantine with ease; the medical men, then under the sway of 'miasmatic theory' and with no '*materia morbis*' or specific causative agent within their comprehension, took an anti-contagionist stance. 'Anti-contagionism was primarily and most significantly a movement against the institution of quarantine and cardon sanitaries which were seen as the unwarranted evil resulting from contagionist theories and which caused unnecessary damage to both health and commerce',[23] and so the anti-contagionist stance was also politically correct and viable. The failure of quarantine measures during the cholera epidemics of 1832 and 1848 in England served to reaffirm anti-contagionism.

As in the metropole, so in the colony, the dominant view among the medical men viewed cholera from an anti-contagionist stance. Sharing this dominant view and in line with the majority of writers on the epidemic in India, Reginald Orton in 1820 discounted the possibility that cholera might be contagious.[24] Similarly, Calcutta physician Francis Balfour stressed the importance of the direction of the wind, especially of the south-easterly, on diseases like fevers and cholera.[25] Sharing the same view, the army surgeon James M'Cabe, for instance, had noticed that the 1818 cholera epidemic in Madras was attended by a south-easterly wind, which carried an unusual amount of rain.[26] Meteorological phenomena, especially variations in monsoon and abnormalities of the atmosphere, particularly heat and moisture, were thought to be responsible for diseases, and hence were linked to the cause of cholera.

Within the 'meteorological theory' of disease causation, the influence of the 'moon' was also taken into cognizance and became important. Many prominent medical men in India in the 1820s, who included Francis Balfour, naval surgeon James Lind and James Johnson, implicated the 'moon' in the causation of fever. Reginald Orton, following the line of these 'lunacists',[27] applied this theory to cholera. Implication of the moon was justified on Newtonian principles and was done within the then-prevailing scientific paradigm.[28]

Adhering to the anti-contagionist stance, James Lawrie, a surgeon with the 53rd Bengal Native Infantry, maintained that cholera was not 'actively contagious' but became an epidemic only at certain times and in certain localities.[29] Stress on 'certain times' and 'certain localities' reflects his adherence to the meteorological theory of disease causation within the then-prevalent climatic paradigm. This was compatible with the 'humoral explanation' of diseases, where atmospheric disorders were thought to generate disorders in the body. Lawrie's stress on 'certain localities' indicated cholera's preference for the lower classes and their unhealthy abodes. Sharing the view of 'atmospheric influences', the role of filth and dirt in cholera causation from an anti-contagionist standpoint, French traveller Victor Jacquemont, who was in India from 1828 to 1831, grasped the differential impact of cholera, i.e. its preference for sepoys and Irish soldiers who came from the lower classes to serve in the British army. Jacquemont emphasized that, in contrast to the indigent and intemperate soldiers, 'gentlemen' were seldom its victims.[30] William Twinning, an assistant surgeon of the Bengal army in 1824 and later a surgeon at Calcutta General Hospital, who also was an active member of the Calcutta Medical and Physical Society, discounted any possibility of cholera being contagious in India. Like Jacquemont, Twinning also stressed the role of sudden changes in temperature in cholera causation.[31]

Among the many who commented and opined on the causation and nature of cholera, there appeared to be a loose consensus on at least three aspects of the disease. First and foremost was the understanding that cholera was non-contagious. Second was the role of atmospheric changes due to temperature variations. Third was the preference which cholera exhibited for the weak, the indigent and the intemperate, who generally inhabited filthy, ill-ventilated, dusty suburbs and had improper diet and insanitary habits. Apart from the larger native population, this included the unhealthy Irish soldiers in the 'lower order' of the British army who, because of their drunkenness and general intemperance, fell prey to cholera.

There was almost no idea as to the specific cause of the disease. All the medical men appeared vague, with the exception of Edmund Alexander Parkes, a famous hygienist of England who in the initial three years of his medical career had served the Army Medical Services in India during the 1850s. Parkes did talk about the presence of a '*material morbis*' or 'specific agent' in connection with cholera.[32] Not discounting the connection between the prevalence of cholera and seasonal variations, a slow but definite cognition of a 'distinct cause of cholera' was emerging. By the end of the 1850s it was understood that this 'distinct poison' had a separate existence which certain conditions of the climate could aggravate or repress.[33]

Optimism

The climatic conditions which aggravated the pestilentiality were to be curtailed by proper sanitary precautions, and the sanitarians thought themselves entitled to proclaim that it was within the power of man to make such pestilence impossible. To attain this greater objective, they exhorted the scientific community to 'search sedulously' for the 'specific poison' of cholera which they thought were propagated by certain special laws, sometimes by what they called contagion and sometimes by other means. The medical men and sanitarians used the word 'poison' only in default of a better term to signify the original cause of the disease, and were clear on the point that these 'poisons' require certain conditions for their development and that by certain conditions their action is modified or destroyed.

Hoping for science to 'succeed in delivering the human race from the terrible scourge of cholera',[34] they, with mixed feelings of optimism and helplessness, understood the limitations of the colonial state to embark on a grand sanitary improvement programme. They realized the practical impossibility of this and so they ardently desired a 'Jennerian discovery' and intervention within the realm of cholera.

> They anticipated that success will not alone be due to the progress of general sanitary improvement. It will be due, if not to the discovery of the actual cause in which the disease has its origin, at least to the knowledge of the manner in which its specific poison can be propagated or can be rendered innocuous.[35]

For them, 'This was a belief which in no manner supersedes or interferes with the conviction of the vast improvement of the public health.'[36]

Simultaneously with the cognition of some 'specific poison' as the causative agent for cholera, fissures began to appear in the anti-contagionist stance. The non-contagionist stance could not reconcile with the erratic nature of cholera. Why cholera attacked a particular place leaving unharmed just the neighbouring place, the 'manner in which places, under apparently identical sanitary conditions, have sometimes been attacked and sometimes avoided'[37] by cholera, and such other contradictions could not be explained by adhering to one particular stance. The non-contagionist stance served to demarcate cholera from other contagious diseases like smallpox and syphilis, which were plainly regarded as contagious. That much efficacy of the non-contagionist stance was conceded, but beyond that 'the older universally accepted belief that cholera was not a communicable disease'[38] was now questioned. In the 1860s, although opinions differed very widely regarding the manner in which cholera was propagated, and although the term contagion still remained rejected, to the medical men of the age 'there remained no question that the weight of authority was decidedly in favour of human intercourse'.[39] In their opinion 'this belief is affected in no degree by the evidence which shows that, under ordinary circumstances, cholera is not directly communicable from man to man by contagion in the same manner which holds good for some diseases.'[40] They attached very different ideas to the term contagion, and were reluctant to use it with reference to cholera. Qualifying their use of the term 'contagion', they made their standpoint clear:

> when we state that the evidence appears to us almost decisive of the

151

fact of the communicability of the disease, we in no way intend to express the belief that it is propagated by actual contact, or through the medium of infected air, or by any particular process, nor that the poison can only be multiplied by the disease itself. We simply concern ourselves with the fact, beyond which our knowledge does not extend, that cholera is, under certain circumstances, communicable by human intercourse.[41]

By the 1860s, nine out of ten medical men were of the opinion that cholera was, under certain circumstances, communicable by human intercourse. 'Yet, in their anxiety not to encourage a belief among the soldiers which, they feared, might be practically mischievous, they not infrequently acted as if they possessed no conviction of the kind.'[42] To curtail fear psychosis among the soldiers the medical men posed as anti-contagionist, but in reality they were contingent-contagionist. Many medical men did not subscribe to this falsehood and, in the words of Dr Budd, it was like 'allowing sentiment into the domain of science'.[43] Such was the importance attached to the health of the army and such was the capacity of cholera to undermine it, that even 'misinformation' was employed to ensure the morale of the soldiers in the wake of cholera epidemics.

Cholera was always depicted by the metaphor of 'wild fire', indicative of a crisis par excellence. The army was the only institution which had the capacity to indulge in such crisis management, more so because the medical men largely belonged to this institution. To implicate the army in the epidemic management was to make the most formidable arm of the empire vulnerable.

Waste from diseases, especially from cholera, among European troops was always high. Almost every war saw deaths by cholera. The Royal Commission on the sanitary state of the army in India, appointed in 1859, recorded a death-rate of 60 per 1,000 among British troops in the years running up to the mutiny (over three times higher than the death-rate of any regiment in Britain), and identified the causes as inadequate sewerage and water supply, poor drainage, and ill-ventilated and overcrowded barracks. In its report of 1863, the commission recommended the creation of distinct areas of European habitation (military cantonments and civil lines), regulated by sanitary legislation similar to that in Britain and situated in accordance with the topographical principles laid down by J.R. Martin, president of the

India Office Medical Board and member of the commission. Martin advocated that the troops be sent by rotation to hill stations about 5,000 feet above sea level.[44] This advocacy was later implemented.

However, the continuing vulnerability of British troops is demonstrated by the fact that they still suffered mortality rates far higher than their Indian counterparts.

> During the cholera epidemic which swept northern India in 1867, European troops experienced a cholera mortality rate of almost 14 per cent per 1000, whereas Indian troops died at a far lower rate of 3 per cent per 1000. In fact, the death-rate from all diseases except fever was lower among Indian troops than among Europeans.[45]

High mortality and morbidity rates among European soldiers, indicating the failure of acclimatization and seasoning in the Indian climate; the baffling and annihilating nature of cholera and the shifting standpoints to understand it; the rurality of the cholera epidemic which made the ambit of endemic area so large that it became difficult to intervene, more so because it entailed interference with the religious and cultural sensibilities of the natives; the real fear of a religious backlash in the form of a second mutiny after 1857; the infancy of the census and the unreliability of metereological registers at least till 1870; the colonial government's unwillingness to provide economic backing to general sanitary precautions; the obsession with the army's health due to high military priorities; the general contempt for the native inhabitants and their landscape, especially in the post-1857 phase when the honeymoon with the 'orient' had ended—all of these and many other factors ensured the 'enclavist' nature of sanitary measures.

The majority of the 'Sanitary Commissioners' acted as 'Epidemic Intelligence officers' who collected data and information from various parts of the country. The epidemiological clues derived from their reports were to be applied in the cantonments to ensure the health of the army. These were not used to forge a sanitary movement in the public domain at least up till 1870.

Health Goes Public

In contrast to the absence of any sanitary movement in India, England saw a full-fledged movement led by Chadwick, Snow and John Simon. As in India, so in the metropole, the exact causality of cholera was not known. There also, generally within the climatic paradigm, the 'miasmatic theory' remained the canonical theory with regard to cholera causation. Still, as a preventive measure, the agenda of sanitation was not only placed but also carried forward on a large scale. Of course, the urban character of the cholera epidemic in England, in contrast to its rural character in India, helped in the initiation and institutionalization of sanitary measures.

In fact, way back in 1817, making a sanitary critique of the ramifications of the industrial revolution, Robert Owen rather naively had linked the filthy insanitary conditions of the working class with the causality of diseases. He tried to induce the government to initiate constructive planning to mitigate the damage caused by the rapid advance of the industrial revolution. Owen, however, failed in his effort. Picking up this strand, Chadwick, through his 'Report on an inquiry into the sanitary conditions of the labouring population of Great Britain in 1842', shook the bourgeois society out of its complacency.[46] Chadwick's report in a sense established the relationship between dirt and disease aetiology, and sanitary measures were initiated. Medical men of the time, with their anti-contagionist stance, manifested contempt for Chadwick's enthusiasm for sanitary measures, but with every epidemic he assumed greater leverage and he was soon able to implement many schemes for clean drinking water and sewage systems.

Soon, in 1849, John Snow and William Budd's epidemiological findings proved cholera to be a water-borne disease. This breakthrough by Snow and Budd validated Chadwick's efforts and gave him an intellectual acquittal. 'John Snow and William Budd not only proved Chadwick's contention that pure water supply and efficient disposal of sewerage is essential to health, but came close to anticipating Pasteur's germ theory.'[47]

Though later on Chadwick's evangelical and dictatorial fervour brought him disrepute, his legacy was carried forward by the persuasive John Simon who, apart from being a sanitarian par excellence, proved himself to be a skilled diplomat, 'lobbying members of parliament, feeding his own ideas into their minds, flattering them into self-delusion that they had themselves conceived his plans'.[48] By and by, Simon convinced the political masters of the day about the efficacy of the entire sanitary movement which he was leading.

Soon newer sanitation techniques were developed. Technological diversification fed into the diversification of sanitation techniques. The efficacy of the pump and the reverence for soap were to soon become the hallmark of urbanity and industrial life. Health became public in England. Medical intervention took cognizance of newer industrial diseases like lung disease, occupational diseases of various kinds, malnutrition, etc. Like Chadwick's sanitary maps, infant mortality maps were produced.

As is generally alleged, Chadwick may have reduced the multi-causality of the disease by reducing disease aetiology to filth and dirt, but the movement which he propelled saw health concerns in a multi-dimensional way and health came on to the national agenda by the 1880s in Britain.

In India, within the climatic paradigm and under the influ-ence of the 'miasmatic theory' of cholera causation, every endemic area of cholera was seen to be so because of its filth, dirt and over-crowding. Slowly, the entire landscape and its natives with their 'pecu-liar social institutions' were made responsible for the disease. But this sanitary critique did not resolve the anti-contagionist and contingent-contagionist tension regarding the nature of cholera. It kept resurfac-ing. It was not resolved even in the metropole but there the sanitary critique produced a Chadwick and a Simon who could lead a sanitary movement. In India the 'dynamism' of the colonial government did not produce any Chadwicks or Simons. Even Snow's epidemiological findings got a very late reception, as the 'meteorological theory' was adhered to by Bryden and Cunningham, the first two sanitary commis-sioners of India after the 1860s. Their epidemiological inquiries tried to link every specificity of the Indian climate to cholera. In doing so, they claimed not only special knowledge of the disease but also pleaded for the epidemiological uniqueness of India.

Contradictions

In the wake of the severe cholera epidemic there was no clear-cut sanitary policy to come to terms with it. Varieties of conjectures with regard to the causality prevailed both among metropole medical men and among colonial sanitary commissioners. Its causation and communicability and the various parameters which defined them were understood differently and led to contestations and dissent, though the influence of Bryden and Cunningham loomed large. The debates around quarantine as the preventive measure for the cholera epidemic gave rise to further contestation and made the epidemic controversial.

There were too many theories regarding cholera and, as will be shown, while some of these theories were compatible with each other sometimes they negated each other. Every theory provided a rationale for one particular mode of sanitary reform. One scientific authority was posited against another. Two different medical men were seen to share the same view on one aspect of the disease and on another aspect of the very same disease they held diametrically opposite views. There was no one-to-one correspondence between the theories that evolved in the metropolis and those that emerged in the colony. The borrowings were selective and considerable autonomy in understanding was manifested by the colonial medical men as regards cholera causation and communicability in particular, and diseases in general.

Due to the shifting standpoints, an element of uncertainty and fluidity characterized the grappling of medical discourse with the epidemic disease. This had its repercussions on the way sanitary reforms were carried out. In the 1860s, Bryden stuck to his rigid position that cholera was an air-borne disease and not water-borne. In his opinion, an unidentified 'pathogenic organism' was transported by monsoonal air currents beyond the endemic area and was responsible for the epidemic. Under the overarching influence of the humoral theory of disease and his own obsession with statistical technique and analysis, Bryden sought to write a 'natural history' of cholera in India, which was to be different from that of Europe because the spreading agencies were different in these countries. Thus, he accorded an epidemiologically unique status to India.

But Bryden had his own contradictions; for him cholera in Britain and India were different because the seasons and meteorological agencies in Britain and India were different. In Europe, according to Bryden, cholera might be spread by contagion instead of monsoonal air currents.[49] J.M. Cunningham (Sanitary Commissioner of India 1866–84) stepped into the shoes of Bryden. He too attempted a 'natural history of cholera', and he too believed in the air-borne theory of its spread. He asked several questions:

> What is the history of this epidemic? What are the facts connected with its spread and how far do they tend to increase our knowledge? Is a specific poison multiplied in those who are attacked, which is capable of being transmitted to, and of producing like symptoms in,

others; and if this were the case, is this poison contained in the discharges, and is it usually disseminated by means of water? Or setting aside the doctrine of contagion, both in the ordinary and modified acceptations of the term, is man the carrier of a specific entity from an infected locality, which germinates and bears fruit, whenever the local conditions are suited to the growth? Is human intercourse the great and indispensable means by which cholera is borne from its home and spread over the earth?[50]

By Cunningham's own confession,

> these were weighty questions which affect the well being not only of India, but of countries in the world, questions which, in these days of rapid and constantly increasing communications between the East and the West have a significance and practical importance very much greater even than they had before.[51]

Was J.M. Cunningham indicating the possibilities of beneficial borrowing of medical knowledge on cholera from the metropole? If this was what he indicated and, on that token, desired, then the whole tenure of Cunningham as Sanitary Commissioner and the various reports he authored fell short of his own ideals. J.M. Cunningham, like Bryden, never showed much enthusiasm or support for John Snow's water-borne theory of cholera causation. '(Snow had already published a pamphlet regarding this theory and a book in 1854)'.[52]

Neither can Cunningham be absolved from the charge of being cold towards those who took a clue from Snow's water-borne theory and wanted to turn preventive measures against cholera in a more specific direction. The dissenters who subscribed to Snow's water-borne theory in some way or the other were Dr Edmund Alexander Parkes (the author of *A Manual of Practical Hygiene*), A.C.C. Derenzy (Sanitary Commissioner of Punjab, 1868), Dr J.M. Coates (Sanitary Commissioner of Bengal), Francis McNamara (Professor of Chemistry at Calcutta Medical School in the 1860s), and S.C. Townsend (Sanitary Commissioner of the Central Provinces in 1869).

There was never a consensus on all aspects of cholera; for example, J.M. Cunningham was more or less an anti-contagionist, but at the same time he was opposed to the pilgrim theory. He opposed quarantine (pilgrim theory) because he thought that 'fear of quarantine compels concealment of cholera cases'.[53] A.C.C. Derenzy opposed

Cunningham's anti-contagionist stance but agreed with Cunningham's opposition to quarantine because 'they (i.e. quarantine) lead the people to conceal the existence of the disease, and, so far tend to diffuse, rather than limit, the contagion'.[54] Clearly, Derenzy was a contagionist unlike Cunningham who was an anti-contagionist. So, from two diametrically opposite standpoints of cholera causation, they were both anti-quarantine as far as preventive measures were concerned. Again, S.C. Townsend, unlike Cunningham, was a contagionist about causation. Interestingly, all three were against quarantine.[55]

Similarly, Dr G.S. Beatson, unlike all the above, was loosely anti-contagionist or was contingent-contagionist. Beatson held that

> in considering the question of expediency of restricting or of not restricting freedom of intercourse, between localities infected or non-infected with cholera, we leave out the word 'contagion' altogether, as no one of those who believe in the diffusion by human intercourse for a moment maintain or think that cholera is contagious in the sense in which we apply that term to smallpox, scarlatina, or the plague. On the contrary they believe that persons in attendance on the sick run in ordinary circumstances and with the ordinary precautions little or no extra risk.[56]

This jelled well with Bryden's and Cunningham's argument for a preventive action in the form of 'general sanitation', or 'practical sanitary action', as against Derenzy's and Parkes' argument for more specific measures against particular diseases like cholera.

Cholera, in Beatson's view,

> therefore in the ordinary sense may be considered to be non-contagious. Certainly it is contagious in the usual acceptation of the term in very limited degree, and probably only under favourable sanitary conditions, and in the case of persons who are at times predisposed to the disease. . . . But notwithstanding the apparent fact that cholera is but very slightly contagious, persons who have been in close attendance on a cholera patient cannot be too careful to observe all necessary precautions as to cleanliness and changing of clothes before they mingle with other individuals; for we have reason to believe that there is sufficient evidence in recorded facts that a person who has been in attendance on a cholera patient, without himself showing any symptoms of the disease, may be the

medium through which a third person (predisposed to take cholera) may take it and die.[57]

It is with such ambivalences as cholera being at the same time 'contagious', 'non-contagious' and 'slightly contagious', that Beatson treads his path of explanation. Interestingly, from this standpoint Beatson argues favourably for the efficacy of quarantine, opposing Derenzy, Townsend and more particularly Cunningham. Cunningham had argued against quarantine stating that there was frequent abuse of regulations pertaining to quarantine. Opposing this, Beatson opined: 'I regard such occurrences were evidence of abuse of regulations, not as any evidence that certain judicious regulations on the subject are in any way to blame for what was not essentially a result.'[58]

Beatson quotes Dr Parkes to validate his opinion on the efficacy of quarantine, but Parkes himself was neither an advocate of quarantine nor its sharpest critic. Beatson cites page 479 of Parkes' book: 'An island or an inland village far removed from commerce and capable for a time of doing without it may practice quarantine and preserve itself, but in other circumstances both theory and actual experiments show that quarantine fails.'[59] Parkes advocates 'practical hygiene', i.e. the use of disinfectants, both against diarrhoeal discharges and to linen.[60] 'In the case of troops coming from infected districts they should be kept in separate buildings for twenty days and ordered to use latrines attached to them in which disinfectants should be freely used.'[61]

The 'quarantine' or 'pilgrim theory' debate itself reflected many dissenting voices. Moreover, the remembrance of 1857 did not give the colonizers the courage to interfere with native customs beyond a limit. Therefore, to implement 'quarantine' as a policy measure, the views of all princely native states, British administrators and chief commissioners, and lieutenant governors of British Indian states were sought, and a consensus was attempted. Many native states frankly admitted their inability to implement it; chief among them were the native states of Rajputana and Hyderabad. 'The opinion both of officiating Resident (Mr Cordery) and Sir Salar Jung seems opposed to any active measures of (quarantine) beyond what was . . . proper sanitary arrangement.'[62] 'In Rajputana the views of the native states are strongly opposed to any measures of prohibition (on pilgrimage).'[63]

Many chief commissioners and lieutenant governors of

British provinces thought that the 'quarantine' would have a 'considerable deterrent effect' and opined that those who disregarded the prohibition should be criminally prosecuted.[64] There was a desire to inflict punishment but also the fear of 'native' backlash. Some administrators argued for its subtler implementation. For example, Mr King, Deputy Commissioner, Partapgurh, thought that it was 'most practical' for 'pilgrims (to) be licensed, and great personages be discouraged from taking large retinues, and especially persons of weak health; that at shrines resorted to by Hindus, a small tax be levied from Mohammedans to discourage resort thither, and vice versa.'[65]

Some administrators were more cautious and argued against quarantine as a general rule. The Lieutenant Governor of Punjab observed that,

> as a general rule, all official action having the appearance of interfering with the religious usages of the people should be studiously avoided, unless the reasons for such interference are potent and unmistakable. Upon this principle, under ordinary circumstances, any official action in the way of dissuading or discouraging people from proceeding to pilgrimage would be impolitical and liable to misconstruction.[66]

Opinions expressed in all the Residents' reports from various native states, small and big, on the whole were consistent as to the inadvisability of authoritatively prohibiting pilgrimage in general: 'as in the days of Chaucer, so now the folk "longen to go on pilgrimages", and it is generally held that to forbid the gratification of this "longing" would be a violation of the promise of religious toleration.'[67]

The administration also underlined the need to discourage pilgrimage by means of a system of tolls. The Chief Commissioner of Oudh opposed this and quoted Maharaja Man Singh in his favour. The maharaja was of the view that 'pilgrim tax, eo-nomine, would be regarded as a *jezia* or poll tax'.[68] This type of opinion went against the desire of the colonial state to demarcate its rule from that of the earlier state.

Just as cholera causation and its communicability were widely debated, so too the efficacy of 'quarantine' as a preventive measure against the spread of cholera remained an unsettled debate. But internationally a consensus was being reached on cholera. An International Sanitary Conference opened at Constantinople on 13 February 1866.

The conclusion of that conference stated the following points:

1. That cholera is communicable from the diseased to the healthy.
2. That it may be communicated
   (i) By the persons in the state of developed Cholera and,
   (ii) By persons suffering from Choleric diarrhoea who can move about and who are apparently in health for some days during the progress of the disease.

Again, 'The transmissibility of Cholera being adopted as a principle, the law of propagation to be deduced from it is evident; Cholera spreads everywhere in proportion to the facility and multiplicity of communication.'[69]

India was famous as a choleric country, so ships moving out of India towards Europe had to face quarantine measures. The colonial government protested against this. The contradiction was that how a government which was against quarantine at the international level was to implement it as a preventive measure in India. How could the colonial state, as a victim of quarantine internationally, victimize its own people with the same measure?

In the post-mutiny phase, as the honeymoon 'with the orient' ended and as the racial arteries hardened, the native body and the native landscape as a source of disease became more prominent. During the phase when acclimatization/seasoning was being advocated, the emphasis was on the British body, to tune itself to the climatic conditions of India. Due to the failure of the older theory of acclimatization, and the racial turn, the blame was squarely put on natives and their filthy mode of living. Indians were thought to be inherently diseased. 'Almost every native face is scarred by smallpox . . . it is common among natives that they accept it as a necessity.'[70] Similarly, in the changed English perception festivity and filthiness were synonymous for the native. The 'pilgrims on the road' as disease-carriers intersected with the army's 'line of march', increasing the vulnerability of the army.

These large movements of 'people on the road' on 'fruit full journeys' and their convergence on a sacred site, were viewed with alarm by the colonial state. A large crowd at an 'autonomous' sacred site with the propensity to spread diseases in a famine-afflicted country challenged the parameters of the colonial rule.

Slowly, in the debates around cholera, the pestilentiality and the choleric nature of Indian plains became prominent. The dissenters who argued against Bryden and Cunningham started taking cognizance of the newer theories of cholera causation in the metropole in particular and Europe in general. As the influence of Bryden and Cunningham receded in the background, Snow's theory of cholera being a water-borne disease gained wider acceptance in India. Now the dissenting medical men in the colony sought vindication in the Max von Pettenkofer's 'sub-soil water theory' of cholera causation. Later, Koch's 'microbial theory' of cholera causation also had considerable influence in the colony. With the acceptance of these new theories advanced by Pettenkofer and Koch, the Indian landscape increasingly came to be considered as a cradle of cholera-causing microbes (*comma bacillus*), spread by the presence of a porous soil with abnormally high levels of ground water and the Indian body as its carrier and agent. Pettenkofer's theory made the chemical and physical analysis of the sub-soil and its humid content important, whereas Koch's theory of cholera causation advanced a move away from chemical to bacterial analysis of water supplies. Both the theories in a way validated Snow's water-borne theory.

The combined effect of Pettenkofer and Koch gave the agenda of sanitation a new meaning. On the one hand, sub-soil drainage for cantonment areas became important; on the other, supply of wholesome water to the cantonment gained importance. Thus, the disease and deaths suffered undermined the initial optimism of acclimatization and seasoning, and consequently gave rise to great anxiety. The matter became worse and tension-ridden because the biologically determined racial turn declared that the Europeans were biologically, i.e. innately, a superior race. Now this superior race had to live up to its own professed superiority.

First of all, it had to save its dying soldiers to instil confidence. Since the British empire was as much founded on the fiction of race as on the Indian soil, there was the need to make the landscape on which the British were to dwell safe, habitable and healthy. The cantonment as the dwelling place was to be made the safest site. The anxiety of the British became all the more acute because of the baffling, teasing and annihilating nature of the diseases. No definite opinion on the origin and spread of these diseases were forthcoming (except in the case of smallpox, there was no major breakthrough). Endeavour towards preventive measures became all the more conflict-ridden because, during

1850–80, we see diseases (like cholera) evading the comprehension of the medical men in both the metropole and the colony. At both places, i.e. at the centre and the periphery, the various conjectures which emerged were debated and contested. Though they influenced each other, one-to-one correspondence was non-existent and, in many cases, was characterized by considerable time-lag. In fact the colonial medical men, or rather the colonial state, was very selective in allowing the metropole to influence indigenous policy-making pertaining to sanitary measures.

Perhaps it was due to this reason that the responses of the two cholera-stressed societies were so different.

Notes and References

[1] Even today, in the north Indian Gangetic plain, at the intersection of summer and the rainy season, when it becomes very humid, sultry and cloudy, when not a leaf flutters due to cessation of wind movement, the people in general characterize these days and its insalubrities by the word *'gumsii'*, and this characterization entails the anticipation of a *mahamari*, particularly cholera. The hovering clouds of these *Gumsii*-filled days are not seen as harbingers of monsoon but bearers of disease and destitution. Besides this general folk wisdom, I am indebted to Mark Harrison for his use of this phrase. He informs us that the idea of 'cholera cloud' as a sinister black presence enhanced the anxieties of British army officers during the 1857 rebellion (Mark Harrison, *Climates and Constitutions: Health, Race, Environment and British Imperialism in India 1600–1850*, New Delhi, 1999, p. 179).

[2] Sheldon Watts, *Epidemics and History: Disease Power and Imperialism*, New Haven and London, 1999, p. 167.

[3] Ibid., p. 67.

[4] David Arnold, *Colonizing the Body: State Medicine and Epidemic Disease in Nineteenth Century India*, Delhi, 1993, p. 159.

[5] Ibid., p. 120.

[5] John Macpherson, *Annals of Cholera from the Earliest Period to the Year 1817*, London, 1812, p. 11.

[7] P. Hehir, 'Historical Note on Cholera in India', *Indian Medical Gazette*, Vol. 46, No. 1, 1911, p. 8.

[8] John Snow, *On the Mode of Communication of Cholera*, London, 1854, p. 1.

[9] Ibid.

[10] Ibid.

[11] Ibid., p. 2.

[12] P. Hehir, 'Historical Note on Cholera in India', p. 8.

[13] T.J. Pettigrew, *Observations on Cholera, Comprising a description of Epidemic Cholera of India, the mode of Treatment and means of Prevention*, London,

1831, pp. 8–10. Also see David Arnold, 'The Indian Ocean as a Disease Zone: 1500–1950' *South Asia* 14, 1991, pp. 1–22.

[14] David Arnold, *Colonizing the Body*, pp. 160–161.

[15] Ibid.

[16] David Arnold, 'The Indian Ocean as a Disease Zone'.

[17] P. Hehir, 'Historical Note on Cholera in India', p. 19.

[18] John Snow, *On the Mode of Communication of Cholera*, p. 2.

[19] Anand A. Yang, *Bazaar India: Markets, Society and the Colonial State in Gangetic Bihar*, New Delhi, 2000, p. 115.

[20] Karlen Arno, *Man and Microbes: Disease and Plagues in History and Modern Times*, New York, 1995, p. 133.

[21] David Arnold, *Colonizing the Body*, p. 159.

[22] F. Frederic Cartwright, *A Social History of Medicine*, London and New York, p. 97.

[23] K. Mishra, 'Productivity of Crisis: Disease, Scientific Knowledge and State in India', *Economic and Political Weekly*, 28 October 2000, pp. 3885–97.

[24] Reginald Orton, 'An Essay on the Epidemic Cholera of India', Madras, 1820, pp. 164–65.

[25] 'Second and Third Sections of the Report of the Commissioners Appointed to Inquire into the Cholera Epidemic of 1861 in Northern India', Calcutta, 1864, pp. 183–84.

[26] Reginald Orton, 'An Essay on the Epidemic Cholera of India', pp. 190- 91.

[27] Mark Harrison, 'From medical astrology to medical astronomy: Sol-lunar and planetary theories of disease in British medicine, *c.* 1700–1850', *The British Journal of History of Science*, Vol. 33, part 1, No. 116, March 2000, pp. 25–48

[28] Ibid., pp. 202–33.

[29] J.A. Lawrie, *Essays on Cholera, Founded on Observations of the Disease in various parts of India and in Sunderland, Newcastle and Gateshead*, Glasgow, 1832, pp. 10–14.

[30] Victor Jacquemont, *Letters from India. Describing a journey in the British Dominions of India, Tibet, Lahore and Cashmere, during the years 1828, 1899, 1830, 1831 undertaken by order of the French Government*, edited by J. Rosselli, London, 1979. See letter dated 7 July 1832, in ibid., Vol. 2, p. 341.

[31] William Twinning, *Clinical Illustrations of the more important diseases of Bengal with the result of an inquiry into their pathology and treatment*, Calcutta, 1832, pp. xvii and 398–400.

[32] E.A. Parkes, *Researches into the pathology and treatment of the Asiatic or Algide Cholera*, London, 1847, p. 156.

[33] 'Second and Third sections of the Report of the Commissioners appointed to inquire into the cholera epidemic of 1861 in Northern India', p. 188.

[34] Ibid., p. 197.

[35] Ibid.

[36] Ibid.

[37] Ibid., p. 195.

[38] Ibid., p. 194.

[39] Ibid., p. 195.

[40] Ibid.

[41] Ibid.

[42] Ibid., p. 197.

[43] Ibid., pp. 197–98.

[44] 'Report of Commissioners appointed to enquire into the Sanitary State of the Army in India' *Parliamentary Papers I and II (1868)*.

[45] *Sanitary Commission Report with Government of India (1867)*, pp. 148, 191; (*1868*), p. 73.

[46] Frederic Cartwright, *A Social History of Medicine*, p. 103; for more details see, Christopher Hamlin, *Public Health and Social Justice in Age of Chadwick: Britain, 1800–1854*, Cambridge, 1998.

[47] Cartwright, *A Social History of Medicine*, p. 109.

[48] Ibid., p. 111.

[49] Mark Harrison, *Public Health in British India: Anglo-Indian Preventive Medicine 1859–1914*, Cambridge, 1994, pp. 101–02.

[50] J.M. Cunningham, 'Annual Sanitary Report for 1872 (Section 1—Report on the Cholera epidemic of 1872 in Northern India)'.

[51] Ibid.

[52] John Snow, *On the Mode of Communication of Cholera*.

[53] J.M. Cunningham, 'Annual Sanitary Report of 1872 (Section 1—Report on Cholera Epidemic of 1872 in Northern India).'

[54] Home/Sanitary, March 1874, No. 14–20(A), National Archive of India (NAI).

[55] Ibid.

[56] Ibid.

[57] Ibid.

[58] Ibid.

[59] Ibid.

[60] Ibid.

[61] Ibid.

[62] Home/Sanitary, March 1870, No. 163–240(A), National Archive of India (NAI).

[63] Ibid.

[64] Ibid.

[65] Ibid.

[66] Ibid.

[67] Ibid.

[68] Ibid.

[69] Home/Sanitary, March 1874, No. 14–20(A), National Archive of India (NAI).

[70] Home/Sanitary, March 1874, No. 13–20(A), National Archive of India (NAI).

An Empire 'De-Masculinized'!

The British Colonial State and the Problem of Syphilis in Nineteenth-Century India

Sabya Sachi R. Mishra

This paper seeks to study the problem of veneral diseases in nineteenth-century India. With shifts in historiography, the question of public health in colonial India has become an important area of research. In recent years many studies have been done on problems such as the relationship between the tropical climate of the country and the diagnostic theories of disease in the nineteenth century; the problem of endemic diseases like plague and cholera in the British period, etc. Syphilis, however, though widely recognized as the most debilitating disease after plague in this period, has not been explored by historians at any extensive scale. By focussing on the variety of ways in which the British medical practitioners and administrators in India perceived the disease, this paper tries to situate the problem of venereal diseases within the wider frame of India's colonial experience.

For the alien rulers in India who had to meet their imperial needs with a limited number of British soldiers, syphilis posed a major threat. It was an incurable menace. It affected the very foundation of the *Raj*—it de-vitalized the British soldier, de-masculinized him, and in no time made him unfit for the purpose. The dominant image of the disease was one of a 'scourge' which the officials desperately sought to contend. Syphilis, by virtue of its aetiology, not only posed a serious health hazard; it had various strategic, financial and cultural ramifications as well.

Syphilis was not typical to the Britishers in India. During the nineteenth century almost every country of the world was wrestling with the problem. In England as well, an array of debates was being carried out to understand the origin, symptoms and diagnosis of the disease. However, for much of the century, answers eluded the questions. And the medical theorists increasingly emphasized preventive measures rather than curative treatment.

This problem of a mystifying aetiology of the disease was compounded by the questions of morality associated with syphilis. In the overtly moral world of the Victorian century, knowledge about the sexual nature of the disease created a moral stigma around it. The rising incidence of syphilis blatantly represented growing promiscuity in an otherwise moral society. The disease became a metaphor which not only reflected the deeper immoral moorings of the society, its control meant public intervention in otherwise private spaces of individuals, and rigid control over and regulation of their sexual activities (specially prostitutes). More importantly, contending with the menace of syphilis involved a social and medical reconstruction of 'sick' and 'healthy', with a focus upon the sanitary state of the sexual organs of individuals.

The patriarchal order of the society produced a specific discourse on the disease. Essentially gendered in nature, the discourse portrayed syphilis as a typically feminine disease. Women, particularly prostitutes, were seen as sole carriers of the syphilitic contagion, and the prevention of the disease got directly associated with their control. This deliberate gendering proved especially fruitful in colonial situations as it gave a free hand to the authorities to put the blame of the disease on the colonized other. It also provided a tool for the extension of the colonizing space through a control of the state over female privacy.

In many cases, as in India, the necessity of controlling the disease led to criminalization of the profession of prostitution, where the prevention of disease became synonymous with retribution. It meant a tight control over the movement of prostitutes, involved hygienic verification of their 'bodies' under the direct gaze of the state, and being sick meant confinement in hospitals for a longer period of time. These measures created a break in the traditional identities of the prostitute, redefined her individuality and the profession, and brought her within the purview of the state on newer terms wherein she came to be looked at and defined through the categories of imperial hygiene. They brought about a radical shift in the very perception of the prostitute as an individual and a professional. Away from the traditional perception of the prostitute as belonging to a marginalized class, staying at the periphery out of necessity and to fulfil certain social needs, she now emerged as a criminal at the centrestage of the colonial rule—as one who infected the colonizer and de-masculinized him. This identity of the prostitute as a criminal was an important transformation brought about by the British rule in India, and was typically colonial in nature. It also had an important bearing upon the treatment of prostitutes as subjects in the preventive discourses of the state. Unlike in England, where prevention of disease through control over prostitutes was closely associated with their rehabilitation in the mainstream society, in India, the entire discourse on the prevention of venereal disease precluded any such responsibility of the state towards rehabilitation of these classes. In its attempt to rescue the soldier from the evil effects of his sexual indulgences, the state, despite recognizing him as equally responsible, spared him, and held the prostitute—the colonized subject and an unequal partner—as solely guilty, and made her pay for it. Almost every colonial society of this period experienced such controlling measures.[1] Despite the number of studies that have tried to look at the history of syphilis within the wider medical history of the nineteenth century, none has been able to see the disjunctions that came in the perception of the disease in colonial settings. A study of the perception of venereal disease in colonial settings is, however, important.

Syphilis and the British Rule in India

Long before venereal disease (VD) became a part of the official discourse in India, it was known as *firungi rog* in the Indian folk tradition. Early Portuguese traders in India were believed to have brought the disease. However, as the British empire in India began its expansionist trail from the late eighteenth century onward, the problem of VD began to figure in a new way. Right from the beginning, officials recognized the incidence of VD to be a result of sexual indulgences between soldiers and prostitutes, an area which, as Ballhatchet writes, was 'most troubling' and 'embarrassing' to the authorities.[2]

The presence of VD among the European troops stationed in India was as old as the colonial rule itself, and there had always been some amount of concern regarding this problem. However the mutiny of 1857 essentially came as a break. It reoriented the concern regarding the disease as, upon enquiry, the officials found that at least one-third of the European troops was perpetually in hospitals on account of this disease alone. The mutiny was a shock that hit at the very foundations of the empire, and such revelations as the number of soldiers afflicted with VD left the rulers unnerved. To look into the deeper aspects of the problem, the government instituted a Royal Commission for enquiry into the sanitary conditions of the army. The commission emphatically argued for stringent legislative measures for prevention of the disease. This facilitated the way for legislations like Act XXII of 1864 and the Indian Contagious Diseases Act, which created a legal framework for the prevention of VD. The official debates carried out during this period around the making of these Acts and towards their operation significantly reveal the wider strategic, financial and cultural fears of the colonizers. They provide us with a context for understanding the newer priorities of the state in the changed circumstances of the post-mutiny era. VD becomes a marker to understand how, in order to overcome its own fears, the authorities came to redefine the roles of the colonizer and the colonized in this period, and sought to control the subject society.

The Soldier and the 'Scourge'

Food, dwelling, conservancy arrangements, occupation both of mind and body, personal hygiene comprising cleanliness, temperance and abstinence from social vice, wrote Special Sanitary Commissioner C. Hathaway, were the five issues affecting the health of European officers and soldiers in India.[3] Among these broader concerns, however, Hathaway rued that the problem of VD among the European troops was of 'vital importance', and accused the writers on military sanitation and the medical officers of evading it 'through false delicacy, or in the hopelessness of suggesting any practical measure'. Emphasizing the importance of the problem, he wrote,

> the question is that of vital importance, it affects the present as well as the future health of thousands of the child unborn, the girl just married and every rank and class of our soldiery, from the recruit recently arrived from England to the broken down and prematurely old invalid, who is being sent out of the country incurably destroyed, at an age when other men are in their prime of life.[4]

Despite the warnings of officials like Hathaway, the British officialdom remained confused about the problem. While most authorities saw the problem of VD as a frightening offshoot of the soldier's sexual indulgence with prostitutes, they found it difficult to put a check on his sexual forays. These uncontrolled sexual overtures of the soldiers, to the dominant military discourse of the time, formed a necessary part of their 'physiological natural instincts'. As one report said,

> for a young man who cannot marry and who cannot attain to the high moral standards required for the repression of physiological natural instincts, there are only two ways of satisfaction, viz., masturbation and mercenary love. The former, as is well known, leads to disorders of both body and mind; the latter, to the fearful dangers of venereal.[5]

There was essentially a duality in the official perception of the soldier's sexuality and its relation with the problem of VD. While, on the one hand, the discourses naturalized the uncontrolled sexual desire of the soldier; legitimized and celebrated his non-monogamous indulgences, yet simultaneously they expressed their fear of what these indulgences always led to. The non-monogamous indulgences of soldiers were seen as markers of their manliness, as Brigadier A. Tucker, Commanding Officer, Rawalpindi Brigade, wrote: 'human nature is human nature, and our men will find means of sexual intercourse other than that authorized, as between husband and wife'.[6] Within this official frame, VD appeared as an 'evil' physical consequence of the 'physiological natural desires' of the soldier. The soldier in these discourses was portrayed as a victim of his natural desires, and this necessitated the need for protecting him from the evil effects of his indulgences.

Protection of the health of soldiers, though vital, was just one of the several reasons that informed the official fear. The discourses on VD point to a number of ideas that accentuated the fear of VD among the British officials in India. For one, as Harrison has argued, it was the incapacitating effect of VD on soldiers that the officials feared the most.[7] The officials described the disease in most distasteful terms, comparing it with 'self-mutilation' by the soldiers, where

> those who are admitted into hospital with primary symptoms, are for a length of time rendered unfit for the performance of any duty, and that the greater number of them after having been discharged

from hospital in due course, return with secondary symptoms, which in almost every instance renders them unfit for the service.[8]

Added to this was the de-masculinizing effect of VD on the soldiers. De-masculinization as the most debilitating effect of the disease often found its way into the official reports, which portrayed 'in unpleasant details cases of soldiers with genital organs "eaten away" by VD'.[9] This de-masculinization of the soldier was, interestingly, the result of the soldier's overtly masculine acts, and realization of this fact created a psychological chasm in the official perception of syphilis. The authorities were confronted with an extremely delicate situation: how to check this gradual yet steady infiltration of the de-masculinizing evil in the army without necessarily tampering with the soldiers' masculinity? Control of the disease through a check on the soldiers' relation with the 'sick' women was perhaps only available option.

The problem of VD had specific cultural attributes as well. Given the hereditary nature of the disease, it was seen as cutting at the 'vitality of the race'. As an official wrote, it was 'impossible to consider without anxiety the enormous extent to which the blood of England is now being tainted with the venereal poison through the country from the Army as its great focus and factory'.[10] The present inefficient state of the soldiery on account of VD got fused with its future effects on the system, 'causing death, broken down constitution and injury to the second generation by a hereditary taint being communicated to the offspring?'[11] Thus VD in an extended form symbolized the fear of the occident from the blood of the orient.

The military authorities in India portrayed fearsome images of the disease as not only keeping

> a large proportion of the Army constantly in Hospital, but the necessary treatment with the ravages of the disease, undermines the constitution, cripples the bodily powers on the march in the field, and predisposes to other diseases, especially rheumatism which affection swells very largely the annual number invalided.[12]

It cut deep into the strength of the army. And particularly in a period when the European soldiers were seen as forming the backbone of the empire, the incapacitating effect of the disease appeared as debilitating the strategic foundation of the British rule in India.

Imperial Survival and the Cost of De-Masculinization

Invaliding of soldiers on account of VD was a major strategic problem for the authorities in India. Contraction of VD meant either keeping the soldier in the hospital for a length of time (and it was never less than three weeks) on account of primary symptoms, or sending him back to England if the disease had reached an incurable stage. The official statistics claimed that almost a third of the British contingent in India was perpetually in the hospital on account of VD, particularly in the post-mutiny period. John Strachey, in his report on VD in the Bengal army, enumerated the percentage of the venereal admission of soldiers, as in Table I:

TABLE I: *Percentage of Venereal Admission among the European Troops in the Bengal Army*

Year	Total Strength of European Troops	Admitted in Hospitals	Percentage in Hospitals
1862	42,980	13,671	31.8
1861	44,879	16,167	36.9
1860	—	—	33.8
1859	—	—	36.0

Source: Letter from John Strachey, the President of the Sanitary Commission for Bengal, to the Secretary, GOI, Military Dept, dated 21 March 1864, Home (Leg.), March 1864, Nos. 11–13, Part B.

On the basis of this data, John Strachey commented: 'we may thus consider that at least one third of the whole European Army passed through the hospitals in the course of the year on account of these diseases alone.' Given the fact that 'the average length of time during which each man remains in the hospital is at least three weeks', the report concluded, 'it may be assumed that on any day in the year a number of men equal to the ordinary effective strength of a Regiment are disabled from this cause.'[13]

A look at the statistics of the pre-mutiny period undoubtedly shows that the disease was always considerably present among the European soldiers. Table II shows the percentage of venereal admissions of the army in India.

Despite such statistical proofs, the authorities avoided the revival of the lock hospitals, which had been closed since 1828.

TABLE II: *Percentage of Venereal Admissions in the Years before the Mutiny*

Year	Percentage of Admission (as against Total Admissions)
1829	11.6
1830	10.6
1831	11.8
1832	14.0
1833	26.8
1834	32.2
1835	28.4
1836	26.2
1837	24.2
1838	26.8
1842	20.5
1843	17.5
1844	16.0
1845	19.6
1846	20.9
1847	29.7
1848	35.9
1849	32.7
1850	28.1
1851	27.1

Source: Prepared by Dr Warning from the Return in the Office of Medical Board, Home (Leg.), March 1864, Nos. 11–13, Part B.

However, the mutiny showed up the importance of the British soldiers in the strategic priorities of the state. As keeping a comparatively larger number of European contingents in India became necessary, VD began to draw fresh attention from the officials. The disease kept a considerable number of soldiers in a state of inefficiency, thus necessarily causing a strategic imbalance. The colonial state in India was desperate to overcome this problem.

Apart from the strategic necessities of the state, the financial implications of the disease also kept the British authorities in a state of quandary. The financial burden on account of this disease was vividly analysed by John Strachey, President, Sanitary Commission of Bengal, who, quoting from the report of the Royal Commission for inquiry into the sanitary state of the army in India, illustrated that 'the annual cost of each soldier in India is 100 Pounds. Assuming this to be correct, the direct money loss caused to the state at the present time by these diseases is not less than 75,000 Pounds per year.'[14] The annual expenditure of 75,000 pounds on inefficient soldiers lying in hospitals, fighting hard to survive the de-masculinizing contagion, was a difficult pill for the officials to swallow.

Besides these strategic and financial implications of the disease, the worst effect of VD, in the overall perception of the officials, was the great drain of manpower from India in the form of invalid soldiers. Every year a number of soldiers had to be sent back home, invalided by the disease. The official records are full of constant references by the supporters of the lock hospital system in India to this incidence. It was recognized fact among the military officials that invaliding from VD was 'greater among the European soldiers in India than in any other class', and the supporters of the lock hospital system argued that

> if this excess is caused in any way (as is shown to be the case) by preventable diseases or defective sanitary arrangements, the expense of renewing the perpetual loss by fresh supply—the sending out of batches of army to fill up the gaps in the ranks of trained and disciplined soldiers, is far more costly than the simple precautionary measure (i.e. lock hospitals) that have been persistently advocated.[15]

This official concern for invaliding of soldiers was also supported by the statistical data. Medical officers claimed that 'fully two-thirds of those who imbibe the disease are invalided within five years'.[16] While individually in some regiments the number of invalid soldiers sent home annually could go up to twelve,[17] an official report analysing the all-India data for the year 1884 concluded that the 'drain on the European Army in India occasioned by ill-health is very considerable'. The statistics for deaths and invaliding in the army for the year 1884 were as in Table III.

About Bengal, the report said,

> this means that every soldier went into hospital one and a half times, 1.1 men out of every hundred men died, and more than three men in every hundred men were sent home invalided. In Madras the admissions to hospital and the deaths are less, but the invaliding is the same. Bombay stands half way between Bengal and Madras for admissions, is very much worse than either in mortality, or slightly better in invaliding.[18]

TABLE III: *Proportionate Ratio of Death and Invaliding in the European Army Stationed in the Provinces of Bengal, Madras and Bombay for the year 1884*

	Bengal	Madras	Bombay
Admission per 1000 (i.e. number of times soldiers were admitted into the hospitals)	1,662	1,109	1,445
Death per 1000	11.68	8.53	19.39
Invaliding per 1000	31.84	31.86	31.36

Source: Quoted from 'Notes on the question of state interference with "Contagious" diseases in Calcutta', Home (Sanitary), Oct. 1887, Nos. 180–197, Part A.

The financial implications of the invaliding, then, the report asserted, was 'of great importance'. As it said,

> the cost of every European soldier put down in an Indian cantonment is reckoned at 145 pounds, and his annual upkeep involves a very heavy expenditure;* he is an expensive machine; he is in fact one of the costly British products, of which despite their comparative expensiveness as compared with the native article, the English have to make use for the administration of the country.

The report added,

> it becomes, accordingly, a financial question of great importance to enquire how far this costly article is economically used: and attention is specially drawn to the unnecessary waste of health and strength involved in the amount of venereal diseases which is at present allowed to exist in the European army.[19]

---

* In Military Proceedings 2361–63, March 1877, the average annual cost of a European soldier in India is taken at Rs 824. The cost of medicine, food, bedding and hospital requisites in Bengal amounted, in 1885–86, to Rs 343 per head of the daily average. In the lock hospitals the average stay of each patient was, in 1885, 79 days. If the same ratio applies in venereal cases in the military hospitals, there would be an annual loss of 1,319,537 days' service.

Syphilis in the Nineteenth-Century Medical Discourse

The official perception of VD was largely shaped by the European aeteology of the nineteenth century, in which syphilis was seen as the root cause of numerous diseases in the human body. As W.J. Moore, Surgeon General with Government of India (GOI), emphasizing the fatality of the disease, wrote:

> primary syphilis may result in a sloughing inguinal sore, or in sloughing phagedena of the penis, which endangers life. And secondary syphilis may result in throat and laryngeal affections, also dangerous to life. It is, however, indirectly and remotely that syphilis proves so very destructive to life. Indirectly there is no disease which causes a greater mortality, as well as all kinds of misery. In questioning patients as to their previous history, how often is it found that the first link of the chain dragging them to the grave is syphilis![20]

Quoting Mon. Record's remarks on VD as 'the terrible contagion which ever threatened mankind', Moore added:

> It is tertiary or remote syphilis which is the most destructive. Diseases of the eye, especially iritis, often ending in blindness; diseases of spinal chord terminating in paralysis; diseases of brain ending in a similar condition; diseases of heart, the forerunner of dropsy,—all result from syphilis. . . . In short, diseases of most internal organs has been fully traced to those degeneration and formations which result from venereal.[21]

The centrality of VD as the root cause for a range of diseases became all the more frightening, as it was believed that the nature of the disease took worse form in a tropical region like India. The medical discourses saw the tropical climate of the Indian subcontinent as particularly conducive for worsening the virulence of the contagion. As Judy Whitehead has shown, the Victorian sanitarians and, following them, the officials in the British Indian medical service, often viewed the diseases as results of environmental decomposition. In India, until about the 1890s, the miasmatic theory of diseases, championed by Edwin Chadwick and Florence Nightingale, was prevalent. The miasmatic theory held that toxic concentrations of vaporous products of decay caused disease. In other words, diseases were caused by 'odours' from rotting substances. Tropical areas were perceived as prime breeders of such miasmatic contagion because organic matter decomposed more rapidly in hot climates than in cold climates.[22] As Surgeon General W.J. Moore wrote:

> Apart from the diagnostic discourse on VD, what made the fear from VD all the more awesome was the lack of any concrete curative medicine during the century. Ballhatchet has shown that the methods of treatment were hazardous, especially for syphilis: mercury and biochloride of mercury were of doubtful efficacy and had unpleasant side effects; iodide of potassium, which was also in general use by the 1850s, was only a little more effective.

He argues that, 'the optimism with which the doctors claimed they could cure patients, both men and women, seems to have been based more on self-confidence than on clinical evidence. Indeed, when the primary lesions disappeared, patients were discharged as cured.'[24] This lack of curative medicine essentially made the state cautious of preventing VD through non-medicinal measures like separating the 'sick' from the 'clean' bodies and regulating the sexual relations of the soldiers with only the latter class of prostitutes, etc. These idioms of 'sick' and 'clean' bodies all through this period were defined through the discourses on lock hospitals which, for all intents and purposes, became the tools for policing the prostitutes rather than curing them of venereal. And, even as late as 1888, when CDA was repealed, the officials deplored the repeal as it was felt that the policing of prostitutes through CDA had well compensated for the lack of curative medicine for the disease.

Given the wide range of strategic, financial and cultural concerns which came to characterize the official perception of VD in the latter half of the nineteenth century, the prevention of the disease came to be a significant 'subject of national importance'.[25] Apart from the immediate need to preserve the health of the army, its prevention got associated with the wider interests of the colonial state in India. As one official aptly put it, 'to the Army VD is a scourge, and the more it is controlled, the more is not only the Army but the state benefited.'[26]

Notes and References

[1] For references see, Joel Best, *Controlling Vice: Regulating Brothel Prostitution in St. Paul, 1865–1883*, Columbus, 1998; David McCreery, 'The Life of Misery and Shame: Female Prostitution in Guatemala City, 1880–1920',

Journal of Latin American Studies, 18, pp. 333–53; Mary Elizabeth Perry 'Deviant Insiders: Legalized Prostitutes and a Consciousness of Women in Early Modern Sevile', *Comparative Studies in Society and History,* p. 20; Jim Zwick (ed.), *The Crowning Infamy of Imperialism,* Philadelphia, 1995; Kay Saunders, 'Controlling (Hetero) Sexuality: The Implementation and Operation of Contagious Diseases Legislation in Australia, 1868–1945', in Diane Kirkby (ed.), *Sex Power and Justice: Historical Perspective on Law in Australia,* Melbourne, 1995, pp. 19–32, etc.

2   Kenneth Ballhatchet, *Sex and Class under the Raj,* Delhi, 1979, p. 10.

3   Memo. by C. Hathaway, Special Sanitary Commissioner, dated Shimla, 14 November 1861, Home (Leg.), March 1864, Nos. 11–13, Part B.

4   Ibid.

5   Quoted in Ballhatchet, *Sex and Class under the Raj,* p. 10. Memo, Oct. 1886, pp. 1888, LXXVII (158), 235ff.

6   Brigadier A. Tucker, Commander, Rawalpindi Brigade, to the QMG of Army, Army Headquarter (No. 216, dated Rawalpindi, 29 January 1863); Home (Leg.), March 1864, Nos. 11–13, Part B.

7   Mark Harrison, *Public Health in British India: Anglo-Indian Perspective on Medicine 1859–1914,* New Delhi, 1994.

8   Letter from Brigadier C. Troup to Asst. Adjutant General, Meerut, No. 262, dated Agra, 27 May 1861; Home (Leg.), March 1864, Nos. 11–13, Part B.

9   Ballhatchet, *Race, Sex and Class,* p. 20.

10   Letter from Asst. Surgeon A.C.C. Derenzy, in Medical Charge B Battery 19th Brigade, Royal Artillery, to Captain A. Callander, Major of Brigade, Mooltan, dated Mooltan, 13 March 1863; Home (Leg.), March 1864, Nos. 11–13, Part B.

11   C. Hathaway, Memo, dated Shimla, 14 November 1861.

12   Letter from Brigadier C. Troup, dated Agra, 27 May 1861.

13   Letter from John Strachey, the President to the Sanitary Commission for Bengal, to the Secretary to the GOI, Military Department, dated 21 March 1864; Home (Leg.), March 1864, Nos. 11–13, Part B.

14   Ibid.

15   C. Hathaway, Memo, dated Shimla, 14 November 1861.

16   Note by the Surgeon General and Sanitary Commissioner with GOI on experimental closure of several lock hospitals during 1885; Home (Sanitary), June 1888, Nos. 102–29, Part A.

17   Lt. Colonel E.B. Johnson, Officiating Adjutant General of the Army, to the Secretary to the GOI, Military Department (No. 236, dated Headquarters Simla, 2 May 1862); Home (Leg.), March 1864, Nos. 11–13, Part B.

18   Notes on the Question of State Interference with 'Contagious' Diseases in Calcutta. Home (Sanitary), October 1887, Nos. 180–197, Part A.

19   Ibid.

20   Memorandum by W.J. Moore, Surgeon General. Home (Sanitary), June 1888, Nos. 102–29, Part A.

21   Ibid.

22   Judy Whitehead, 'Bodies Clean and Unclean: Prostitution, Sanitary Legisla-

tion, and Respectable Femininity in Colonial North India', in *Gender and History*, Vol. 7, No. 1, April 1995, pp. 41–63.

23 Memorandum by W.J. Moore.

24 Ballhatchet, *Race, Sex and Class*, p. 18.

25 Ibid., p. 86.

26 Letter from J.B. Harrison, Surgeon, 27 P.I., in Medical Charge, Meean Meer, dated 11 February 1863; Home (Leg.), March 1864, Nos. 11–13, Part B.

Medical Missionaries at Work

The Canadian Baptist Missionaries in the Telugu Country, 1870–1952

Raj Sekhar Basu

I

The study of medical missionary enterprise in India has long been a neglected area of historical research. Medical missionaries in India, as in the other underdeveloped parts of Asia and Africa, performed roles almost similar to that of 'change agents'. Historians specializing in Asian social history have very often stressed that as 'change agents', medical missionaries facilitated certain innovations. In fact, by promoting a western innovation in the form of western medical science, European medical missionaries undertook efforts to change the health standards and behavioural attitudes of the Indians with whom they came into contact.[1]

Significantly, by the mid-decades of the nineteenth century, the basic worldview of the missionaries underwent a profound change. To be precise, the missionary characterization of the cultural regions of the world came to be expressed in terms of two broad divisions—'Christian' and 'Heathen'. The heathen population was further subdivided into two distinct categories—the 'cultured people' and the 'savages'. India, to many missionaries, resembled Africa in terms of backwardness and ignorance. The missionaries frequently pointed out that undernourishment, overpopulation and lack of proper sanitation facilities were responsible for the high incidence of diseases like tuberculosis, cholera and smallpox.

Western medical missionaries also believed that prevalence of superstitions and unflinching faith in quack remedies led to heavy loss of lives. Consequently, India came to be perceived by the missionaries as a strange land reverberating with stories of mysteries and of deaths and horrors.[2] Presumably, their bizarre experiences in a heathen land also influenced the missionaries to endorse ideas relating to

Europe's cultural superiority and its civilizing mission in the world. The western medical missionaries supported the imperial claim that European colonization had brought western medical science close to the doors of the unfortunate nations. The British official classes in India frequently responded to such adulation by acknowledging the missionary work among the natives under colonial rule.[3]

However, by the last years of the nineteenth century, western medical missionaries in India realized the implications of their 'care and cure' policy vis-à-vis the complex process of Christianization. In this context, as late as the 1920s, a European medical missionary observed:

> for the continued preservation of Christianity to Hindus and Muslims, there is no more potent agency than the work of Medical Mission. The successful evangelization of a block of 320,000,000 may be regarded as the dream of an enthusiast. But the idea of let us say 320 medical missionaries, each ministering and witnessing to 1,000,000, no longer seems wildly impracticable.[4]

In a sense, it was argued that the missionary medical enterprise that had developed out of 'Christian humanism' could be utilized to promote Christianity in lands professing diverse faiths and culture.[5]

Yet, throughout much of the nineteenth century, medical missionaries occupied a rather subdued position in the entire missionary enterprise in India. The attitude of the missionaries, nonetheless, underwent a change from the 1870s onward. The onset of famine and wide-scale loss of human lives convinced the missionaries that medical missions needed to be recognized as powerful adjuncts of missionary work in the subcontinent. The missions felt that medical missionaries would not only broaden the contacts with non-Christian communities, but also provide a momentum to the Gospel enterprise. Furthermore, the humanitarian opinion within the missions stressed that the Christian premise to 'heal the sick' justified an honoured place for medical missions in every missionary programme.[6] Thus it became imperative on the part of the missionaries to develop medical work as an essential part of the ministry of the Christian church, emulating the example set by the founder Jesus Christ himself.[7]

In the present essay, I seek to unravel the ways and means through which the Canadian Baptist missionaries utilized medical missions to gain new followers in the coastal Telugu-speaking districts of erstwhile Madras Presidency, in the late nineteenth and early twentieth centuries. The narrative will be essentially based on the records relating to Canadian Baptist medical mission work in south India. For all practical purposes, the essay will broadly deal with developments between 1870 and 1952. This sort of periodization is relevant since the Canadian Baptist missionaries devoted their energies towards medical relief only towards the end of the nineteenth century. In the following century, the Canadian Baptists competed with the government-run medical institutions in providing sanitation and medical relief to the people. The Canadian Baptists, despite being understaffed and poor in terms of finances, proved to be pioneers in the treatment of influenza, cholera and leprosy. The sincerity and devotion displayed by the missionary doctors in the maternity health-care dispensaries and the leper asylum homes, made them particularly popular amongst the lower castes. As a consequence, their immense popularity accounted for the conversion of a sizeable number of outcastes and loosening of caste rigidities. Thus, by the early 1930s, the Canadian Baptists were able to reveal beyond all doubt the efficacy of medical mission work in the spread of the Gospel in a non-Christian land.

II

The American Baptist missionary activity in India in the early decade of the nineteenth century paved the way for the later indirect contacts between the Canadian Baptists and the Telugus. In the mid-1830s, Rev. Samuel Day of the American Baptist Missionary Union laboured in the southern part of the Telugu country, and laid the foundations on which Christian churches were established in the following decades.[8] The Baptists in central Canada from then on sent individual financial contributions to assist their American brethren in their venture.

In 1866, during the Convention of Ontario and Quebec Baptists at Beamsville, the Canadian Baptists consolidated themselves by forming the Canadian Auxiliary to the American Baptist Missionary Union. A.V. Timpani, a missionary volunteer of this Auxiliary, was finally selected by the Ontario and Quebec Convention in 1867, to work among the Telugus in south India.[9]

Towards the end of 1868, after a few months of language study, the Timpanis decided to settle in a new American Baptist mission outpost at Ramapatnam, 150 miles north of Madras. Rev. and

Mrs John McLaurin soon joined them, after a long sea voyage from Ontario to India through the newly-opened Suez Canal. Thereafter, in October 1870, the Foreign Missionary Society came to be formed, replacing the Auxiliary that had worked alongside the American Baptist Missionary Union in India.

The Canadian Baptists in the subsequent years continued to cooperate with the American Baptist missionaries. But in 1874, they decided to have their own mission. Meanwhile, certain unexpected events transpired to bring the missionaries from central Canada into close relationship with the Baptist missionaries from the Maritime Provinces.[10] Interestingly, in the northern Circars, or districts of the Telugu country along India's east coast, the two Canadian missions functioned harmoniously side by side. Although they were supported and supervised by two different conventions in Canada, they developed close collaboration. In fact, as early as 1876, they began to organize joint annual conferences to discuss their common problems and programmes. In the following years, they sent resolutions to their respective home constituencies for undertaking serious efforts towards unification. In 1912, finally, their pleas were heard, when the Canadian Baptist Foreign Mission Board was organized with dominion-wide representation and the two mission fields in India were unified. Thus, the region comprising mostly of the northern Circars or districts of the Telugu country came to be recognized as an exclusive area of Canadian Baptist missionary work.[11]

III

In the mid-1870s, the Canadian Baptist missionaries mostly devoted their energies to finding new followers in localities in and around Vizagapatnam. In course of time, they organized churches and mission stations in Bobbili and Tuni. However, within the space of a few years, Coconada became the centre of their activities.[12] In these years, the Canadian Baptists mainly employed women missionaries in preaching the Gospel and opening schools for both the upper and lower castes.[13] By the early 1890s the Canadian missionaries were able to draw several women medical missionaries for setting up dispensaries and hospitals for the cure of the sick, belonging mostly to the untouchable communities.[14]

The real opportunity for the Canadian Baptist missionaries to relieve the sick of all their troubles, came during the famine of 1897.

183

The famine, which was followed by devastating epidemics of cholera and smallpox, created panic in places such as Peddapuram, Chicacole and Tekkali. The Canadian Baptist mission station in Tekkali sent some of their medical missionaries to boost the government's relief programmes. The medical missionaries, in most cases, involved themselves in providing medical support to the untouchables among the Telugus.[15] .

The widespread effect of the famine, especially in the last decade of the nineteenth century, afforded more opportunities to the Canadian Baptists for medical work. In this situation, the missionaries felt that by making arrangements for medical relief, they could substantially increase the number of their followers. Presumably with such objectives in mind, the mission authorities deputed experienced medical missionaries to set up hospitals and dispensaries in the interior. In 1898, under the instructions of the mission, Dr E.G. Smith and his wife, a trained nurse, set up a small hospital at Yellamanchili, close to Vizagapatnam. This hospital, within a short period of time, earned a special reputation for the successful treatment of female patients. The successful treatment of female patients also led to some conversions from the socially ostracized and indigent sections of the society.[16]

However, by the early years of the twentieth century, Pithapuram became the focus of Canadian Baptist medical enterprise. In 1901 Dr E.G. Smith made a short visit to Pithapuram to cure the sick and disease-affected people. This visit turned out to be an important affair, since it substantially broke down the caste opposition to the missionaries. Dr Smith's success in curing the people of their ailments earned a great deal of popularity for the missionaries. Consequently placed in a far more comfortable position compared to that in previous years, the missionaries became more seriously involved in efforts to establish hospitals and dispensaries.[17]

In the following years, the Canadian Baptists were able to enhance their presence at Pithapuram by laying the foundations of the Bethesda hospital. The funds for this hospital were largely provided by two women missionaries from Canada. In the years between 1904 and 1910, construction of missionary and maternity wards on the basis of donations from both India and Canada, added greatly to the size of the hospital. Furthermore, the rise in the number of patients led to the construction of more wards, the funds for which largely came from Indian sources.[18]

The hospitals at Yellamanchili and Pithapuram, apart from serving as centres of medical and evangelical work, also proved to be training institutions for paramedical personnel—for compounders and medical assistants. The compounders, who generally provided medical relief to the lower castes, were made to undergo a vigorous training programme in health care and sanitation. Moreover, they were also imparted special training in spreading the message of the Gospel and the humanitarian aspects of Christianity, particularly among the untouchable communities. Incidentally, such programmes to a large extent accounted for the popularity of the Canadian Baptist missionaries among the socially ostracized communities in the Telugu-speaking eastern coastal districts of Madras Presidency.[19]

The expansion of medical work, however, posed a few challenges to the Canadian Baptists. Their close connections with the 'untouchable' castes made them increasingly aware of the need to start strong campaigns in favour of temperance. At the same time, there was also a realization that hospitals and dispensaries under women medical missionaries needed to be established, in order to gain wider acceptability among women. In other words, it was felt that through the successful treatment of female patients, women medical missionaries could open up the possibilities for an absolutely limitless field of 'medical evangelism'. Moreover, the mission authorities also entertained a belief that women medical missionaries alone could break down the caste Hindu opposition towards the treatment of leprosy, that mostly affected people belonging to the untouchable communities.[20]

Interestingly, apart from such ground realities, certain developments in Canada too prepared the ground for the deployment of young women as mission volunteers in India. For instance, the New Women Movement in Canada in the last years of the nineteenth century greatly inspired young women to aspire for careers in mission stations located in different parts of the world.[21] But, most of the women who preferred to serve in the Canadian Baptist mission stations in India in these years seemed to be more interested in *zenana* work, bible missions and educational programmes. Dr Pearl Smith and Miss D'Silva were possibly the lone exceptions in this regard. Dr Pearl Smith, who later married Rev. Jessie Chute, was one of the pioneer Canadian Baptist women medical missionaries in south India.[22]

While the debate over the deployment of women medical

missionaries continued, some women medical practitioners expressed their preference to serve in mission stations in India. In 1904, Dr Gertrude Hulet, a Canadian Baptist woman medical missionary, on her own initiative, began medical relief operations in Vuyyuru in Krishna district. She purchased land with financial assistance from a friend for the purpose of setting up a hospital and a dispensary. Later, this hospital turned out to be a centre of medical relief and Gospel work.[23]

Dr Hulet's efforts were emulated in the following years by several women medical missionaries. In fact, the rising number of female patients encouraged a substantial number of women medical missionaries to seek positions in the hospitals run by the Canadian Baptists in the eastern coastal Telugu-speaking districts. In 1910, the Canadian Baptist mission authorities, in keeping with the sentiments of the women medical missionaries, appointed Dr Jessie Allyn as in-charge of the Bethesda hospital. She was also instructed to undertake programmes that would be of benefit to the female patients. Dr Allyn's sincerity attracted the attention of both upper- and lower-caste women in Pithapuram. The services rendered by her to the Rani during her childbirth also brought her into close contact with the Rajah of Pithapuram. As a mark of appreciation for her services, the Rajah and Rani presented a purse of $3000 to start a Women's Hospital and Home for Nurses.[24] Financial assistance and support from the Rajah were also utilized by the Canadian Baptist women missionaries to set up training centres for imparting the techniques of western medical science to Indian nurses.[25]

By the 1910s, the active support and encouragement of the mission authorities enabled the medical missionaries to emerge successful in their ventures. The efficient functioning of the surgical and out-patient departments in the hospitals also evoked a great deal of public support for the missionaries. The expertise displayed by the medical missionaries in diagnosing and treating various types of diseases led to a breakdown of popular superstitions and prejudices. In most cases, as advocates of western medical science, the missionaries successfully countered the challenges posed by 'sorcerers' and traditional medical practitioners. The women medical missionaries mounted a spirited campaign among the outcaste demon worshippers to vindicate the point that, as followers of Jesus Christ, they had the power to protect the people from the evil designs of the spirits.[26] The efforts of the missionaries sometimes bore fruit since, after successful treatment of diseases, the 'outcastes' promised to use western medicine and made pledges that they would not worship village goddesses in the future.[27]

The devotion displayed by the Canadian Baptist medical missionaries, thus, accounted for their popularity particularly among the Muslims and the untouchable communities. These communities, which for long had been treated with contempt by the upper-caste Hindus, received a great deal of care and support from the missionaries. The sincerity with which the missionaries served the patients from these communities influenced some of the 'untouchable' families to turn to the Gospel for relief and support. In the mission hospitals, many of the 'untouchables' who had been cured of diseases felt strongly about the 'humanitarian aspects of Christianity'. In a sense, the medical missionaries through their services made the socially ostracized communities realize that Christianity represented 'a new God and a new love'.[28]

IV

The First World War years, 1914–18, witnessed a few experiments in the field of higher education. In the beginning such experiments were mainly conducted by individual Protestant denominations. But, within a short period of time, there was a realization in the missionary circles that a single denominational board could not maintain an efficient faculty and provide funds for running schools. Faced with these very practical difficulties, several women's boards of foreign missions decided to come together to cooperate in providing for Union Colleges for women. Such cooperation, it was believed, would make it possible to establish well-equipped institutions. The women's boards in Canada and the United States as well as those from England displayed their eagerness to promote such common projects. By the time the war came to an end, such efforts had led to the establishment of the Vellore Union Medical Missionary School. European missionaries from several Protestant denominations felt that since there were only 150 doctors to serve around 150,000,000 women, such medical schools could turn out a larger number of doctors and medical assistants for the service of humanity. Moreover, it was believed that these institutions could train Indian Christian women, who could act as doctors for their own people.[29]

The Canadian Baptist women, apart from making small

contributions to the Vellore Medical School, sent lady doctors to serve in the Indian mission stations. In 1920, the Women's A.B.F.M. Society sent two sisters, Dr Jessie and Bessie Findlay, who had graduated in medicine from Manitoba University, to serve in India. Subsequently, the initiatives aimed at building up an efficient team of doctors brought the Canadian Baptist women into much closer contact with the American Baptist missionaries. Close relations between the American and the Canadian Baptists were witnessed in 1922 when Dr Allyn temporarily took charge of Vellore from Dr Ida Scudder.[30]

The beginning of the 1920s witnessed a further expansion in the medical relief work of the Canadian Baptists. Both foreign and Indian funds were utilized to construct new buildings, acquire new instruments and promote advanced methods in treatment. Moreover, electrification work was undertaken to improve the efficiency of the hospitals. The Canadian medical missionaries also took the help of Indian and Canadian doctors to carry out temperance and leprosy mission campaigns.[31]

In the early 1920s Canadian women medical missionaries also became greatly involved in efforts to establish outdoor dispensaries. These dispensaries, which were mostly built in temporary sheds, acted as feeders for the hospitals run by the missionaries. The medical missionaries also attended long-distance calls to provide medical relief to the distressed. As a result of such efforts, the caste Hindu opposition that had prevailed over a long period of time underwent a remarkable decline. In most places of the eastern coastal Telugu-speaking districts, racial hatred for the missionaries gave way to a feeling of brotherhood. The selfless service provided by the medical missionaries to the people, irrespective of caste and religious affiliations, proved to be one of the most important factors behind this sort of transformation in the social environment.[32]

The change in the social attitude of the caste Hindus was particularly noticed in the villages of the Ramachandrapuram field of the Canadian Baptist missionaries. In villages like Kotipalli, situated within the field, Indian Christian doctors along with Canadian medical missionaries used western medicines and advanced clinical techniques to cure patients suffering from chronic stomach ailments and diseases like leprosy. The success of the missionaries in healing these diseases sometimes brought about a change in the social scenario, which the missionaries often described as 'revolutionary'. In this context, a

Canadian missionary, drawing an interesting contrast between the medical missionaries and the brahmin priests, observed,

> On one side of the tank are the Brahman priests, modern pirates, washing their hands in the sacred waters to be rid of their sins; on the other side is the Christian doctor, modern representative of the Great Physician, cleansing putrefying sores, healing diseases and treating ills of all sorts, for all conditions of people, then pointing them to the Lamb of God, who takes away the sins of the world.[33]

By the late 1920s, the involvement of the medical missionaries with the treatment of diseases like tuberculosis and leprosy became much more pronounced. The Canadian medical missionaries constructed a big tubercular sanatorium at Rajahmundry to improve the health standards of the rural labouring classes, who mostly came from a depressed-class background.[34] The medical missionaries also renovated the Ramachandrapuram and Vizianagaram leper homes to protect the diseased from all forms of social discrimination. The Ramachandrapuram Leper Home, which received $15,000 as financial assistance from Canada, became a sort of 'model' institution for the treatment of leprosy. The field of service covered by these homes was very large, but they turned out to be surprisingly effective. These homes together accounted for the daily treatment of 175 inmates. Interestingly, the Ramachandrapuram Leper Home, in these years, proved to be one of the most important centres of medical evangelism.[35]

The successes enjoyed by the medical missionaries in the treatment of leprosy paved the way for the large-scale conversion of untouchables to Christianity. In fact, several factors may have been responsible for such a development. Presumably, most of the leprosy-infected patients who were diagnosed as 'burnt-outs' preferred to accept Christianity to escape from social oppression. At the same time, it also needs to be stated that many of the 'cured' embraced Christianity to secure a guaranteed livelihood. In other words, the decision on the part of the Canadian Baptists to employ the 'cured' as mission workers seems to have largely encouraged this trend of conversion.[36]

The closing years of the 1920s witnessed efforts on the part of the Canadian Baptist mission to build up a large body of medical personnel, from among men and women belonging to Indian Christian families. Several educated Telugu Christian women were selected for medical training in Vellore. Also, four Christian men as well as a woman, M. Eviamma Benjamin, were provided financial assistance to complete the graduate medical programme offered by the Union Medical School at Vellore.[37]

V

The economic depression in the early 1930s posed several problems for the Canadian medical missionaries. The hospitals run by them faced severe financial crisis. Their functioning too was affected because of the paucity of trained Indian nurses. Moreover, the normal activities of the medical missionaries was often hampered because they suffered from long periods of illness, caused mostly by the spread of typhoid fever. The widespread effect of cholera epidemics also posed difficulties to the medical missionaries, who were suffering from financial crisis as well as shortage of staff.[38]

However, within a short period of time, the Canadian Baptist mission adopted a series of measures to overcome these problems. Realizing the shortage of trained medical personnel, they recruited some Indian Christian doctors to bring back normalcy in the functioning of their hospitals. The Indian assistant doctors were mostly employed in the hospitals dealing with cases of cholera and maternity. At the same time, in order to curtail the expenditure incurred due to full staffing of hospitals with graduate nurses, the mission instructed women missionaries to introduce practical nursing courses. This measure proved to be of great success in later years.[39]

The onset of the Second World War, however, exposed the missionaries to a new set of problems. Scarcity of materials and high prices made it difficult for them to undertake repair and construction work in the hospitals and dispensaries. In some cases, the missionaries tried to overcome such problems by hiring buildings on rent. Further, in order to meet the shortage of Indian doctors, the medical missionaries tried to mobilize rural women in support of midwifery training programmes. The mission also utilized free trained workers to carry out specialized duties.[40]

Despite these problems, the medical missionaries did commendable work in several spheres. The Canadian missionary nurses utilized the facilities available at the Bathesda hospital in Pithapuram to train a large number of Indian boys and girls in nursing. The Canadian medical missionaries, supported by the health nurses, arranged house-to-house visitations to eradicate leprosy and other forms of skin infection.[41] But it was in the sphere of temperance that they had most success. The medical missionaries, supported by fellow missionaries mostly involved with educational work, undertook temperance propaganda in the villages. They also took the help of Indian pastors and churchmen attached to the field councils, to implement decrees condemning the consumption of alcoholic drinks.[42]

From 1944 onwards, the activities of the Canadian Baptist medical missionaries underwent a decline. With the war showing signs of coming to an end in Europe, many of the medical missionaries expressed their desire to return to Canada. The Canadian missionary nurses and medical technologists serving in the coastal Telugu-speaking districts too expressed similar desires. But, more importantly, it was the huge financial drain caused by the war that impeded much of the humanitarian activities of the medical missionaries. The severe financial crisis of the late 1940s made it difficult for the medical missionaries to provide medical relief almost free of cost. They also faced difficulties in procuring stocks of medicine and linen. As a consequence, the medical facilities in the hospitals run by them declined. Subsequently, with the Government of India introducing special rural health-care programmes, the missionary hospitals faced a stiff challenge from government-run institutions. Thus, in order to survive in this situation, the Canadian medical missionaries preferred to amalgate their hospitals and pool their resources in closer unity.[43]

VI

The narrative dealing with the activities of the medical missionaries belonging to the Canadian Baptist mission reveals beyond all doubt the importance of 'medical evangelism'. In fact, the mission literature of the Canadian Baptists, since the early decades of the twentieth century, are replete with stories of medical mission work, which was believed to be 'the most humane and the most necessary of all social service'.[44] Apart from such stout defence of medical mission work, there were frequent assertions that medical missionaries combining the rare elements of religion and medicine could be the most effective catalysts for mass conversions.

However, it is extremely doubtful as to whether the Canadian medical missionaries endowed with such double qualities could act as effective facilitators in the complex process of mass conversion. It needs to be understood that in India medical mission work rarely succeeded in creating situations for mass conversions.[45] In most cases, the Canadian medical missionaries, like their Protestant counterparts, had to be content with a few cases of conversions that took place within the mission hospitals. The Canadian medical missionaries, it may also be recalled, met with very little success in converting the upper castes to Christianity. Their successes by and large were confined to the leprosy-infected patients undergoing treatment in their leper homes.[46]

Nevertheless, the Canadian Baptist mission sent well-qualified doctors, started medical training centres, and established hospitals and dispensaries, particularly in areas that needed medical relief from infectious and contagious diseases like typhoid and cholera. At the same time, they achieved considerable success in the spheres of maternity and child care.[47] But, despite their usefulness, the scale of medical relief provided by the missionaries was far smaller than that of government institutions. For instance, in the early 1920s, the numerical strength of the Canadian Baptist medical institutions was indeed minuscule compared to the government-run institutions. To be precise, compared to 2,500 government hospitals and dispensaries, the Canadian Baptists maintained eight hospitals and nearly 100 small dispensaries.[48]

Despite their limited scale of operations, however, the medical missionary-run hospitals outshone the government-run institutions in terms of treatment and health care, and in the use of modern medical techniques and equipment. The increasing number of appointments of women medical missionaries also gave the Canadian Baptists a distinct edge. The qualities of sympathy, motherliness and self-forgetting service demonstrated by the women missionaries accounted for their remarkable success in treating patients.[49] Significantly, without the financial contributions of the missionary women's societies in Canada, the Canadian Baptist mission would not have been able to undertake large-scale programmes in favour of temperance and eradication of leprosy.[50]

More importantly, it needs to be understood that the Canadian medical missionaries had to toil hard to gain social recognition for their work. In the early years of the twentieth century, traditional aversion to western medicine and the vituperative anti-missionary campaigns launched by the brahmin priests and lower-caste 'sorcerers' too often impeded their progress. In the subsequent decades, the successful treatment of infectious diseases on the part of medical missionaries considerably countered the popular aversion towards western medical science. By the early 1920s, the sincerity and devotion displayed by the medical missionaries attracted a substantial section of the rural population of the Telugu-speaking eastern coastal districts towards the mission hospitals. There were an increasing number of patients willing to undergo treatment in the mission hospitals, which practised the principles of western medical science.[51] Although the Canadian medical missionaries only touched the peripheries of the Telugu society, they were able to establish that they too, like the Indian seers, believed in soul-service and in the universal brotherhood of man.[52]

Notes and References

[1] Yuet-Wah Cheung, *Missionary Medicine in China: A Study of Two Protestant Missions in China*, Lanham, 1988, p. 3.

[2] For more details see, Mary Pauline Jeffrey, *Ida S. Scudder of Vellore: An Appreciation of Forty Years of Service in India*, Mysore, 1939, pp. 13–17; D. Clarke Willson, *The Story of Dr Ida Scudder of Vellore*, London, 1959, pp. 83–87.

[3] Rosemary Fitzgerald, 'Clinical Christianity: The Emergence of Medical Work as a Missionary Strategy in Colonial India, 1800–1914' in Biswamoy Pati and Mark Harrison (eds.), *Health, Medicine and Empire: Perspectives on Colonial India*, Hyderabad, 2001, p. 89.

[4] Dr Ernest F. Neve, *A Crusader in Kashmir: Being the Life of Dr Arthur Neve, with an account of the Medical Missionary Work of Two Brothers and its later developments down to the present day*, London, 1928, p. 14.

[5] Incidentally, since the early decades of the nineteenth century, missionaries had tried to establish a relationship between Christianization and Civilization. The missionaries essentially based their analysis on the biblical concept of sin. The backward state of non-European cultures was interpreted in terms of sin. It was widely felt that the Gospel alone could not only transform individuals, but make communities, societies and states happy. In a sense, according to this sort of thinking, the hope of the backward non-European peoples lay in conversion to Christianity. For more details see, Dr Ernest F. Neve, *A Crusader in Kashmir*, pp. 68–70. Also see, J. Simensen, *Norwegian Mission in African History, Vol. I. South Africa, 1845–1906*, Oslo, 1988, pp. 36–38.

[6] Sundararaj Manickam, *The Social Setting of Christian Conversion in South India*, Weisbden, 1977, pp. 169–70.

[7] The Christian missionaries believed that since Christ had been deeply involved with the suffering humanity, hospitals and refuges needed to be built for the care of people infected with different diseases. In this context, the missionaries were greatly influenced by one of the sermons of Christ—

'Heal the sick and say unto them, The Kingdom of God is nigh to you.' For more details see, Dr Ernest F. Neve, *A Crusader in Kashmir*, pp. 71–72; Sundararaj Manickam, *The Social Setting of Christian Conversion*.

[8] Orville E. Daniel, *Rising Tides in India* (*A profile of the past and present*), emphasized the compelling need and opportunity to consolidate the Christian church in India, with particular reference to an area on the southeastern coast, where Canadian Baptist missionaries have served for nearly a century. Also see *The Calcutta Christian Observer*, Vol. V, 1836, p. 362.

[9] For more details see, Rev. M.L. Orchard and K.S. Malaurin, *The Enterprise* (*The Jubilee Story of the Canadian Baptist Mission in India 1874–1924*), Toronto, 1924, p. 147; Orville E. Daniel, *Rising Tides in India*, p. 71; T.S. Shenston, 'Teloogoo Mission Scrap Book' [microfilm], Brantford, 1888, p. 45.

[10] Rev. W. Gordon Carder, *Hand to the Indian Plow*, Vishakapatnam, 1976, p. 44; also see, M.B. Diwakar, 'An Investigation into the Historical Antecedents of the Crisis in the Convention of the Baptist Churches of Northern Circars during 1972–74' (unpublished dissertation, United Theological College, Bangalore), 1978, p. 1.

[11] Orville E. Daniel, *Rising Tides in India*, pp. 74–75.

[12] Rev. W. Gorden Carder, *Hand to the Indian Plow*, pp. 60–61, 84.

[13] In the 1880s, the women missionaries laid the foundation of *zenana* work in towns like Coconada and Samalkot. The *zenana* mission was considered to be an effective mechanism for the evangelization of the rural areas of south India. For more details, see Rev. W Gordon Carder, ibid., p. 125. Also see, Rev. M.L. Orchard and K.S. McLaurin, *The Enterprise*, p. 59.

[14] *Mission Handbook*, Baptist Foreign Missionary Society, Toronto, 1895, p. 13.

[15] For more details see, *Report of the Canadian Baptist Telugu Mission*, Coconada, 1897, p. 23.

[16] The Canadian Baptists reported that those who were cured believed that the changes in their fortune had been brought about by Christianity. Interestingly, at the time of their discharge from the hospital they carried away tracts and Gospel portions, and even requested the medical missionaries to write a verse of the scripture on their prescriptions. See Rev. M.L. Orchard and K.S. McLaurin, *The Enterprise*.

[17] Ibid.

[18] Ibid., p. 249. Also see, Rev. W. Gordon Carder, *Hand to the Indian Plow*, p. 145; *Among the Telugus and Bolivians—Report of the Canadian Baptist Foreign Mission Board on the Indian and Bolivian Fields with Directory and Statistics*, Toronto, 1943, p. 12.

[19] Rev. M.L. Orchard and K.S. McLaurin, *The Enterprise*.

[20] Rev. M.L. Orchard, *Canadian Baptists at Work in India*, Toronto, 1922, pp. 143–45; Report of the Canadian Baptist Telugu Missions for 1899 (Twenty-Third Annual Conference held in Coconada, 12–16 January 1900) Madras, 1900, p. 38.

[21] For more details see, Ruth Compton Brouwer, *New Women for God:*

Canadian Presbyterian Women and Indian Missions, 1876–1914, Toronto, 1990, pp. 19–21.

22 Rev. W. Gordon Carder, *Hand to the Indian Plow*, p. 145. Also see, Rev. John Craiq and Miss Helena Blaackador, *Beacon Lights*, Toronto, 1914, p. 110.

23 Rev. M. L. Orchard and K.S. McLaurin, *The Enterprise*, pp. 251–52.

24 Rev. W. Gordon Carder, *Hand to the Indian Plow*, pp. 251–52.

25 Ibid., p. 250.

26 Rev. M.L. Orchard, *Canadian Baptists at Work in India*, pp. 132–33.

27 Ibid., p. 133.

28 Ibid., p. 135. For more details, see Seventh Annual Report of the Canadian Baptist Foreign Mission Board, Covering the Work of the Year 1917–18, n.d. (Divinity School Archives, McMaster University, Canada), p. 31

29 Rev. M.L. Orchard, *Canadian Baptists at Work in India*, p. 146.

30 Ibid., p. 147.

31 The successes of the Vizianagaram Leper Mission encouraged the Canadian Baptists to start leper homes in Ramachandrapuram. The Canadian Baptists utilized the services of an Indian Christian doctor, Dr Joshee, to provide medical support to the lepers. Dr Joshee, who had been trained in the Agra Medical School, was ably assisted by Dr Massee of the National School of Medicine at Calcutta. The Canadian Baptists also utilized the services of Indian doctors Jarvis and Krupa Rao Chowdhuri, to bring about an improvement in the functioning of the surgical departments in the hospitals. For more details, see Eleventh Annual Report of the Canadian Baptist Foreign Mission Board Covering the Work of the Year 1921–22, n.d. (Divinity School Archives, McMaster University, Canada), p. 30; Canadian Baptist Missionary Conference in India, Eighth Annual Conference (held at Coconada, India, 31 December 1919 to 9 January 1920) Madras, 1920, p. 25; Rev. M.L. Orchard, *Canadian Baptists at Work in India*, p. 137.

32 Rev. M.L. Qrchard and K.S. Mclaurin, *The Enterprise*, p. 302.

33 Rev. M.L. Orchard, *Canadian Baptists at Work in India*, p. 139.

34 Mary S. Mc Laurin, *25 Years On, 1924–1949* (with an introduction by Mrs Albert Mathews), Toronto, n.d., pp. 95, 103. Also see, Canadian Baptist Missionary Conference in India, Eighteenth Annual Conference (held at Coconada between 28 December 1929 to 3 January 1930), Madras, 1930, p. 21.

35 Rev. M.L. Orchard and K.S. McLaurin, *The Enterprise*, p. 303. For more details see, Canadian Baptist Missionary Conference in India (Twentieth Semi-Annual Conference held at Coconada between 3–9 July 1931), Madras, 1931, pp. 15–16.

36 In the Ramachandrapuram Leper Home a Canadian woman missionary, Miss S.I. Hatch, with the help of a mission doctor, Dr Augustine, spread the message of the Gospel among the lepers. In fact, about 400 out of the 1,000 who had passed through the Ramachandrapuram institutions accepted Christianity. In Vizianagaram, eight from different castes were baptised. At the same time, the missionaries also stated that relatives of the several high-

caste people who had been saved carried the message of Christianity to the villages that had been out of the reach of the missionary preachers and bible women. For more details see, Rev. M.L. Orchard and K.S. McLaurin, *The Enterprise*, p. 304. Also see Canadian Baptist Missionary Conference in India, Twentieth Semi-Annual Conference, p. 16.

37 Nineteenth Annual Report of the Canadian Baptist Foreign Mission Board, 1929–30 (Divinity School Archives McMaster University, Canada), n.d. p. 15. For more details see, Canadian Baptist Missionary Conference in India (Seventeenth Semi-Annual Conference held at Coconada, between 11–18 July 1928), Madras, pp. 2–3.

38 Mary S. McLaurin, *25 Years On*, p. 100.

39 Ibid., p. 101.

40 Ibid., p. 102.

41 Ibid., p. 104.

42 Minutes of the Telugu–Oriya Council of the Canadian Baptist Mission (Tenth Annual Meeting, No. 10, held in Coconada between 9–14 July 1943), Coconada, 1943, p. 4.

43 Mary S. McLaurin, *25 Years On*, p. 105.

44 Rev. M.L. Orchard, *Canadian Baptists at Work in India*, p. 129.

45 Historians like Dick Kooiman have pointed out that one should not be misled by the missionary accounts dealing with conversions, arising out of medical mission work. He argues that famines and other cases of emergency merely created a kind of 'rush hour' in situations where religious transgressions were believed to have been frequent. More recently, scholars like Rosemary Fitzgerald and Koji Kawashina have pointed out that missionaries hardly succeeded in generating large-scale conversions, involving both the higher and the lower castes in the society. For more details see, Dick Kooiman, 'Mass Movements, Famine and Epidemic: A Study in Interrelationship', *Modern Asian Studies*, Vol. 25, No. 2, 1991, p. 299; also see, Rosemary Fitzgerald, 'Clinical Christianity', p. 129; Koji Kawashima, *Missionaries and Hindu State, Travancore: 1858–1936*, Delhi, 1998, p. 147.

46 The Canadian missionaries, it needs to be argued, rarely disclosed the names of their upper-caste converts and the upper-caste inhabited villages which had embraced Christianity. In most cases, the information relating to the conversion of the upper castes remained scanty. This is well brought out in the narratives left behind by the Canadian Baptist missionaries, notably M.L. Orchard and K.S. McLaurin. For more details see, Rev. M.L. Orchard and K.S. McLaurin, *The Enterprise*; also see, Rev. M.L. Orchard, *Canadian Baptists at Work in India*.

47 During the First World War years, the Canadian missionaries devoted their energies especially towards child care. In these years, since the annual child mortality rate was close to 1,500,000, the Canadian missionaries became involved in setting up child welfare departments, with government assistance. Canadian medical missionaries like Dr Cameron also started milk depots. See, Rev. M.L. Orchard, *Canadian Baptists at Work in India*, p. 143.

[48] For more details see, Rev. M.L. Orchard, ibid., pp. 130–31; also see, Mary S. McLaurin, *25 Years On*, p. 25.

[49] The slogan of the Canadian Baptist mission, 'Women's work for women', not only broadened the scope of missionary propaganda, but also brought women missionaries into closer contact with women in the rural areas. See, Rev. M.L. Orchard and K.S. McLaurin, *The Enterprise*, p. 225.

[50] In the years between 1876–77 and 1921–22, the women's societies raised a total of $611, 692. At the same time, during these years they also sent thirty-five missionaries. For more details see, Rev. M.L. Orchard and K.S. McLaurin, ibid., p. 226.

[51] In the early 1920s, hospitals run by the Canadian medical missionaries catered to more than 3,000 in-patients. They also provided medical relief to 49,000 out-patients. See, Rev. M.L. Orchard, *Canadian Baptists at Work in India*, p. 131.

[52] Interestingly, the missionaries, in order to compete with Gandhi's campaigns in favour of 'soul-service', wrote couplets:

'In Christ there is no East or West
In Him no South or North,
But one great fellowship of love
Throughout the whole wide earth
In Him shall true hearts everywhere
Their high communion find,
His service is the golden cord
Close binding all mankind.'
See Rev. M.L. Orchard, *Canadian Baptists at Work in India*, p. 141.

Disciplining the Body?

Health Care for Women and Children in Early Twentieth-Century Bengal

Sujata Mukherjee

Gender-specific imperial medical intervention in colonial India was given a new direction in the period following the First World War. Apart from the curative practice of hospital medicine, intrusive health education for mothers and children, organization of baby shows, and publicity and sale of medical literature developed as part of the programme for making individuals aware of health issues. As has been pointed out, 'after an earlier focus on the medicalization of child-birth which sought to provide scientific training for midwives and to establish facilities such as maternity hospitals with specialized obstetricians, the emphasis was now shifting to the extension of ante and post natal care to mothers and children.'[1] Although this health programme was initially launched and funded by non-government organizations run predominantly by wives of viceroys and other European ladies, the involvement and cooperation of local governments were gradually forthcoming. The post-World War period saw popularization of health education through celebration of health weeks, health talks by supervisors who often visited homes of school children, medical inspection (at schools, etc.), film shows, exhibitions, etc.

This paper is a preliminary attempt at examining the health conditions of women and children and the activities of private organizations of Europeans, as well as the administrative measures adopted by the government in the sphere of health care for mothers and children in early twentieth-century Bengal. Official health intervention for providing maternity benefits in mines, jute mills and plantations have received some amount of scholarly attention.[2] The work of wives of viceroys in the sphere of maternal and child care have been interpreted by scholars as examples of racist benevolence which served to provoke nationalist resentment.[3] Yet, an analysis of these activities in the sphere of health care for women and children in early twentieth-century India may provide important insights into the question of how far perspectives on health issues for women (and children) changed, and whether this was related to the larger question of a transformation and shift in the nature of imperial medical intervention in colonial India.

Indian Women and the Growth of Western Medical Care

Nineteenth-century India witnessed the growing patronage of western medicine and a gradual undermining of indigenous medical systems by the colonial state.[4] It has been argued by scholars like Radhika Ramasubban that western medicine, as it developed at least until 1900, remained largely confined to a small enclave of white residents and soldiers.[5] David Arnold has suggested that in the first half of the nineteenth century, in an essentially male-oriented and male-operated system of medicine, the primary areas of concern were the army, jails and hospitals—exclusively male domains.[6] Hospitals and dispensaries partly funded by the state and also sponsored to a large extent by enthusiastic Indians, became—albeit in a limited way—centres for vaccination against smallpox and for the dissemination of western ideas about sanitation and hygiene.

The triumph of the Anglicists in 1835 led to the abolition of teaching in indigenous medicine in the Native Medical Institution (founded in 1822), Sanskrit College and the Calcutta Madrasa, but the colonial state continued to utilize the services of medical personnel acquainted with native drugs. Indian compounders were appointed in almost all the charitable dispensaries in Bengal. The government of Bengal, from time to time, drew up schemes for employing the native male *kaviraj* to popularize western medicine (alongside the use of indigenous drugs) at the village level. There were about ten to fifteen *tikadars* (inoculators) who practised in 1830. Their number rose to thirty in 1844, and to 68 by 1850.[7] In 1907, the Director General of the IMS agreed to the proposal of giving commissioners of different districts all over India a free hand to permit municipal and local boards to choose and employ *vaids* and *hakeems*. There is, however, no evidence of any attempt on the part of the colonial government to utilize the services of female practitioners of traditional medicine in the growing sphere of public health services, though Indian women depended on these practitioners for medical care on a large scale.[8] The Census of

1881 recorded the number of such practitioners to be 812.

From 1870 there was a change in government policy and dispensaries were left to depend increasingly on local revenues. Hospitals were established through private initiatives of persons like Pestonji Hormusji Kama, a wealthy Parsi, who offered huge subscriptions to establish a hospital for women and children. In 1883 Dr Edith Pechey came to India from England to join the new hospital; she was followed by Dr Annette Benson and Dr Eliza Turner Watts.[9] In the 1880s different medical colleges in the three Presidencies opened their doors to female students. During the same time, in Bengal, 'there were attempts to make dispensaries more acceptable to Indian women otherwise prevented from attending by the seclusion of purdah'.[10] The total number of dispensaries in Bengal rose from 61 in 1867 to over 500 in 1900; but in 1871, only 18 per cent of the patients attending dispensaries were women. According to modern researchers, although the number of women attending dispensaries rose by the turn of the century, it was 'simply a function of the growing number of such institutions in the province'.[11] The total number of female patients treated at the indoor and outdoor departments of Calcutta medical institutions rose from 41,217 in 1886 to 44,370 in 1899. The number of children treated fell from 65,003 to 53,022 during the same period. Female beds in indoor departments rose from 428 in 1891 to 473 in 1897, while the number of male beds rose from 1,248 to 1,662 in 1897.[12]

The colonial state's first intervention in the field of Indian women's health came in 1868, in the form of the Contagious Diseases' Act, which was designed to protect the soldiers from venereal diseases by regulating the treatment of prostitutes.[13] While the state's role in the sphere of providing health care for women in India remained marginal, the hegemonic ambitions of western medicine were represented by the activities of women missionaries from England and the United States, who came to India from the 1860s onward, and established hospitals, dispensaries and training centres for midwives and nurses. The 1880s also saw the entry of Indian women in medical colleges in India and abroad. A Brahmo lady Kadambini Basu, one of the first women graduates in the British empire (the other was Chandramukhi Basu), took admission in the Calcutta Medical College in 1883 and was awarded the GBMC (Graduate of Bengal Medical College) degree in 1886.[14] Anandibai Joshi graduated in the same year from the Women's Medical College in Philadelphia.[15]

The first systematic and regular attempt to provide western medical help to Indian women started in 1885, with the establishment of the Dufferin Fund or the National Association for Supplying Female Medical Aid to the Women of India. Mary Scarlieb and Elizabeth Bielby (a missionary doctor at Lahore) personally met and informed Queen Victoria about the lack of medical care for Indian women, and the queen asked Lady Dufferin, the new vicereine, to investigate into the scope for providing medical help to Indian women. The Dufferin Fund was established in August 1885, with three aims: to provide medical teaching and training to women; to organize medical relief; to supply female nurses and midwives to hospitals and private homes.[16] The wives of other viceroys followed the example set by Lady Dufferin. The Victoria Memorial Scholarship Fund was set up by Lady Curzon in 1903.

It has been pointed out that the work of women missionaries, wives of British officials and western-educated Indians brought the issues of women's health and reform of the indigenous process of birthing onto the public arena.[17] The medical model which developed in late nineteenth-century India treated female patients mainly for problems associated with generativity;[18] moreover, it mainly tried to extend medical help to respectable , *pardanashin* women, who were unlikely to seek medical help provided by men.[19] Meredith Borthwick has argued that even respectable women, or Hindu *bhadramahila*, were treated by *vaidyas* or Ayurvedic physicians.[20] It has been pointed out that Duff hospitals 'were to be staffed and run by women, and out-fitted with the necessary curtains, partitions, and separate entrances to allow the *pardanashin* to observe all rules of sex segregation'.[21] By 1907, more than two million women a year were being treated at institutions wholly or partly funded by the Dufferin committees.

Disease and Mortality among Women and Children

The health of European women (and children) in India commanded special attention since the early nineteenth century, as their condition was considered as a marker of European vulnerability to the Indian climate. It was thought that European women had to endure greater physical hardships than their Indian counterparts because of the destructive effects of a tropical climate on the European constitution. They were thought to be particularly susceptible to the influence of tropical climates. High mortality among European children was also a constant source of anxiety among the Anglo–Indians. The chief causes of death among European children appear to have been 'convulsions', diarrhoea and 'debility'.[22] Recent researches have pointed out that environmental sanitary measures, including supply of pure water, removal of excreta and refuse, checking overcrowding and providing ventilation, meant for 'creating little islands of purity in the miasmatic landscape of India in order to protect the health of both soldiers and administratively important civilians therein', had considerable effect on reducing sickness and mortality among soldiers as well as women and children of the British army in India from the late nineteenth century.[23] The death rate for soldiers, children and women recorded a considerable decline between 1870 and 1903. Mortality figures among European women were however higher than among men; in 1889 the death rate among European women in India was just over twenty per 1,000, and among children, just over forty-eight per 1,000. In comparison, the mortality rates of European soldiers declined to sixteen per 1,000. Official records show that the diseases that most affected the death rate of European women in India were puerperal fever, phthisis and enteric fever.[24]

From the late nineteenth century onwards, the high rate of infant mortality in India drew the attention of the press in Britain. Journalist Mary Frances Billington wrote in the 1890s that infant mortality was very high in India mainly due to the ignorance of the *dais*. The infant death rate in England around 1870 was 162. It came down to 96 in 1917, and in 1920 it was as low as 80 per 1,000. In contrast, during the first two decades of the twentieth century in Bengal, one in five babies died before the first birthday. In many of the large towns in England the infant death rate was below 70 in 1919, and in some of the smaller towns even below 50. In contrast to this, it was found that in India 'there is scarcely a large town in which the infant mortality rate is not higher than 200 and in many of the larger towns it is more than 400'.[25] The report of Dagmer Curjel recorded in 1920 a 49 per cent survival rate among infants in Bengal. In 1921 infant mortality rates were still on the increase and were, even among the *bhadralok*, double the corresponding proportions in European countries.[26] It was reported in 1940 that infant mortality was higher in Bengal than in any other province except the Central Provinces, Orissa and Burma.[27] The British officials claimed that the practices of traditional Indian mid-

202

wives and unhygienic environment were mainly responsible for the unusually high rate of infant mortality in Bengal.[28] British critics also focussed on the prevalent practices of child marriage and consummation immediately after puberty as other reasons behind the high maternal and infant mortality in Bengal. In 1909, Major W.W. Clemensha, Sanitary Commissioner of Bengal, pointed out: 'Out of 2,700 children that die within the first month (in Calcutta), more than 1,200 or nearly 50 per cent come under the hands of premature birth and debility at birth . . . probably early marriage is the preponderating factor.'[29] In 1920–21, female mortality was over 5 per cent as against the male mortality rate of 3.3 per cent. It was also noted that 'there is a phenomenal excess of female mortality in Bengal during the first part of a woman's reproductive age period'.[30]

The Age of Consent Committee (1928–29) found that the birth rate in Bengal was considerably lower than in any other province, and came to the conclusion that this was due to early sexual intercourse and the subsequent emaciation of women. British administrators, who emphasized poor hygiene and 'curious' practices, however admitted that poverty was important among the causes of infant and maternal deaths, particularly among the labouring classes. Women who were malnourished and overworked could not give birth to or bring up healthy and strong children. Anaemia during childbirth and chronic calcium deficiency resulting from strenuous pregnancies were major problems.[31] Diseases such as lung infections, bronchitis, diarrhoea and measles—which caused most of the deaths of children between one month and one year—were closely related to poverty, especially to inadequate housing, clothing and sanitation. In some official reports, the causes of maternal and juvenile deaths and poor health were traced to social customs, unhygienic environment, malnutrition, dirty midwifery and untrained midwives.[32]

There was also a clear link between the survival of the infant and the occupation of the father. It seemed that children of professional fathers had a 'clearly higher chance of survival' than children of peasants. Among non-middle-class people, direct access to land and food was important for infant health. Those without access, such as artisans and, in particular, domestic servants, suffered higher rates of infant motality—20 per cent higher than the average in the latter case.

The Bengali witnesses before the Age of Consent Committee, including women doctors and health workers, pointed out that the low birth rate accompanied by high infant mortality was due to the malnutrition of overworked women and the economic decline of the province. In addition, they argued, it was not the mother's age at birth that exhausted women but the high frequency of births. Scarcity and the high price of cow's milk were also blamed for infant mortality. The nationalist press criticized the government for supply of poor-quality milk to places like the Calcutta Medical College Hospital, and also for their reluctance to do anything to reform the bad housing conditions in Calcutta.[33]

Medical Care and Health Education for Women and Children in the Early twentieth Century

The concept and pattern of medical care seems to have undergone a shift in India in the twentieth century. In the nineteenth century, the predominant model for public health was hospital medicine, concentrating on symptoms and signs that together configured a pathology. This model maintained its influence in twentieth-century British India, but gradually a new paradigm, surveillance medicine, developed. Surveillance medicine moved the attention of medicine from pathological bodies to each and every member of the population. Health education developed as an important aspect of the public health care system and as a component of surveillance medicine. It has been argued that

> professional health visitors represented the movement of western medical care and the state into Indian homes; maternal and child welfare centres, often collaborators of local governments and private philanthropists, were be permanent sites for primarily preventive and only secondarily curative work for infants and education of their mothers, primarily of lower social and economic classes.[34]

In the changing international scenario of the early twentieth century, improvements in maternal and infant health became matters of worldwide interest. Increasing imperial rivalries and anxieties about the future health condition of the children of the army, to some extent, prompted certain measures aimed at improving the health of mothers and children. England witnessed a steep downward trend in infant mortality between 1903 and 1908. According to scholars, these years of transition coincided with 'the real take-off of the health visiting movement, and it is reasonable to conclude that the movement did have a sizeable impact on the infant death rate.'[35] High rates of sickness amongst British soldiers during the Boer War pointed to the necessity of adopting health measures to reduce infant mortality and diseases among the working class (since most of the army recruits belonged to this class), in order to increase the efficiency of the troops and the workforce in the face of steep international rivalries.

The twentieth century also witnessed the growing importance of personal or individual hygiene in place of older ideas of macro-sanitation and public hygiene in public health measures. While in the later model individuals were considered as irrational beings incapable of inculcating healthy domestic practices or pursuing elevated standards of personal or domestic habits, in the twentieth century a strong effort was made towards health education of individuals for improving personal hygiene. One important fall-out of this hygienic model was the increased influence of eugenics societies, which placed stress on biological fitness and purity of race. Women's role as natural biological reproducers and conscious mothers of healthy children was strongly emphasized. It has been pointed out by scholars that the expansion of the middle-class family ideal, with the mother as the home-maker and father as the provider, was at the core of public health projects of the early twentieth century, including the Child Welfare Movement.[36]

In India, organization of baby shows and welfare exhibitions, and distribution of prizes and rewards for childcare became part of the programmes arranged by Dufferin hospitals and of some vicereines, including Lady Reading.[37] Private philanthropic organizations as well as public health administration were geared to meet the supposedly crying needs of Indian women and children for maternal and infant benefits. Public health education, child welfare centres and baby shows were patterned on the western model which would supposedly provide better health and a longer life-span for women and children. The Lady Chelmsford All India League for Maternity and Child Welfare, established in 1919, coordinated the maternal and child benefit activitites in all the provinces of British India. With its headquarters at the Viceregal Lodge in Simla, it was intended to act as a central agency for collecting information regarding child welfare and to train lady health visitors. In July 1923, the Public Health Commissioner of the Government of India sent out the programme for a National Health Week, as formulated by Professor Bostock Hill in England with the suggestion that such a programme be adopted in India and held in October 1923, when National Health Week was observed in England.[38] Although there are references to scattered baby weeks being held in India during the late 1910s, the first National Health and Baby Week occurred in 1924. The Baby Week Movement was inaugurated in 1924 throughout Bengal as part of an all-India movement. The Indian Red Cross Society Welfare Division, opened in January by Lady Lytton, took part in it. Lectures and exhibitions were organized in different districts to celebrate baby weeks. In the same year, the government of Bengal formed a Child Welfare Committee by a resolution of 1919; it was made permanent in 1921. The committee recommended, among other things, education of *dais*. The government made annual grants to the local authorities for providing training to nurses and *dais* in different hospitals.

One of the most important activities of the Lady Chelmsford All India League for Maternity and Child Welfare was publication of literature for sale on maternity and child welfare subjects; it was the only organization involved in this kind of publication. Another important activity of the League was supporting health schools in different provinces. The Bengal School for Welfare Workers was started in 1924 and eight students were trained in the inaugural year. The Countess of Lytton, as president of the League, in her address on the occasion of the inauguration of the school and a hostel, emphasized the importance of selection and training of suitable people to become health visitors, 'as the establishment of Welfare Centres was in its infancy and pioneers had to be especially capable'. Of the eight students who successfully completed their training in the first year, 'two students of the English course will have charge of Welfare Centres being opened up in jute mills, one has charge of a Calcutta Indian Baby Clinic. Of the students of the vernacular course, three have charge of Calcutta Indian Baby Clinic, one has returned to Dacca.' The school budget was met entirely by voluntary contributions and it was regretted that the local government did not come forward to give financial help.[39]

The 1920s also saw inauguration of school hygiene work in Bengal. In 1920, a School Hygiene Branch of the Bengal Sanitary Department was opened to look after the health of school boys and girls. It comprised one deputy sanitary commissioner, one medical inspector, and one medical inspectress of schools. Medical inspection and diagnosis of sick school children were carried out from 1928 in Calcutta by school medical officers. A large number of students were found to be suffering from malnutrition, eye problems, throat problems, skin disease, enlarged spleens, etc. As part of school hygiene work, visits by health workers to school children's homes were introduced. It was reported in 1945 that a nurse attached to the students' clinic opened during 1934–35 by the administrative office of the School Health Division visited the homes of school children and notified the parents about the health of the children and also delivered health talks.

In the 1920s, the Health Publicity and Propaganda Branch of the Public Health Department of Bengal gradually expanded to carry out extensive works including organization of magic lantern shows, film shows, etc. By 1928 films were regarded as the best propaganda instrument. The Ward Health Associations of the Calcutta Corporation arranged lantern lectures and exhibitions to educate mothers on health care for themselves as well as their children. Health films dealing with, among other subjects, maternity and child welfare, were produced and shown by the Bengal Public Health Department.[40] Health talks were broadcast from the Calcutta station of the All India Radio on subjects like diseases among women, infant mortality and nursing.

The Public Health Department of the government of Bengal, apart from carrying out publicity and propaganda work, assisted in the activities of different organizations involved in arranging Calcutta Health Week Exhibitions, focussing on subjects like women's health and child welfare. Government financial aid was given to some of the voluntary associations, like the Bengal Health Welfare Committee of the Provincial Branch of the Indian Red Cross Society and the Saroj Nalini Dutt Memorial Association, connected with maternal and child welfare work.

Internationally, debates on maternity benefits were initiated at the Convention of the International Labour Conference held in Washington in October 1919. It suggested several maternal benefits for the female workforce in industrial and commercial establishments. In the jute mill areas of Bengal, a novel scheme was introduced to educate pregnant women as well as midwives about child care. In March 1928 the Maternity and Child Welfare Centre of the Titagar mills offered the service of a qualified health supervisor, and started instruction classes for expectant mothers and midwives, as well as baby clinics. Following this example, other jute mills also started similar educative classes during the 1920s.

Initially, events like baby shows were condemned as being an insult to Indian motherhood by a section of the nationalist Bengali press. However, in the period following the first World War, nationalist politics encouraged Indian women activists to organize baby shows and work for improvements in the conditions of childbirth. As has been argued by Judy Whitehead, through their social reform proposals, the colonized middle classes sought, by the 1920s, 'to project themselves as the legitimate heirs of "the nation", pitted against a colonial bureaucracy increasingly wary of alienating its narrowing base of political support'.[41] Associations formed by middle-class women organized social work including child and maternal welfare in different parts of the province. At an all-India level, the Women's Indian Association was formed in 1917 in Madras by Margaret Cousins, an Irish feminist, theosophist and musician, and Dorothy Jinarajadasa, also an Irish feminist. Membership was opened to both Indians and Europeans. The WIA's monthly journal, *Stri Dharma*, launched in 1918, was published in English but included articles in Hindi and Tamil. Between 1917 and 1922, the WIA, through articles in *Stri Dharma*, stressed the necessity for educating girls, apart from other subjects, in child welfare, first aid, hygiene, biology and the sciences, to make them aware of their future duties to the nation as caretakers of healthy, strong children. Women doctors like Mary Scarlieb (Mary Scarlieb received her medical degree from Madras in 1875 and set up private practice there until ill-health forced her to return to England, where she became a noted eugenicist, active in the Infant Welfare Movement) and Muthulakshmi Reddy (the second president of the WIA, the first female medical graduate of Madras Presidency, and a president of the AIWC in the 1930s) supported training of women in domestic or personal hygiene, sanitation, child and maternity welfare.

The activities of women's associations as well as the ideals promoted by them might seem, at first glance, an extension of the nineteenth-century agenda of reforms, but despite similarities there were important differences as well. The Bengali male intelligentsia's agenda of social reform in the nineteenth century (as is well known) was immediately aimed at improving the lot of women, but was also promoted by an urge to address the need for reshaping the norms and functions of middle-class family life as a site for the moral and cultural restructuring of the nation. The main social utility as well as commitment of women's education—which in a way formed the key area in the agenda of reform of women's condition—was seen to lie in the constructive role expected to be played by the new women in bringing about moral and social welfare of family members.[42]

A large number of pedagogical texts written in this period produced a normative discourse on the family which framed new rules and laid down guidelines for an ideal housewife, for proper home management, scientific nurturing of children, regulation of dietary habits, creation of hygienic environment, etc. Lack of knowledge and education amongst women was seen as causing harm not only to the family but even to the nation.[43] It was pointed out that women who were ignorant of the rules of the body would not only harm themselves but, by producing weak and deficient children, would also destroy the nation. Thus, with the emergence of the family as a site where national-ist restructuring was to be carried out, women were awarded a special, augmented status in remodelling the private domain of the nation. In the twentieth-century reconstruction of ideal motherhood, and in the activities of women's organizations, we find a broadening of the class basis of future mothers of the nation and incorporation of the poorer classes as being in need of education in mothercraft.

In 1925, Gurusaday Dutt founded the Saroj Nalini Dutt Memorial Association (SNDMA), an umbrella organization for *mahila samitis*, village or municipal women's groups. In 1913, follow-ing the days of the Swadeshi Movement, the first such group had been founded by his wife, Saroj Nalini, in Patna. This and subsequent groups had provided the social space for middle-class women who ventured to leave their *zenanas*, and impart instruction on health and hygiene to women in the local district towns and surrounding villages.

By 1929 there were about 250 autonomous groups all over Bengal. One of the primary aims of these associations was to improve the conditions of birth. Classes on hygiene were arranged and baby shows were also organised. In 1925 the *mahila samiti* of Bankura celebrated a baby week which included the screening of a film titled *The Cry of the Baby*.[44]

It has been argued that events like baby shows indicate the desire of both British officials and Indian political leaders to move from private to public spaces and relationships. Their role was basically edu-cative but they were designed to create clients for maternal and child welfare centres, and to open the doors to lady health visitors. It must also be remembered that health education was no doubt developed as part of the machinery of surveillance medicine, and that many health education practices involved the imposition of 'truths' about health, in which the patient lost control of her or his own body. Instead of choice, the patient experienced government control over her or his body or family from the outside. Therefore, health education certainly contributed to the management of social and individual bodies. Traditionally, health education has been considered as an asset within health care, because it provides information and suggests alternatives to individuals, families or groups, to prevent disease and promote health. From this perspective, health education seems to be a healthy practice and a weapon for the empowerment of patients. Many historians have challenged this assumption and provided a critique of health education which employs the concept of bio-power (as developed by Michel Foucault in the first volume of his *History of Sexuality* [1990]).

TABLE 1: *Maternal and Infant (under one year) Deaths in Bengal during 1929–45*

Year	Total Deaths (Maternal)	Death Rate per mille of births (Mother)	Total Deaths (Infant)	Death Rate per mille of births (Infant)
1929	9770	7.2	244864	179.9
1930	9515	7.7	231872	187.3
1931	10687	7.7	242552	174.0
1932	11525	8.7	237593	178.9
1933	14228	9.6	294975	200.1
1934	13692	9.3	277194	189.2
1935	15608	9.5	259036	158.5
1936	16581	9.9	285956	170.9
1937	17857	10.0	300770	176.2
1938	17438	10.9	280923	184.7
1939	15792	9.5	234301	146.6
1940	15758	9.2	267894	159.3
1941	14803	8.9	248226	155.7
1942	13503	8.99	223500	154.3
1943	10732	9.01	224998	195.4
1945	11824	8.8	186355	143.2
1945	11824	8.8	186355	143.2

Source: Bengal Public Health Reports of relevant years.

TABLE 2: *Statistics for all Hospitals in Calcutta*

Year	No. of male indoor patients	No. of female indoor patients	No. of male outdoor patients	No. of female outdoor patients
1891	16486	4875	49748	12911
1892	16957	4787	53587	16016
1893	17418	4996	60485	17383
1894	16229	4939	63860	17734
1895	17986	4623	65354	17997
1896	16789	5116	62510	17925
1897	19574	5697	66248	20628
1898	15968	4883	48523	16608
1899	15994	4877	60706	18407
1900	19374	5439	66930	17802
1901	17187	5191	68716	18275
1902	19069	5483	72957	19085
1903	17548	5412	73224	19707

Source: *Twenty Years Statistics.*

Bio-power refers to the mechanisms employed to manage the population and discipline individuals. According to Foucault, biological life is essentially a political event: population reproduction and disease are central to economic processes and are therefore subject to political control.

The work of professional health visitors undoubtedly represented a movement of western medical care and the state into Indian homes. The propaganda efforts of maternal and child welfare centres, work of school inspectors, etc., meant that the health system was turning from repressive approaches to constructive approaches aimed at participation of clients, which would at the same time lead to better and more professional control of the population. From another point of view, the benefits derived from efforts at improving hygienic knowledge or domestic health behaviour in the case of the general population in British Bengal was not very noteworthy. It seems that campaigns for adopting better individual health practices could bring about dramatic health improvements only when it was preceded by a macro-sanitary and administrative infrastructure, better nutritional status and, moreover, when applied to a relatively well-fed and well-housed population, like the Indian army.[45] As shown in Table 2, the maternal death rate in

Bengal showed an upward trend between 1929 and 1938, rising from around 7 per cent to nearly 11 per cent. Between 1939 and 1944 it fluctuated between nearly 9 per cent and more than 10 per cent. The infant death rate also presented a dismal picture, fluctuating between nearly 150 per cent and more than 200 per cent during the same period.

Notes and References

1 Barbara N. Ramusack, 'Motherhood and Medical Intervention: Women's Bodies and Professionalism in India after World War I', paper presented at the Wisconsin Conference on South Asia, 1996. I am indebted to Geraldine Forbes for directing my attention to this paper and to Barbara Ramusack for giving me permission to cite and quote from her paper.

2 Samita Sen, *Women and Labour in Late Colonial India: The Bengal Jute Industry*, Cambridge, 1999, pp. 142–76. Also see Dagmer Engels, *Beyond Purdah? Women in Bengal 1890–1930*, Delhi, 1999, pp. 123–51.

3 D. Engels, ibid.

4 At the time of the British conquest, India's medical system had a pluralistic structure, incorporating Ayurvedic, Unani, Siddha, as well as folk medicines of different kinds. The early nineteenth century witnessed an enthusiastic rediscovery of India's past therapeutic knowledge by orientalist scholars. See Charles Leslie, 'Ambiguities of Revivalism in Modern India', in C. Leslie (ed.), *Asian Medical Systems: A Comparative Study*, Berkeley, 1976, pp. 356–67; D. Arnold (ed.), *Warm Climates and Western Medicine*, Clio Medica 35, The Welcome Institute Series in the History of Medicine, Amsterdam, 1996. Also see Deepak Kumar, 'Unequal contenders, uneven ground: medical encounters in British India, 1820–1920', in Andrew Cunningham and Bridie Andrews (eds), *Western medicine as contested knowledge*, Manchester, 1997, pp. 172–90; Abhijit Mukherjee, 'Natural Science in Colonial Context: The Calcutta Botanic Garden and the Agri-Horticultural Society of India, 1787–1870', unpublished Ph.D. dissertation, Jadavpur University, Calcutta, 1996.

5 Radhika Ramasubban, 'Public Health and Medical Research in India: Their Origins under the Impact of British Colonial Policy', *SAREC Report,* Stockholm, 1982; 'Imperial Health in British India, 1857–1900', in Roy Macleod and Milton Lewis (eds), *Disease, Medicine and Empire: Perspectives on Western Medicine and the Experience of European Expansion*, London, 1988.

6 David Arnold, *Colonizing the Body: State Medicine and Epidemic Disease in Nineteenth Century India*, Delhi, 1993, p. 254. Hospitals and dispensaries, partly funded by the state and also sponsored to a large extent by enthusiastic Indians, became—albeit in a limited way—centres for vaccination against smallpox and for dissemination of western ideas about sanitation and hygiene.

7 Poonam Bala, *Imperialism and Medicine in Bengal: A Socio-Historical Perspective*, New Delhi, 1991, p. 57.

[8] See Sujata Mukherjee, 'Women, Medicine and Empire: Female Practitioners and Patterns of Health Care in Colonial Bengal' in *Modern Historical Studies*, Vol. 2.

[9] Anil Kumar, *Medicine and the Raj: British Medical Policy in India, 1835–1911*, New Delhi, 1998, p. 59.

[10] Mark Harrison, *Public Health in British India: Anglo-Indian preventive medicine 1859–1914*, New Delhi, 1994, p. 89.

[11] Ibid., p. 90.

[12] *Report on the Calcutta Medical Institutions, 1887–99*, Calcutta.

[13] Kenneth Ballhatchet, *Race, Sex and Class under the Raj: Imperial Attitudes and Policies and their Critics, 1793–1905*, New York, 1980, p. 44.

[14] Malavika Karlekar, 'Kadambini and the Bhadralok', *Economic and Political Weekly*, 21, No. 19, 26 April 1986, pp. WS-25–31; Geraldine Forbes, *The New Cambridge History of India*, IV, 2: *Women in Modern India*, Cambridge, 1998, pp. 161–62.

[15] G. Forbes, ibid.; Meera Kosambi, 'Anandibai Joshee: Retrieving a Fragmented Feminist Image', *Economic and Political Weekly*, Vol. XXXI, No. 49, 7 December 1996, pp. 3189–97.

[16] See Maneesha Lal, 'The Politics of Gender and Medicine in Colonial India: The Countess of Dufferin's Fund, 1885–1888', *Bulletin of History of Medicine*, 68, 1994, pp. 29–66.

[17] Geraldine Forbes, 'Managing Midwifery in India', in Dagmer Engels and Shula Marks (eds), *Contesting Colonial Hegemony: State and Society in Africa and India*, London, 1994, pp. 152–72.

[18] Geraldine Forbes, 'Medical Careers and Health Care for Indian Women: Patterns of control', *Women's History Review*, Vol. 3, No. 4, 1994, pp. 515–30.

[19] According to Margaret I. Balfour and Ruth Young, strictly *pardanashin* women would never go to male doctors, while respectable sections of female patients might go to male physicians for health problems not connected with women's diseases or childbirth. See M. Balfour and R. Young, *The Work of Medical Women in India*, London, 1929, p. 34.

[20] Meredith Borthwick, *The Changing Role of Women in Bengal, 1849–1905*, Princeton, 1984, pp. 216–17, 159.

[21] G. Forbes, *The Memoirs of Dr Haimabati Sen, from child widow to lady doctor*, translated by Tapan Raychaudhuri, edited by Geraldine Forbes, p. 30.

[22] *Report of the Sanitary Commissioner with the Government of India* (1890), p. 58. Henceforth, *SCGI*.

[23] Sumit Guha, *Health and Population in South Asia: From Earliest Times to the Present*, New Delhi, 2001, pp. 123–37.

[24] *SCGI* (1890) p. 58; (1899), p. 61.

[25] 'Lecture on the Responsibility of Man in Matters Relating to Maternity', read by Dr A. Lankester, M.D., at the Maternity and Child Welfare Exhibition held at Delhi in February 1920, revised and reprinted in 1924.

[26] *Census of India, 1921*, V, 1, pp. 209, 230.

[27] Resolution no. 1176 P.H. dt. 23 July 1940, of the Government of Bengal,

28 *Census of India, 1911*, VI, 1, p. 30.

29 Ibid., p. 31; cited in D. Engels., *Beyond Purdah?*, p. 130.

30 *Census of India, 1921*, V, 1, p. 255.

31 GOI, *AoC Evidence 1928–1929*, pp. 14–15, 40; cited in D. Engels, *Beyond Purdah?*.

32 Dr M.I. Belfour, *The Indian Year Book, 1922*, p. 483; cited in Kabita Ray, *History of Public Health: Colonial Bengal 1921–1947*, Calcutta, 1928.

33 Reply by the Minister-in-Charge, Local Self Government Department, to a question in the Bengal Legislative Council, on 7 Feb. 1921, F. No. P.H.Q–22, progs. A 24–25, April 1921. *Dainik Basumati* (Cal.), *RNNB*, for the week ending 5 November 1921, No. 44, p. 770; *Hitavadi*, 9 April 1920; *RNNB*, 17 April 1920.

34 B.N. Ramusack, 'Motherhood and Medical Intervention', pp. 2–3.

35 F.B. Smith, *The People's Health 1830–1910*, London 1979, p. 114; cited in Sumit Guha, *Health and Population in South Asia*, p. 133.

36 A. Davin, 'Imperialism and Motherhood', *History Workshop Journal*, 5, 1978; cited in Judy Whitehead, 'Modernizing the motherhood archetype: Public health models and the Child Marriage Restraint Act of 1929', in *Social Reform, Sexuality and the State*, ed. Patricia Uberoi, New Delhi, 1996, pp. 187–209.

37 D. Engels, *Beyond Purdah?*, pp. 146–48.

38 B.N. Ramusack, 'Motherhood and Medical Intervention', p. 7.

39 *Annual Report of the National Association for Supplying Medical Aid by Women to the Women of India*, 1925.

40 During 1927 a film named *Debdut* was made by the Public Health Department on the subject of maternal and child welfare. It became so popular that it had to be run six times in the course of a day at some exhibitions. The film was also shown at Calcutta during the Congress of the Far Eastern Association of Tropical Medicine, at the request of the authorities. Delegates from Korea, Java and Japan interviewed the publicity officer and expressed their willingness to have a copy of the film. *Bengal Public Health Report*, 1927, p. 70.

41 Judy Whitehead, 'Modernizing the motherhood archetype', pp. 187–209.

42 Himani Bannerji, 'Fashioning a Self: Educational Proposals for and by Women in Popular Magazines in Colonial Bengal', *Economic and Political Weekly*, 26, 43, 1991.

43 Pradip Kumar Bose, 'Sons of the Nation: Child Rearing in the New Family', in Partha Chatterjee (ed.), *Texts of Power: Emerging Disciplines in Colonial Bengal*, Calcutta, 1996, p. 123.

44 D. Engels, *Beyond Purdah?*, p. 149.

45 Sumit Guha, *Health and Population in South Asia*.

Social History of Western Medical Practice in Travancore

An Inquiry into the Administrative Process

Sunitha B. Nair

In this study we intend to analyse the processes by which the hegemony of western medical practice over indigenous health-care practices followed widely in Travancore[1] for centuries was achieved.[2] Vaccination was introduced for the first time in Travancore in the year 1811, while in British India it was introduced only in 1830.[3] The paper starts with a brief review of the literature relating to the history of socio-cultural processes that led to the domination of western medical practice in Travancore in this period. Subsequently, it deals with the social history of the introduction and enforcement of western medical practice in Travancore. It also analyses the roles played by the state machinery and the Christian missionaries in promoting western medical practice, thereby sidelining the various indigenous medical practices. Further, the relation between western medical practice and the process of colonization is also looked into.

Introduction

The introduction of western medicine was not an altogether easy and smooth process. There was resistance from the people. Still, the domination of western medical practice was enforced through state intervention by various means. Imposition by the state machinery alone could not have been successful in propagating western medicine. It was the missionaries who popularized western medical practice. Missionary activities created a new habitat as well as new notions about health and hygiene in the society.

We seldom come across any comprehensive work that recounts the historical development of western medicine in colonial Travancore. However, a few research papers have shed light in the field.

215

Kabir M. and T.N. Krishnan explain the historical development of western biomedical practice, by using the concept of social intermediation.[4] They emphasize the importance of social policies and programmes of selective social change, without which the health transition would not have taken place. K.N. Panikkar refers to the domination of western medical practice over indigenous medical practices, while referring to the revitalization of Ayurveda in Kerala.[5] Benny Varghese has attempted to analyse the discourse of western medical practice as it unfolded in Travancore.[6] Kawasaki gives a historical outline of the arrival of western medicine in Travancore and its development under royal patronage.[7] Another study which focusses on the material processes and developmentalism in colonial Thiruvithamkur consider the introduction of western medicine to be part of the colonial project of modernity.[8] Koji Kawashima, in his book *Missionaries and a Hindu State: Travancore, 1858–1936*, devotes one chapter to western medicine. It mainly discusses the role of Christian missionaries in popularizing this practice in Travancore.[9] Vineetha Menon gives a brief note on the history of biomedicine in Kerala as a background to her study of the spread of the modern health-care system in the settlement of Kannikkars, a hill tribe of Travancore.[10]

In the period 1800–60, the interface of colonialism and traditional political–social processes set forth the elements in the making of the metropolitan political–cultural hegemony in Travancore. The military and political subordination of the Thiruvithamkur state to the British paramount power had been completed by the first decade of the nineteenth century. The political and, to some extent, socioideological 'reconstitution' of the state followed this.[11] The state as well as the missionaries did their best towards the introduction and further expansion of western medical practice in the region, as part of carrying out the colonial project of modernity.

Introduction of western medical practice, which was alien to the socio-cultural milieu of the natives, was considered a major social change in the first half of the ninteenth century. As with schooling and printing, in the case of western medicine too, the state and the missionaries acted in unison to attain their goal.[12] Now let us analyse how western medical practice became a system and exercised its power over all sections of society without any caste/class differences.

Western Medicine as Preventive Care

Before the official introduction of western medicine, Christian missionaries had propagated it way back in 1811 itself. Rani Gauri Lakshmi Bai, the then ruler of Travancore, had formally permitted its introduction in the region. Western medicine was introduced first as preventive care—as vaccination against smallpox, to be specific. Widespread occurrence of smallpox and continuous pressures from Colonel Munro (Resident and Diwan of Travancore) forced Her Highness to start a small unit for vaccination, with a resident doctor. This was considered as the starting-point of the formal acceptance of western medicine.[13] Since then the state continued to promote western medicine for curing various epidemics that occurred frequently. From the administrative reports of various years in the colonial period, it is clear that the outbreak of epidemics was a major public health problem faced by the state. The people were reluctant to accept western modes of treatment. However the state supported the introduction of western medicine and gave maximum patronage to further advancement and wider implementation of the system.

Vaccination was the first preventive measure propagated by the state. Although vaccination was introduced in Travancore in 1811, smallpox spread in a severe form in 1871 and lasted for nearly a year, causing heavy mortality. As a result there was a sudden increase in the rate of vaccination from 1864–65 to 1874–75 (see Table 1). Further, there was a significant increase in the total number of vaccinations.

Table 2 shows that the lower castes were being vaccinated more than the upper castes. This means the state was able to create a consensus among the lower castes about the efficacy of this practice. It is in this context that the role of missionaries becomes significant,

TABLE 1: *Number of Persons Vaccinated*

Year	Vaccination
1864–65	16,626
1874–75	72,289
1884–85	78,783
1894–95	NA
1904–05	1,55,655
1914–15	2,19,631

Source: *Administrative Reports of Travancore*, various years.

217

TABLE 2: *Caste-wise Vaccination*

Caste	1884	1890
Brahmins	892	658
Kshatriyas	108	36
Malayali Sudras	14,708	20,269
Pandy Sudras	3,731	4,995
Mahomodans	4,067	3,806
Christians	24,854	25,543
Inferior castes	37,638	44,613

Source: *Administrative Reports of Travancore*, 1884–85 and 1890–91.

whose main project in the region was conversion. Those who were converted were to lead a totally different life armed with a new world-view and different values.[14]

Through a proclamation in 1880, vaccination was made compulsory for all government servants, pupils in schools, *vakils*, persons seeking medical help from the hospitals, inmates of jails and persons depending on state charities.[15] Vaccination was made compulsory in the rural as well as urban areas of Travancore, by rules and regulations.

Vaccination against smallpox was made compulsory throughout the state in the rural areas of Travancore with the help of temporary rules passed by the Government under the Epidemic Diseases Act and in the urban areas with the help of rules under the City Municipal Act and the District Municipalities Act.[16]

Even under these circumstances some vaccinators were not ready to vaccinate the lower castes. For instance, two Pulaya vaccinators were appointed for the vaccination of hill tribes.[17] Vaccination was carried on under the supervision of the medical officers of health epidemiology and vital statistics. According to the standards already laid down at the commencement of the vaccination campaign, each vaccinator had to perform at least 50 vaccinations a day.

Social Resistance

Initially the majority of the people seem to have resisted vaccination attempts for various reasons. For instance the brahmins feared that by vaccination they would lose their *brahmanyam*.[18] Since they

218

considered the cow to be sacred, use of cow lymph for vaccination went against their religious values. Many of them feared that by vaccination they might acquire certain features of the cow, say, its sound, body structure, etc.[19] Some of them thought that vaccination would turn their heads into cow-heads. There was resistance from educated people too. They were confused by the differences of opinion about the efficacy of the practice. For instance, a report of the Royal Commission had argued that mere vaccination could not prevent smallpox in India, and that good sanitary measures alone could reduce its occurrence. Again, some people argued that vaccination will lead to other diseases like leprosy, syphilis, etc.[20]

These different opinions among the Britishers as well as natives created utter confusion among the common people about its efficacy. Fear was the main reason for the common people to resist vaccination. It is reported that in the year 1950–51, 552 persons objected to get themselves vaccinated, of whom eighteen were prosecuted and thirteen convicted.[21]

The officials, realizing the resistance of the public, tried to persuade the people in various ways to get vaccinated—propagating vaccination as a package with curative care; giving *battas* to vaccinated subjects as well as parents/guardians of vaccinated subjects; increase in the payments to vaccinators, etc. This is very clear from Dr Andy's recommendation towards the reconstitution of the Vaccination Department:

> It is essential to give training to vaccinators for treatment of ordinary diseases along with vaccination to gain more acceptance from the public. Again it is recommended that small grant or *batta* of 1 *chakram* should be given to subjects of vaccination on the first day of operation and 2 *chakrams* on the eighth day of successful cases. It is also recommended that *battas* should be given to parents/guardians of the vaccinated subjects who follow the vaccinator from village to village to supply lymph. Further an increase in the payments to vaccinators is also desired.[22]

In order to contain the public resistance to western medicine, Mr Patterson (a government official) suggested that treatment of diseases should be printed in Tamil and Malayalam and distributed among the people. He argued that this would promote interest in His Highness as well as among the public.[23]

An epidemic of cholera was the next important occasion and

context for the imposition of western medicine. The earliest record of the ravages of cholera in Travancore dates back to 1869–70. The next outbreak of the epidemic was in 1876–77, in all the divisions of the state and at the capital, and in 1881–82 it broke out in an unusually severe form at Nagarcoil and Sucheendram. In spite of all the preventive measures taken by the state, deaths due to cholera were increasing. This reveals the inefficiency of preventive measures; at the same time, native preparations became more effective. For instance, a native physician called Moothu Swamy Pillai developed a medicine for cholera, since the deaths due to cholera were increasing day by day.[24]

Plague was another important epidemic that broke out during the period. In the midst of the epidemic, inoculation was an important preventive measure. Usually, influential leaders of the people, heads of castes, teachers of religion and village headmen were approached by the people for help. The advantages of inoculation were explained to them. The assistance secured by the beneficiaries was in turn used to persuade their less-educated brothers to protect themselves from plague through inoculation.[25] In this case too, the people were forced to accept western medical treatment. Considering the paramount interests of public health, His Highness the Maharaja of Travancore enacted a regulation in 1897 to provide better prevention against the outbreak of dangerous epidemics—the Epidemic Disease Regulation of 1898.[26] Accordingly, a local authority was appointed in every infected area to order immediate evacuation of the infected houses.

Towards Institutionalization

The Travancore government was keen on institutionalizing western medical practice from the very beginning of its propagation, through constitution of departments and appointments of officials. The first hospital was opened around the year 1817 and the appointment of a *durbar* physician also dates back to this period. The Medical Department was gradually developed and by 1860 there were seven medical institutions in the state.[27] In 1819 two small dispensaries were opened up, one in the palace and the other within the premises of the Nair Brigade Barracks. Sri Uthram Thirunal Maharaja took a special interest in western medical science. He studied the subject and found pleasure in treating cases in the dispensary attached to the palace. Earlier the people, especially *savarna* Hindus, were not ready to buy medicines from the medical stores, but later, when the Maharaja himself started a medical store, the resistance was minimized. The Maharaja also used to explain the efficacy of English medicines. This medical store was known as 'Elayaraja Dispensary'.[28]

In 1865, Ayilyam Thirunal Maharaja laid the foundation-stone of the Civil Hospital, which subsequently became the General Hospital. In addition to general hospitals and dispensaries, specialized hospitals also began emerging during the period. In 1896–97 the Women and Children's Hospital was opened and placed under the charge of a lady doctor. A hospital for chronic cases was established in 1897. In the years 1898–99, a medical school was opened at the capital for training hospital assistants, and this institution was expected not only to supply the personnel required for the medical service of the state but also to bring into existence a number of private practitioners who would carry the blessings of European medical services to parts of the country which were not within easy reach of state interventions.[29] An ophthalmic hospital was founded in 1906. An X-ray branch was opened in the General Hospital in 1903 and a new X-ray apparatus of the latest model was installed there in 1927.[30] Tuberculosis being on the increase in Travancore, the opening of a T.B. hospital in the state engaged the attention of the government in 1930. Lady Linlithgow laid the foundation stone of the T.B. Hospital on 11 January 1939 at Asaripalam, three miles west of Nagarcoil.[31]

With institutionalization in progress along with social education through literature and other means, the social acceptance of western medicine gained momentum. There was a steady rise in the demand for the western medical system, as shown by the growth in the number of patients treated in various government hospitals in Travancore (see Table 3).

TABLE 3: *Number of In-patients and Out-patients in various Government Hospitals in Travancore*

Year	In-patients	Out-patients	Total
1904–05	15,574	6,15,861	6,31,435
1914–15	21,131	7,30,557	7,51,688
1924–25	NA	NA	NA
1934–35	70,071	2,183,422	2,263,493

Source: *Administrative Reports of Travancore*, various years.

The table shows that the number of people who were treated in the allopathy hospitals was continuously increasing. By 1950–51 the number of in-patients and out-patients rose to 1,57,906 and 3,894,735 respectively.

Even though the total number of patients treated in government hospitals was increasing, the lower castes and upper castes were treated in an unequal manner. For instance, due to untouchability, Pulaya patients were segregated from others in the General Hospital. A separate shed was constructed for Pulaya patients at one corner of the hospital compound, alongside a shed for the carriages and animals of the medical officers attached to the hospital.[32] Further, one portion of the Thycadu Hospital was allotted exclusively for the treatment of brahmins.[33] Again, the state sanctioned a request for a special ward for Europeans in the General Hospital.[34]

Surgery was the most terrifying aspect of western medicine as far as the people were concerned. It was a subject of alarm because of the risk factor involved in it. People seem to have avoided surgery as much as they could. However, the overall acceptability of the western treatment system encouraged many to undergo surgery in cases that were otherwise uncurable. According to a statistical assessment, a total of 4,677 persons underwent surgery in 1935, of which 870 were major operations. In 1936 the number rose to a total of 7,506, and out of this 1,534 were major operations and the rest minor—a marked increase from the figures of the previous year.

A total of 2,338 patients were admitted to the X-ray and electro-theraputic sections of the hospital in the year 1935, as against 1,461 patients in 1934. The dental section and the ear, nose and throat sections of the hospital attended to 5,686 and 5,386 cases respectively. In the Women and Children's Hospital, there were 2,675 obstetric cases distributed among 2,382 in-patients and 293 out-patients.[35]

Except, vaccination, constructive public health work did not start in Travancore until 1895, when the Sanitary Department was established. It was organized to conduct vaccination, to collect vital statistics and to look after sanitation. The department was placed under the charge of an officer called the Sanitary Commissioner. The Rockefeller Foundation appointed Dr W.P. Jacocks to take up public health work in Travancore, as per the request of the Royal Government, in 1928. The working programme of Dr Jacocks comprised of hookworm treatment campaigns, public health education, epidemiological and vital statistical investigations , health unit work, medical entomology and plague control measures.[36]

In 1934, with a view to coordinate the public health activities of the state on an up-to-date and scientific basis under a single direction, the Sanitary Department was amalgamated with the public health organization, and a permanent Public Health Department was constituted under the control of a deputy director. Subsequently, in 1935, the designation of the head of the department was changed to Director of Public Health. A public health laboratory was also started in the new department, embracing the sections of the government bacteriologists, the chemical examiner, the public analyst under the food adulteration regulation, the hookworm laboratory and the vaccine depot. The preparation of cholera vaccine on a large scale was a notable feature of the work in the public health laboratory in the year 1935. A total of 40,508 cc of this vaccine was prepared, besides 4,537 cc of typhoid vaccine and 305 autogenous vaccines. A total of 60 samples of vaccine lymph and 1,291 samples of water were bacteriologically examined.[37]

Public health education was also an important part of the public health work in Travancore.

> The health educational officer undertook an intensive lecture programme in various parts of the state in aid of vaccination campaign, cholera preventive measures, anti-malarial operation and mosquito control, accompanied by demonstrations of cinema films, lantern slides, charts, etc. Further 1,041 lectures were delivered to an estimated audience of over two lakhs of people. Over 64,000 copies of public health bulletin, pamphlets and posters in English and vernacular were distributed among the people.[38]

So far, the Municipal Act, the Village Panchayat Act, the Village Unions Act, the Epidemic Diseases Act and the Food Adulteration Act had contained some provisions to deal with the public health problems of specified areas. But as per the Public Health Act of 1121 ME , a new Bill was proposed to invest the Director of Public Health with certain statutory powers for controlling and supervising all public health measures throughout the state. It enabled the government to apply the rule to issues like drinking water, drainage, latrine, milk trade, lodging, food control, etc.[39] The Rockefeller Foundation continued to give honorary advice to the state in matters of public health.

Professionalization and Government Control

The colonial government tried to regulate the medical practice in the state. The introduction of the Travancore Medical Practitioner's Act of 1944 was meant to protect the public from treatment by unskilled medical men. It was an Act intended to regulate the qualifications of practitioners and to provide for the registration of practitioners of various systems of medicine with a view to encourage the study and spread of such systems. Accordingly, the Travancore Medical Council was established for carrying out the provisions of this Act. Every member of the council was to be a registered practitioner and the holder of a recognized qualification under the Act. No practitioners other than a practitioner registered under this Act could practise medicine, surgery or midwifery. Many additional provisions were later introduced, by which unregistered practitioners were prohibited from practising under any system. Any breach of the prohibitions was made punishable.[40]

The state persuaded the native society in different ways to accept western medical practice. Sensing the reluctance of women patients to appear in a public space such as a hospital to seek treatment, the Travancore government encouraged more women to enter the medical profession. Their decision to recruit trained nurses and midwives as well as *dais*, i.e. untrained women practising midwifery, in the medical profession was to attract women to this public space.

> Provision was made for the registration of all persons who followed the profession of midwifery and nursing. Even untrained women were allowed to register, provided they were certified to be in the practice of the profession and they were to apply for registration within the time specified in the Bill.[41]

In order to give them sufficient opportunity for practising midwifery, the British government found it necessary to increase the patient capacity of the maternity hospital. They appointed fourteen Nair women in the medical department for practising nursing and midwifery, to attract the upper-caste women.[42]

The Beginnings of Privatization

In order to reduce congestion in government hospitals, it was decided that deserving private medical practitioners should be encouraged to start nursing homes on payment of subventions. The award of grants-in-aid to private medical institutions began in 1887. However, a regular system of awarding grants-in-aid to encourage private agencies was sanctioned only nine years later, in 1896.[43] Accordingly, Rs 1,500 was granted as subvention to the hospital attached to the Sri Ramakrishna Ashram, Travancore, and Rs 1,000 to Mr N. Padmanabhan, retired assistant surgeon, who had started a private dispensary at Vaikom.[44]

So far we have discussed in detail how the state promoted western medical practice and thereby institutionalized this practice. But the task of popularizing western medical practice among the lower castes was taken up by the Anglican missionaries.[45] In this too the missionaries were helped with financial grants by the Travancore government.

Of the missionary societies, the London Missionary Society (LMS) had the most substantial medical mission in Travancore, even though the number of patients it treated was much less than the number treated in government institutions (see Table 4).

The first medical missionary sent to Travancore was A. Ramsay.[46] In 1838 he began medical work at Neyyur, one of the mission stations in south Travancore. But he left the mission in 1842 and Dr Charles Leitch was sent to Travancore in 1852. After his death Dr John Lowe took charge in 1861, and there was a substantial increase in medical work after his arrival. A medical training class, undoubtedly one

TABLE 4: **Number of Patients Treated in Government and LMS Institutions**

Year	Govt. Institutions	LMS Institutions
1870–71	66,757	12,046
1880–81	92,419	NA
1890–91	120,883	NA
1900–01	438,433	66,996
1910–11	543,345	113,203
1920–21	940,170	118,144
1930–31	1,975,328	145,532

Source: *Travancore Administration Report* for 1870–71, 1880–81, 1890–91, 1900–01, 1910–11, 1920–21 and 1930–31; *South Travancore Medical Mission Annual Report* for 1937 in *Travancore Report CWMA* (quoted from Koji Kawashima)

225

of the most important activities behind the expansion of the medical mission, was started by Lowe in 1864. The first batch of students finished their course in 1867 and they were posted to the newly-established dispensaries at Attur, Santhapuram and Agashteessapuram in 1868, Nagarcoil in 1871, and Tittuvilei in 1874. In 1902, it had seventeen outstations. The Neyyur hospital offered a high standard of treatment with up-to-date equipment.[47]

In 1930 the LMS had twenty-three medical mission stations which treated about 372,410 patients world wide, while the medical mission in Travancore alone treated a total of 163,121 patients. This means that it treated 43.8 per cent of the total number of patients treated by all the medical missions of the LMS. Meanwhile, as the medical mission developed, it came to depend more and more on sale of medicines, fees or offerings collected from the patients. The income from sale of medicines, fees and offerings in 1914 was about Rs 18,660 in total, which means that more than 65 per cent of the total income was collected from patients as of the year 1914. The medical mission thus became increasingly independent on the Travancore government financially, though it still received considerable sums in the form of grants from the government.[48] In short, the church and the state worked in collaboration with each other in Travancore to spread western medicine. British administrators' accounts as well as missionary writings criticized native health-care practices as 'unscientific as well as traditional thus creating the condition for introducing western medicine'.[49] Neither the British administrators nor the missionary establishments were concerned about the socio-culutral milieu within which native practices were performed.

Modernization of Indigenous Systems

The indigenous health-care practices in colonial Travancore were well-entrenched in social and cultural milieu. Of the varied medical systems like Ayurveda, Siddha, Unani and folk medicines, Ayurveda was the most organized and systematized branch of medical knowledge. But with the introduction of modern medicine indigenous medicine, particularly Ayurveda, lost its supremacy. During the 1890s the nationalists began to claim the effectiveness and superiority of Indian systems of medicine, and a movement began which aimed at recognition and patronage of indigenous medicine by political authorities. The All-India Ayurvedic Congress established in 1907 was one of the results of this movement. This movement influenced state policy towards indigenous medicine in Travancore.[50]

In 1889 the government opened an Ayurveda *pathasala* (school) in Trivandrum and sanctioned a system of medical grants to *vaidyans* (doctors) in 1895–96. The grants were generally given to those who passed out of the Ayurveda *pathasala*. In 1917–18, an Ayurveda Department was created , which revised the curriculum of the Ayurveda *pathasala* on an up-to-date scientific basis to suit modern equipment. It was headed by an officer designated Director of Ayurveda. The number of in-patients in the government Ayurveda hospitals and dispensaries rose from 227 in 1934 to 260 in 1935, of whom 194 were men, forty-eight women and eighteen children. But the strength of the Ayurveda college fell from 125 in 1934 to 119 in 1935.[51]

The colonial government also showed some interest in the development of the Ayurvedic system of medicine. A report presented by Dr Ravi Varma regarding the functioning of the Ayurveda Department suggested that none of the existing Ayurvedic schools was working in a satisfactory manner to impart knowledge in the field of medicine.[52] He criticized the department for not having a manual or code, showing the *modus operandi* of its working. According to him, the department needed the services of experts having comparative knowledge of the western and eastern systems. He further argued that these persons should be graduates in the western system and should study Ayurveda in a critical manner. The report continued:

> Rather
> i. filling lacuanae with collations from Charaka, Sushruta and . . .
> ii. incorporating from the western systems details as in anatomy
> iii. bringing out the rationales underlying the original teaching by intensive study of the texts and from comparative knowledge
> iv. fully describing operative and other procedures from the western system as well as from experience, and
> v. re-identifying the various drugs and habilitating them on to the binomial nomenclature.[53]

This report was an exemplary site of the legitimization of western medicine and the process of de-legitimization of the culture of the subjected.

Even though the Ayurveda Department developed only

gradually, it functioned very much within the system of western medicine. Probably the British government found it necessary to promote at least one native medical practice to satisfy the demands of the native people. T.K. Velupillai's speech represented the voice of the natives against the indifferent attitude of the government towards Ayurveda. He criticized the government for low grants to the Ayurveda Department and comparatively high grants to the Allopathy Department. He argued:

> Although, Allopathic medicines are powerful and useful, Ayurvedic medicines are found to be keeping with our mode of life; and that is why we find that the Ayurvedic physicians are still able to maintain their hold on the public confidence, although the Allopathic and Unani systems have been in this land for centuries.

He further says, 'Europeans live on beef, ham, apricots and champagne. They have the habit of smoking cigarette. But we live on rice, tapioca, pickles and perhaps a little milk or buttermilk. We have the habit of taking oil bath.'[54] He clearly cited the differences in the socio-cultural milieu into which western medicine was introduced.

Some of the native practices for curing various diseases which seemed to be very effective were totally discouraged, and any such attempts were quashed by the application of the standards of western medicine to them. For instance, a mass petition for popularizing 'cholera powder' prepared by Moothuswami Pillai was rejected by the *durbar* physician on the ground that it was an unscientific preparation. The *durbar* physician, in his letter to the Maharaja of Travancore, stated that it is purely a native preparation and its contents are unknown. Therefore it cannot be popularized through the medical department.[55]

Concluding Observations

The present study argues that western medical practice became a dominant system of curing in Travancore by the second half of the nineteenth century. The system provided treatment for all types of diseases, along with preventive measures. The institutionalization and professionalization attempts continued throughout the nineteenth century. They included the building up of a hierarchy among the providers of treatment; creating specialized departments for various parts of the body, age-groups and gender; fixing standards for practitioners; classifying different stages of treatment, etc. Further, this new way of curing was accompanied by new notions about health and hygiene in the society as well as about one's own body. Missionaries also played an important role in this process.

Besides these efforts by the state and missionaries, those of the educated and powerful sections of people in the native state influenced the common people. All these together constituted natives as bearers and objects of this non-rooted system of curing. Thus the acceptance of the western system of medicine in Travancore can be situated in the context of the internalization of the newly-circulated notions on body. As a result of this, though western medicine was initially enforced by the government, in course of time different segments of the society demanded access to this new system of treatment.

Notes

1. Travancore (Malayalam: Thiruvithamkur) occupied the south-west portion of the Indian peninsula. It was bounded on the north by the state of Cochin and the British district of Coimbatore; on the east by the British district of Maudura and Tinnevelly; and on the south and west by the Indian Ocean. The population of the state, according to the census of 1911, was 34,28,975. Hinduism was the predominant religion and its followers constituted about two-thirds of the entire population while the Christian formed over a fourth and the Mahomedans one-fifteenth—quoted from *Administration Report of Travancore, 1092 M.E.* Government of Travancore, 1918, pp. XI and XII.

2. Ayurveda, Siddha, Unani, folk medicines, etc., are examples. For details see N.V. Krishnankutty Varier, *Ayurvedattinte Charitram*, (Malayalam), 1993.

3. Vaccination was the first preventive measure that was introduced in India and practised on a large scale. It was introduced first into Bombay in the year 1830 and a Vaccination Department was formed in 1858. For details see *Report of the Health Survey and Development Committee*, Vol. 1, 1946.

4. M. Kabir and T.N. Krishnan, 'Social Intermediation and Health Transition: Lessons from Kerala', paper presented at India International Centre, New Delhi, 24 January 1992.

5. K.N. Panikkar, 'Indigenous medicine and cultural hegemony: A case study of revitalization movement in Keralam', *Studies in History*, Vol. 8, No. 2, 1992.

6. Benny Varghese, 'Indigenous Health Care and Introduction of Western Medicine', unpublished M.Phil. dissertation, School of Social Sciences, Mahatma Gandhi University, 1993.

7. Kawasaki, seminar paper, International Seminar at the Institute of Social Science, New Delhi, 1993.

8. K.T. Rammohan, 'Material Processes and Developmentalism: Interpreting

Economic Change in Colonial Thiruvithamkur, 1800–1945', Ph.D. thesis, unpublished, Kerala University, Trivandrum, 1996. Here 'Thiruvithamkur' is used as the Malayalam equivalent of Travancore.

9 Koji Kawashima, *Missionaries and a Hindu State: Travancore 1858–1936*, Delhi, 1998 , pp. 114–48.

10 Vinitha Menon, paper presented at the International Seminar of Interdisciplinary Centre, Kerala University, Trivandrum, 2000.

11 K.T. Rammohan, 'Material Processes and Developmentalism'.

12 Ibid.

13 P. Bhaskaranunni, *Pathonmpatham Noottandile Keralam* (Malayalam), Kerala Sahitya Akademy, Trichur, 1988.

14 For more details of conversion in Travancore, see Dick Kooiman, *Conversion and Social Equality: The London Missionary Society in South Travancore in the Nineteenth Century*, Delhi, 1989.

15 T.K. Velupillai, *The Travancore State Manual*, Vol. IV, Government of Travancore, 1914, pp. 208–36.

16 *Travancore and Cochin Administration Report, 1950–51*, Government of Travancore, 1952.

17 Cover file, Bundle No. 55, File No. 15767, 1890, Vaccination to the hill tribes and appointment of two Pulayas as vaccinators, Kerala State Archives, Trivandrum.

18 See, Herman Gundert, *Malayalam and English Dictionary*, New Delhi, 1872, p. 755.

19 K.C. Veerarayan Raja, 'Vasuri Keerivekkal' (Malayalam), *Mangalodayam*, No. 6, 1085 ME, pp. 209–48.

20 T.P.R. Menon, 'Vasuri Keerivekkunnathu Kondulla Chila Doshangal' (Malayalam), *Mangalodayam*, No. 3, 1088 ME, pp. 29–60.

21 *Travancore and Cochin Administration Report, 1950–51*.

22 Cover file, Bundle No. 42, File No. 16152, 1866, Dr Andy's recommendations regarding vaccination department, Kerala State Archives, Trivandrum.

23 Cover file, Bundle No. 19, File No. 15766, 1844, Mr Patterson's suggestions about the vaccination department, Kerala State Archives, Trivandrum.

24 For details refer Cover file, Bundle No. 147, File No. 707, 1890, Kerala State Archives, Trivandrum.

25 *Rules and proclamations of Travancore*, Vol. III (1082–1091 ME), 1928.

26 Ibid.

27 *T.K. Velupillai, The Travancore State Manual*, Vol. IV.

28 Ibid.

29 Nagam Aiya, *The Travancore State Manual*, Vol. I, New Delhi, 1989.

30 *Administrative Report of Travancore, 1930–31*, Governmeent of Travancore, Trivandrum, 1932.

31 Tuberculosis Hospital Nagercovil, Confidential file, Bundle No. 1185, File No. 477, 1946, Kerala State Archives, Trivandrum.

32 Cover file, Bundle No. 152, File No. 3181, 1890, Construction of a shed in

the General Hospital for the treatment of Pulaya patients, Kerala State Archives, Trivandrum.

[33] Ibid.

[34] Cover file, Bundle No. 139, File No. 2530, 1889, European ward in the General Hospital, Kerala State Archives, Trivandrum.

[35] *Administrative Report of Travancore, 1934–35*, Government of Travancore, Trivandrum, 1936.

[36] Ibid.

[37] Ibid.

[38] Ibid.

[39] *The Travancore Public Health Act*, 1121 ME, Legislative file, Bundle No. 139, File No. 271, Kerala State Archives, Trivandrum.

[40] For details, see, Travancore Medical Practitioners Act, 1119 ME; The Acts and Proclamations of Travancore, 1119–1120 ME, Vol. XIV, Part I, Government of Travancore, Trivandrum, 1946.

[41] Legislative file, Bundle No. 143, File No. 262, The Travancore Nurses, Midwives and Dais Act, 1121 ME, Kerala State Archives, Trivandrum.

[42] Cover File, Bundle No. 51, File No. 369, 1869, Medical Department Midwifery Classes, Kerala State Archives, Trivandrum.

[43] *Administrative Report of Travancore, 1930–31.*

[44] *Travancore Cochin Administrative Report*, 1122 ME, Government of Travancore, Trivandrum, 1948.

[45] K.T. Rammohan, 'Material Processes and Developmentalism'.

[46] Dick Kooiman, *Conversion and Social Equality.*

[47] Koji Kawashima, *Missionaries and a Hindu State.*

[48] Ibid.

[49] *Making of Modern Keralam*, Report of the UGC Major Research project, 1993–96, unpublished, School of Social Sciences, Mahatma Gandhi University, Kottayam.

[50] Koji Kawashima, *Missionaries and a Hindu State.*

[51] *Administrative Report of Travancore, 1934–35.*

[52] Confidential file, Bundle No. 187, File No. 543, Ayurvedic Department reorganization: certain reports by Dr Ravi Varma, Kerala State Archives, Trivandrum.

[53] Ibid.

[54] T.K. Velupillai, *Speeches in the Travancore Legislative Council,* 3 November 1925, 1st session, Vol. I, Trivandrum, 1926.

[56] Cover file, Bundle No. 147, File No. 707, 1890, Kerala State Archives, Trivandrum.

References

*Administrative reports of medical and public health department, Travancore (1904–05)
 – (1950–51),* Trivandrum: Government of Travancore.

Aiyya, Nagam (1989). *The Travancore State Manual,* Vol. II, New Delhi (rpt).

Arnold, David (1989). *Imperial Medicine and Indigenous Societies*, Delhi: Oxford University Press.

Bala, Poonam (1991). *Imperialism and Medicine in Bengal: A Socio-Historical Perspective*, Delhi: Sage Publications.

Bhaskaranunni, P. (1998). *Pathonpatham Noottandile Keralam,* Trichur: Kerala Sahitya Akademi.

Epidemic Diseases Regulations Act of 1073. Trivandrum: Government of Travancore.

Foucault, Michel (1973). *The Birth of the Clinic.* New York: Vintage Books, New York.

Kabir, M. and T.N. Krishnan (1992). *Social Intermediation and Health Transition: Lessons from Kerala,* New Delhi: India International Centre, 24 January.

Kakar, Sudhir (1980). *Shamans Mystics and Doctors: Psychological Inquiry into India and its Leading Traditions,* Delhi: Oxford University Press.

Kawashima, Koji (1998). *Missionaries and a Hindu State: Travancore 1858–1936,* Delhi.

Kooiman, Dick (1989). *Conversion and Social Equality: The London Missionary Society in South Travancore in the Nineteenth Century,* Delhi: Manohar.

Kumar, Anil (1998). *Medicine and the Raj: British Medical Policy in India 1835–1911,* Delhi: Sage Publications.

Lesley, Doyal (1979). *Political Economy of Health,* Pluto Press.

Making of Modern Keralam, Report of the UGC Major Research Project 1993–96, unpublished, School of Social Sciences, Mahatma Gandhi University, Kottayam.

Mateer, Samuel (1993). *Native Life in Travancore,* London.

Menon, K. Padmanabha (1987). *History of Kerala,* 4 volumes, Delhi: Asian Educational Services.

Panikkar, K.N. (1992). 'Indigenous Medicine and Cultural Hegemony: A Study of Revitalization Movement in Keralam', *Studies in History,* Vol. 8, No. 2.

Ram Mohan, K.T. (1996). *Material Processes and Developmentalism: Interpreting Economic Change in Colonial Tiruvithamkur, 1800–1948,* Ph.D. Thesis, unpublished, Kerala University, Trivandrum.

Report of the Health Survey and Development Committee, Vols I and II, 1946.

Somerwel, Howard (1940). *The Knife and Life in India: History of Surgical Missionary of South Travancore,* London.

Travancore Administrative Reports (1865–66)–(1950–51), Government of Travancore.

Varghese, Benny (1993). *Indigenous Health Care and Introduction of WesternMedicine,* unpublished M.Phil. dissertation, School of Social Sciences, Mahatma Gandhi University,Kottayam.

Veluppillai, T.K. (1996). *The Travancore State Manual,* Vol. IV, Trivandrum: Government of Kerala.

Gauging Indian Responses to Western Medicine

Hospitals and Dispensaries,

Bombay Presidency, 1900–20

Mridula Ramanna

For an analysis of Indian responses to western medicine, both attendance at hospitals and dispensaries, and public reactions to public health and sanitary measures, are equally important. Indian initiative and funding had led to the establishment of medical institutions in nineteenth-century Bombay.[1] While this could be seen as buying patronage, it could also be regarded as an indication of the acceptance of western medical facilities, albeit limitedly. Donors made the initial endowments and expected the government to maintain the institutions and pay the salaries of medical personnel employed therein. However, this was done reluctantly because, as David Arnold has shown, the British had a narrow view of their own responsibility towards the health and welfare of Indians.[2] State intervention came whenever diseases became epidemics and threatened to cross over from the European to the Indian quarters. While only one-tenths of the population availed of western medicine even in the cities by the end of the century, fear of hospitalization had only increased after the plague epidemic and the forcible segregation measures. Dr Thomas Blaney, a popular English private practitioner of Bombay, observed that plague patients died of fright rather than of plague when taken to hospitals.[3] Given this background, this paper attempts to gauge the extent of the acceptance of western medical facilities, on the basis of records of hospitals and dispensaries in Bombay Presidency, for the first two decades of the twentieth century. This study will focus on the period between the aftermath of the plague epidemic and the introduction of dyarchy at the provinces by the Government of India Act 1919, when health was made a transferred subject, and will analyse some questions of health care.

First, the varied dimensions in the funding of these

institutions are explored. Public benefactions were made both for the extension of existing facilities and for the establishment of new ones. What was the colonial response to the donations? Second, the patient profile is studied. The number of patients did increase, though fears of ritual pollution persisted. What were the diseases for which patients went to hospitals and dispensaries? An answer to this is attempted with the help of tables. How were diseases categorized in the records? While in the previous century relapsing, remittent and enteric types were included under the head of fevers, now distinctions were known and made. The nomenclature reflected the changing knowledge of the typology and the views of the colonial medical establishment. Another issue examined is the nature of medical facilities then available for women. Was there an awareness of women's health, per se? The staffing pattern in hospitals and dispensaries is looked at. Though the monopoly of top positions by the Indian Medical Service (IMS) continued, was there any Indian involvement in health matters?

Funding of Institutions

Public donations continued to fund hospitals and dispensaries, as did British unwillingness to subsidize them. Arnold has shown that private philanthropy funded hospitals and dispensaries in Britain, and the British expected the same here.[4] Hospitals and dispensaries were classified into four types. The first and second were funded with provincial revenues. In 1910, out of a total of Rs 12,02,000 allotted as provincial revenues, the share of hospitals and dispensaries was Rs 81,000.[5] In addition to hospitals like Jamsetji Jeejeebhoy (J.J.), St George's, Goculdas Tejpal (G.T.) and Cama in Bombay city, David Sassoon in Poona, Hutteesing and Premabhai in Ahmedabad, Sir Cowasji Jehangir (C.J.) in Surat, founded with Indian funds in the previous century, civil hospitals were located in twenty towns of the Presidency, including Aden and Muscat. The third type, mainly dispensaries, were financed by municipalities and district local boards. The municipalities were in constant financial distress and government found itself being called upon to pay the salaries of personnel who manned them. Under law, the local boards were expected to maintain the dispensaries, and received a grant share from the Government of India.[6] The fourth type of medical institutions were established by private subscribers; they occasionally received government or local funds.

Evidences of governmental reluctance to provide financial support at the turn of the century are to be found in the records. Thus, in 1899, grants to the Ranchodlal and Victoria Jubilee (V.J.) dispensaries in Ahmedabad were decreased and had to be supplemented by private contributions.[7] The Collector pointed out, in vain, that these dispensaries were availed of by women patients from outside the city.[8] In 1901, a number of grants-in-aid dispensaries, which had been established in the previous century by donors paying for the building, furniture and sometimes even the salary of the medical officer, were sanctioned lower grants. A proposal for an endowed dispensary in Nipani was not approved because the municipality was in debt and could not bear its share.[9] Similarly, the municipalities of Ratnagiri, Karwar and Belgaum were in dire financial straits and could not support hospitals and dispensaries in the early 1900s, and the Bombay government did not want to support them. On the other hand, the compulsions of a malarial location and the distance from medical help led to sanction being granted for the establishment of a dispensary at Sujawal in Sind. The reactions of officials to the request from the American Marathi Mission, Ahmednagar, for a grant to fund the building of their hospital, are interesting. The local Collector suggested that the grant be made conditional to the hospital being opened to all castes, without distinctive treatment to Indian Christians. He also recommended that the hospital staff should be recruited solely on merit, and that the Civil Surgeon and Collector be included in the management. The Surgeon General, G. Bainbridge, held that government hospitals and leper asylums had greater claim to these funds. The application was consequently rejected, with a small token amount being sanctioned.[10] In the case of Nadiad, the people obviously wanted western medicine and maintained a dispensary without government assistance. They unsuccessfully called for aid from government only when they found the municipality-appointed doctor's performance in medico–legal cases unsatisfactory.[11] In Chiplun, a grant-in-aid dispensary was sanctioned in response to the observation made by the additional sessions judge, Ratnagiri, about the absence of facilities for post-mortem examination. The Civil Surgeon, while endorsing the necessity, pointed out that the lack of a dispensary led to concealment of crimes such as criminal abortion and death from poisons.[12]

Most donors to hospitals and dispensaries in the Presidency were Parsis, indicating higher receptivity of western medicine by them.

Nagar Brahmins, Banias and Jains in Ahmedabad, Bohras in Surat, Sindhis in Karachi and Hyderabad, Marathas in the Konkan, Jews in Poona, and local Muslims in Aden also made endowments. Benefactions were made for different purposes. Thus, Kakkirapa Timappa Mudiraddi donated Rs 1,000 per annum for diets of poor patients in the Hubli dispensary. Rustamji Byramji Jejeebhoy not only donated towards building a hospital at Matheran, but also made a separate contribution for the purchase of dispensary labels and books. Nasserwanji Jehangir Wadia endowed a dispensary at Andheri, Bombay, Sir Dinshaw Manekji Petit at Panvel, Bomanji Ardeshir Dalal in the Panchmahals, and Khan Bahadur Nowroji Pestonji Vakil an ophthalmic hospital at Ahmedabad. Bai Alibai, the sister of a western-educated doctor, B.H. Nanavatty, provided funds for an aseptic operating table and aseptic instruments, for use in the C.J. Hospital, Surat. Sir Chunibhai Madhavlal, grandson of Ranchodlal Chotalal, the pioneer of public health in Ahmedabad, contributed Rs 1,15,000 for a training school for nurses and midwives in Ahmedabad. The Western India Turf Club's donations improved facilities for the treatment of military patients, and enabled the installation of electricity and remodelling of the X-ray room at Sassoon Hospital. Jerbai Wadia offered to build and maintain a permanent dispensary at Khandala, provided the government gave the land. The dispensary had been started by her husband at the request of the villagers in 1896.

To what extent were the donors involved in the running of these institutions? Jerbai had her son included in the management committee of the dispensary and recommended that the hospital assistant, who had been serving on a temporary basis, be absorbed into government service.[13] Again, the move to shift the Rukminibai dispensary in Kalyan was dropped in deference to the wishes of the donor's (Mangaldas Nathubhai) family.[14] The Bombay Municipal Corporation had a committee of Indians including Sir Pherozeshah Mehta, Doctors Bhalchandra Krishna Bhatavadekar and N.N. Katrak, among others, to scrutinize donations offered to build dispensaries.

The paucity of beds in hospitals is repeatedly recorded. By 1922, 6,717 beds are said to have been available in the Presidency.[15] Bombay city had only 1,557 beds for a population of 9,79,445 persons, and of these, 638 were specially for accident cases and sudden illnesses.[16] The urgent requirement for another hospital in the mill area led to the construction of the King Edward Memorial Hospital in 1926, in Parel.

Patient Profile

The reports collated statistics about the patients, community-wise under the following heads: Hindu, Muslims, 'Others', and Europeans, which included Eurasians. In 1907, Hindus constituted 63.3 per cent, Muslims 30 per cent, 'Others' 6 per cent, and Europeans 0.7 per cent, of the total number of patients in hospitals and dispensaries. In the same year, men patients constituted 49.2 per cent, women 20.6 per cent, male children 17.5 per cent, and female children 12.7 per cent of the total. These figures would be representative for the two-decade period of this study.[17]

An issue which the authorities found objectionable was that the well-to-do took gratuitous medical treatment, meant for the poor. Rules were issued to put a stop to this practice and when municipalities refused to comply government grants were withdrawn, as in the case of the Raipur dispensary in Ahmedabad. Requests to set up hospitals for women at Surat and Karachi were rejected for similar reasons. Subsequently, it was laid down that income-tax payees, persons earning more than Rs 40 per month, 'servants' of municipalities or of private firms, and those paying land revenue upwards of Rs 300 per annum were to be charged for treatment. The charges were fixed at 8 annas for consultation, 3 annas for medicines and 4 annas for subsequent consultations.[18] The Bombay government observed that the law, which made the maintenance of these institutions obligatory on municipalities, discouraged private contributions.[19]

In 1910, there were debates among the senior British IMS officers about free medical assistance being used irrespective of the patient's circumstances. One suggestion made was that, like in England, public hospitals should be closed to the rich. These discussions also reveal differing perceptions within the medical establishment about the extent of the acceptance of western medicine in this first decade of the twentieth century. While Major Evans, Senior Surgeon, J.J. Hospital, maintained that Indians of all shades appreciated 'our therapeutics and surgery at its value', his counterpart at Poona, Lt Col. Smith averred that 'well-educated England-returned' Indians used western medicine in alternation to the treatment provided by *hakims* and *vaids*. Private practitioners found that they had to lower their fees to compete with free dispensaries, besides having to compete with indigenous practitioners, failed students, ex-compounders and dressers. Lt. Col. Collie, of St George's Hospital, contended that private practitioners were to be found in every small town of the Presidency. Indians went no more to *hakims* and *vaids* than all classes in Europe patronized quacks, bone-setters and chemists. Where in Europe or America would state-run institutions receive well-to-do patients on Rs 4 per diem, he asked. He also observed that in Ratnagiri, *vakils* and *sirdars* attended along with labourers and fishermen. European private practitioners charged Rs 5–10 per visit, while their Indian counterparts charged Rs 3–5 per visit, and hence it was remarked that Europeans from 'every walk of life' went to the latter. They found health care cheaper in India, an operation in a provincial town in England costing the equivalent of Rs 1,000, while at Sassoon Hospital, Poona, it cost only Rs 150.[20]

Diseases Treated

The hospital and dispensary reports for the nineteenth century collected statistics of admissions mainly under the heads of smallpox, cholera and fevers. Till 1910, the categories included, besides the first two mentioned above, respiratory diseases, malarial fevers, rheumatic fevers, dysentery and diarrhoea, diseases of the eye, and venereal diseases. The largest number of patients were treated for malarial fevers, while the smallest number were treated for smallpox (Tables 1 and 2). Quinine was sold at cheap rates in malarial districts, particularly in Sind. A large number of dysentery and diarrhoea cases were either among pilgrims or the destitute. However, it was noted with satisfaction that people were beginning to realize the advantage of protecting their water supply with potassium permanganate, which was freely distributed. The major hospitals, like J.J, which had limited beds, only took in cases of serious illness and accidents.

Even in the previous century, patients had resorted to hospitals for surgery, despite reservations of ritual pollution. The use of anaesthesia had made surgery acceptable. The number of admissions for 'injuries' followed those for malaria. These included industrial accidents, which were found to be growing with the 'introduction of mechanical appliances'.[21] The largest number of surgeries were for the

Indian Responses to Western Medicine

TABLE 1: *Number of In-Patients at Hospitals, Bombay Presidency, 1911–22*

Year	Small-pox	Malarial fevers	Tuber-culosis	Other tuber-culosis	Cholera	Dysen-tery	Diarr-hoea	Labour cases	Leprosy
1911	460	6,380	1,049	966	103	1,157	1,280		1,844
1912	810	6,727	1,035	1,193	735	1,793	1,706		1,757
1913	457	6,736	1,108	1,247	94	1,496	1,314	3,556	1,627
1914	390	7,193	1,179	1,156	290	1,529	1,476	5,378	1,502
1915	583	6,879	1,164		30	1,279	1,189	6,195	1,590
1916	1,348	7,919	1,119		202	1,482	1,202	6,723	1,546
1917	554	8,757	1,158	970	146	1,469	1,148	7,559	1,525
1918	1,798	6,844	1,058	990	598	1,303	1,066	7,245	1,968
1919	1,116	8,149	1,428	1,223	1,474	1,948	1,668	6636	1,730
1920	686	8,529	1,297	1,302	189	1,666	1,468	7,857	1,724
1921	636	9,768	1,589	1,044	105	1,720	1,362	8,291	2,461
1922	260	7,980	1,298	1,007	72	1,385	1,450	6,936	1,531

Source: *Report of Civil Hospitals and Dispensaries, Bombay Presidency,* relevant years (the blank spaces indicate non-availability of statistics).

TABLE 2: *Statistics of Out-patients at Hospitals and Dispensaries, Bombay Presidency*

Diseases	Mean for Triennium, 1911–13	Mean for Triennium, 1914–16	Mean for Triennium, 1917–19	Mean for Triennium, 1920–22
Smallpox	440	162	351	302
Malarial fevers	383,919	443,460	462,057	450,047
Tuberculosis	5,246	4,8498	4,532	5,419
Other tuberculosis	4,765	4,634	4,123	4,595
Cholera	1,829	1,291	1,734	524
Dysentery	39,742	39,425	39,139	35,410
Diarrhoea	51,184	50,780	49,137	50,413
Leprosy	679	621	573	598
Injuries	152,365	173,533	165,562	190,209

Source: *Report of Civil Hospitals and Dispensaries, Bombay Presidency,* relevant years.

removal of 'vesical calculi' (stones in the kidney), followed by extraction of the lens for cataract. Other surgeries included abdominal operations, operations for hernia, abscess of the liver, removal of cysts and tumours, and amputations. Surgical work was commended for its high standard, and was facilitated by 'improved means of carrying out aseptic work'.[22] That treatments were by and large successful is evident from the decline in the ratio of deaths to total patients treated. In fact, during the World War, serious surgical cases from East Africa and Mesopotamia were treated at St George's. The level of progress was high in the large hospitals, where much was done to update the operation rooms and provide aseptic instruments, but these facilities were wanting in the mofussil areas. It was observed that acute surgical cases were received in hospitals after being treated by indigenous practitioners, narcotics having been given to stifle the pain. Chronic cases came, expecting to be relieved of the pain, and the surgeon often operated not to save or prolong a life but to relieve the unbearable symptom. It was further noted that Hindus would remove patients against medical advice, in order to perform the last ceremonies at home.[23]

From 1911, the reports distinguished between tuberculosis of the lung and other tuberculars. Tuberculosis attracted frequent notice in the reports, since the number of admissions of these cases increased. The proposal to have separate wards was deferred in 1916, owing to war expenses. Venereal diseases were another challenge. They constituted 30 per cent of the cases among out-patients and 18 per cent of in-patients at J.J. Hospital, and 11 per cent of the general practitioners' clientele. 30 per cent of infant deaths were due to infantile syphilis. When influenza broke out in epidemic form in 1918, not only was the disease not recognized promptly but there was no head under which cases could be recorded, and hence they were registered under 'other infectious diseases'.

Supplementing the work of curative medicine were the voluntary efforts to contain and prevent diseases. The King George V Anti-Tuberculosis League was established in 1912, due to the collaborative efforts of J.A. Turner, Executive Health Officer, Bombay city, and Dr N.H. Choksi, who had done commendable work at the Infectious Diseases Hospital during the plague outbreak of 1896–97. The League aimed at spreading information about the disease through lectures and distribution of pamphlets, conducting visits by health visitors and medical inspection at mills, schools and factories. It did not fund a hospital for advanced cases, but set up a dispensary.[24] Lectures and magic lantern demonstrations were also given by the Director of the Bombay Bacteriological Laboratory and by Indian medical officers of the District Sanitary Associations of Dharwar and Bijapur. Sanitaria were founded in Devlali. Dr B.S. Kanga, who was in charge of the Lingoobai Tuberculosis Dispensary, and Dr F.N. Moos, who was qualified in public health, called for greater involvement of municipalities in providing parks and gardens.[25] Yet it was felt that there was general apathy and lack of consciousness of the infectiousness of the disease, consumption being looked upon as a matter of luck and unavoidable.

The other area where voluntary organizations worked was with persons afflicted with venereal diseases. These were the Anti-Venereal League, under the charge of Dr Socrates Noronha, the Salvation Army, the Presidency Women's Council, Pandita Ramabai's Home at Khedgaon, and the Hubli Criminal Tribes Women's Home.

Facilities for Women

Hospitals and dispensaries were classified as 'general and female'. The need for increasing the numbers of the latter was repeatedly emphasized. Cama Hospital, set up in 1886 for the exclusive use of women and children, increased the number of beds and opened a separate ward for septic cases.[26] Grants were given to the Lady Dufferin Hospitals in Sholapur and Sukkur, Baker Hospital in Larkana, and King Edward Memorial Hospital in Poona. The number of adult females seeking medical relief was 20.8 per cent of the total in 1909.[27] The establishment of facilities for particular communities would have helped overcome inhibitions. 1887 saw the founding of the Parsi Lying-in Hospital; the Masina (1902), Khoja (1918) and Bhatia (1922) Maternity Hospitals were established in Bombay city in the next century. Endowments were also made for lying-in facilities in other cities. The Naoroji Maternity Hospital, Ahmedabad, was set up for Parsis and Europeans.[28] The forty-two-bed Jacob Sassoon General Hospital was opened in 1909 in Poona for Europeans, with ten beds reserved for Jews; the family of Padamji offered to put up a lying-in ward attached to the Pestonji Sorabji dispensary, Poona; and Chinubhai Madhavlal funded a new lying-in ward at the V.J. dispensary.[29]

Surgeries on women included mainly obstetric operations, like the removal of fallopian tubes, fibroids, ovarian cysts and uterine appendages. Interestingly, inducement of premature labour and abortion, and hysterectomy were also recorded. While in the first decade it was observed that there was high mortality among parturient women, being brought in after every other measure had been tried, an increase in the number of 'labour' cases was reported by the second decade of the century. Of these, an increase of 31.3 per cent was noted in the municipal dispensaries in Bombay city and 19.9 per cent in the mofussils.[30] It was found that better maternal health care was not only required but also appreciated. Yet, mortality at childbirth was 5 per 100, against 5 per 1,000 in England.[31] The views of two contemporary women doctors are to be seen in this connection. Dr Jerbanoo Mistry made a forceful plea for more maternity homes, ante-natal care for expectant mothers, and training of midwives and *dais*, in her paper presented at the All-India Social Service Conference, Bombay. She pointed out that not only poor but upper- and middle-class women were ignorant of hygiene and the care of infants. 'Many women who are childless and permanently disabled are so from maltreatment received during delivery.'[32] She also made the pertinent observation that the training provided thus far had not succeeded because it had adopted European methods without altering them to suit Indian needs. Dr J.R. Dadabhoy, in her paper on infant mortality at the same conference, suggested 'preventive obstetrics', which was the supervision of women from early pregnancy till lying-in was over, as the solution to combat maternal and foetal morbidity. Her contention was that 70 per cent of infant deaths could be prevented with proper measures for infant feeding, including breast-feeding.[33]

Voluntary work was done for maternal and infant welfare. This comprised visits by lady health visitors, and publication of booklets on maternal and child care. It was recorded that the percentage of women being attended by untrained women had fallen. The Bombay Sanitary Association campaigned for the reduction of infant mortality and the Lady Willingdon Scheme provided for more maternity wards in Bombay.

Staffing of Institutions

While dispensaries were manned by underpaid Indian assistant surgeons and hospital assistants, the top positions in the larger hospitals were still held by British doctors of the IMS. The IMS was meant to furnish medical men for the army, but the fact was that they held civil appointments in sanitary and medical departments. There was no chance for anyone, Indian or even European, however able or brilliant, to get this appointment. It was this monopoly that was the basic issue of the medical reform movement which was spearheaded by the Bombay doctors Atmaram Pandurang and K.N. Bahadurji, in the 1890s.[34] Even after thirty years there was no change. Most western-educated Indian doctors, for over half a century, had successful private practice. The medical profession of the Bombay Presidency, under the aegis of the Bombay Medical Union (BMU), submitted a memorial to the Secretary of State under the chairmanship of Dr Bhatavadekar in 1909, protesting the anomalies and abuses of the monopoly by the IMS.[35] The BMU claimed with satisfaction in 1912 that, as a result of their long struggle, the posts of honorary physicians and surgeons at J.J. Hospital and the professorships of bacteriology and physiology at Grant Medical College (the only medical college then in the Presidency) had been thrown open to Indians.[36] In the 1919 IMS Commission, the only Indian medical representative was Sir T.B. Nariman. While conceding that the IMS had done good work, the *Indian Social Reformer* remarked that it was an anomaly with no parallel in any civilized country.[37] As the *Servant of India* pointed out: 'Competent Indian talent has been iniquitously excluded. The millions of the population have been allowed to suffer from the absence of an independent medical profession, since the prizes of the service and the opportunities of hospital practice are monopolized by officers lent from the military.'[38]

During the war, the Lady Hardinge War Hospital was set up in Bombay, where Indian doctors served as honorary physicians and surgeons.[39] Though it was noted that the proportion of medical officers to patients was lower in Bombay than in London, the fact that the subordinate positions were held by Indians doubtless created confidence in those who came to hospitals and dispensaries. By 1918 the health officer in Karachi was Dr E.D. Shroff, who had a degree in public health, and in Ahmedabad, Dr R.K. Mhatre. The paucity of women doctors to attend to women patients was repeatedly noted in the reports. Jerbanoo Mistry observed that they would rather die than let male doctors attend on them.[40] It was under the direction of Dr Motiben Kapadia that the V.J. dispensary became popular. In the 1920s, Indian doctors like Avabai Mehta, Jerusha Jhirad and Cecilia D'Monte were appointed medical officers at Cama Hospital, Avabai having been house surgeon for two decades.[41] A gradual Indianization of services took place when health came under the charge of Indian ministers in the third decade of the century.

Nursing services in Bombay city had been provided by the All Saints Sisters, Anglican missionaries, from 1884–1902. However, it was observed that most of the medical establishment did not appreciate the need for nursing. In the 1900s nursing was promoted first for Europeans. Consequently, St George's Hospital, which catered exclusively to Europeans and Eurasians, received three times the government grant given to the J.J. group of hospitals, which was the largest in western India.[42] This anomaly seems to have been removed by 1911. A total provision of Rs 1,16,977 was made as grants to nursing, of which Rs 40,000 was allotted to J.J.[43] A committee including Dr Annette Benson, who served at Cama Hospital from 1894–1918, recommended the training of nurses.[44] It was pointed out that modern methods of treatment required constant skilled attention, and the testimony of doctors who had trained nurses to assist them pointed to the value of this measure. At the same time, the apathy of Indians in contributing to the G.T. Hospital Nursing Association was noted, even though the committee included Indians: Sir Dinsha Petit, Dr Bhatavadekar, Ibrahim Rahimtula and Gordhundas Goculdas Tejpal. The Bombay Presidency Nursing Association was established in 1910 and conducted qualifying examinations. Associations were also set up at Belgaum, Dharwar and Matheran.[45] These organizations mainly provided European or Eurasian nurses to war hospitals, hospital ships and private nursing. By 1917, facilities for training nurses were available at J.J., Cama, and St George's, and civil hospitals in Poona and Karachi, at the King Edward VII training institute, Ahmedabad, and the Morarabhai Vribhukandas dispensary, Surat.[46]

Conclusion

This paper has explored aspects of colonial policy and Indian attitudes. While the former revealed contradictions, the latter showed ambivalence in Indian responses towards this area of public health. Though governmental reluctance to provide financial support to institutions is evident, there were instances when the authorities initiated the establishment of dispensaries, in malarial districts, or when it was a necessity for judicial cases. Various issues appear in the correspondence between the government and local bodies. The latter often pleaded that plague measures added to their expenditure and applied for increase in grants, but the former expected greater fiscal discipline and recommended collection of arrears, noting in one instance that municipal councillors were defaulters.[47] It also seems clear that the government felt that it was obliged, if at all, to support facilities for the poor. Thus it dissociated itself from the Prince of Wales dispensary at Aden, established in 1875, funded by voluntary contributions and attended by well-to-do Arabs, Muslims and Parsis who did not attend the local civil hospital.[48] The policy of funding medical missionary work only if their institutions were open to all was pursued.

As indicators of receptivity to western medicine, the statistics of attendance at hospitals and dispensaries show a marginal change in Indian attitudes towards medical institutions. In his paper presented at the Bombay Medical Congress in 1909, Turner attributed the aversion to hospitals to the plague epidemic, and the unpopular measures of segregation and isolation. Indians knew of cholera and smallpox but the great mortality of plague was an unknown experience, and they ascribed this to doctors and hospitals and not to the disease. This led to protests against the Infectious Diseases hospitals in Bombay in 1897 and 1899. Forty caste and community hospitals, in the city of Bombay alone, had been established during the epidemic and had ceased to exist in 1900, when the policy of isolation was abandoned. Turner regretted that though thousands of patients left the hospitals cured, they did not advise their caste men to resort to them. He believed sanitary knowledge to be the only remedy to overcome inhibitions.[49] Yet, Indian financial support of these institutions continued to be considerable. On occasion, the paucity of funds postponed the establishment of dispensaries till Indian donors came forward, as in Khed district.[50] Endowing public welfare was in keeping with the Indian tradition. Thus the Ranchodlal home medical relief institution was set up at Ahmedabad to provide relief to those who were unable to attend hospitals and dispensaries. Not only were Indian civic leaders and doctors associated with hospital and nursing associations, but there was involvement in discussions pertaining to hospitals. Gokuldas Kahandas Parekh protested in an informal budget conference about the allotment of a grant to the Church of Scotland, on the grounds that the latter would use the hospital to proselytize. Subsequently this was sanctioned on the basis of an undertaking from the mission that the hospital would be open to all classes.[51] Non-governmental organizations supplementing state medical facilities were Indian-directed and financed. This was apparent during the influenza epidemic of 1918–19, when the government threw up its hands in despair and voluntary funding and effort saved lives, at least in the cities, by distributing flu mixture, milk and blankets.[52]

Notes and References

[1] Mridula Ramanna, 'The Establishment of Medical Education and Facilities for Women in the City of Bombay', *Indica*, 31, No. 1, March 1994, pp. 41–50. For a discussion on the promotion of hospitals and dispensaries see Mridula Ramanna, 'Western Medicine and Public Health in Colonial Bombay, 1845–1895', Hyderabad (forthcoming).

[2] David Arnold, *Colonizing the Body*, Berkeley, 1993, p. 270.

[3] 'Report on Native Papers, Bombay Presidency' (hereafter RN), *Mumbai Vaibhav*, 4 May 1899.

[4] David Arnold, *Colonizing the Body*, p. 270.

[5] General Department Volumes, Maharashtra State Archives, Mumbai, (hereafter GD), 12, 1910, No. 1253, 14 March 1910.

[6] *Proceedings of the Council of the Governor of Bombay*, Vol. xlii, Bombay, 1904, p. 51.

[7] Mridula Ramanna, 'Ranchodlal Chotalal: Pioneer of Public Health in Ahmedabad', *Radical Journal of Health*, 11, 2/3, 1996, pp. 99–111.

[8] GD, 38, 1899, Ahmedabad Collector/Commissioner, Northern Division, No. 4331 of 1898. The Bombay government had formulated the following rules regarding dispensaries in the 1860s: (1) a dispensary had to be located in a place of sufficient importance as regards the wants of the people, (2) the people were to erect a building at their expense, and (3) an assistant surgeon or hospital assistant was to be appointed in charge of the dispensary.

[9] GD, 48, 1901, No. 4404, 2 August 1901.

[10] GD, 49, 1902, No. 6983,15 December 1902

[11] GD, 58, 1910, No. 6226, 13 December 1910.

[12] GD, 40, 1907, Govt. Resolution (hereafter GR), 10 Janunary 1907.

[13] GD, 7, 1901, No. 6878, 7 December 1901.

[14] GD, 58, 1910, Letter No. 4907, 5 October 1910.

[15] *Triennial Report on Civil Hospitals and Dispensaries*, Bombay Presidency, 1920–22, Bombay, 1922, p. 2.

[16] *Report of Civil Hospitals and Dispensaries*, Bombay Presidency (hereafter RCHD), Bombay, 1916, p. 2

[17] RCHD, 1907, p. 6.

[18] GD, 49, 1903, No. 2870,21 September 1887.

[19] GD, 38, 1899, GR, 5792, 14 December 1899.

[20] GD, 75, 1910, Accompaniment to GR No. 5001, 11 October 1910.

21 RCHD, 1909, p. 3.

22 Ibid., 1908, p. 2.

23 GD, 11, 1908, Surgeon General/Govt of Bombay, No. s b/1925, 17 September 1908.

24 *Report of the Bombay Medical Union, 1911–12,* Bombay, 1913, pp. 141–42. While Ratan Tata gave Rs 15,000 per annum, the government and the municipality donated Rs 10,000 each, and the public subscribed Rs 1,35,000.

25 *Report and Proceedings of the All India Social Service Conference,* Bombay, 1924, pp. 125–41.

26 *Fifty Years of the Cama and Albless Hospitals,* Contemporary Medical Archives Centre, Wellcome Institute for the History of Medicine Library, London, p. 5.

27 RCHD, 1909, p. 2.

28 Ibid., 1908, p. 3

29 Ibid., 1907, p. 10.

30 Ibid., 1914, p. 2.

31 Ibid., 1917, p. 1.

32 Jerbanoo Mistri, 'Training and Provision of Dais and Midwives', in, *Report and Proceedings of Social Service Conference,* p. 57.

33 J.R. Dadabhoy, 'Infant Mortality, its causes and how to remedy it', in *Report and Proceedings of Social Service Conference,* p. 65.

34 Mridula Ramanna, 'Professional Reform: The Efforts of Dr K.N. Bahadurji', *Journal of the University of Mumbai,* 54, 1997, pp. 95–109.

35 *British Medical Journal,* 29 January 1910, p. 271.

36 *Report of the Bombay Medical Union for 1911–12,* Bombay, 1913, p. vi.

37 RN, *Indian Social Reformer,* 23 March 1919.

38 RN, *Servant of India,* 4 July 1918.

39 RCHD, 1916, p. 9. They were Drs R. Rao, S.R. Shrigaonkar, V.N. Bhajekar, D.D. Gilder, G.V. Deshmukh and D.N. Duggan.

40 Jerbanoo Mistri, 'Training and Provision of Dais and Midwives', p. 57.

41 *Fifty Years of Cama,* pp. 6–7.

42 GD, 45, 1905, financial dept (hereafter FD), No. 3198, 21 September, 1905. Motlibai Hospital for women, Petit for children and the Dwarkadas Lallubhai dispensary were founded in 1892.

43 GD, 74, 1910, GR No. 6049, 2 December 1910.

44 GD, 45, 1905, Letter No. 723, 6 February 1905. Benson had a reputation as a surgeon, attracting patients from different parts of India. *Fifty Years of Cama,* p. 6.

45 RCHD, 1910, p. 6

46 Ibid., 1917, p. 1.

47 GD, 58, 1910, Letter No. 4224, 1 September 1910.

48 GD, 69, 1911, Letter No. 3954, 29 June 1911.

49 J.A. Turner, 'Sanitation in India', in *Proceedings of the Bombay Medical Congress,* 1909, p. 471. He described the practices followed to elude the vigilance of the plague officials, like hiding the sick with the dead or under

mattresses, or even tying up corpses in sitting positions near the cooking places.

[50] GD, 58, 1910, FD No. 440, 5 February 1910.

[51] GD, 74, 1910, letter No. 1513, 3 February 1919.

[52] See Mridula Ramanna, 'Coping with the Influenza Epidemic: The Bombay Experience', in Howard Phillips and David Killingray (eds.), *The Spanish Flu*, London (forthcoming).

Public Health Issues and the Freedom Movement

Gandhi on Nutrition, Sanitation, Infectious Diseases and Health Care

Amit Misra

The provision of basic health care to all citizens is one of the important goals of a welfare state. It seems worthwhile, therefore, to examine how far the freedom movement under the tutelage of Mahatma Gandhi was informed of the need to include basic health care in its agenda. It is hoped (albeit fondly) that an understanding of the agenda that has received the most widespread endorsement in recent Indian history would enable the channelization of our health policy along more democratic and humanitarian lines. In contrast to a disturbing contemporary movement in our country to deify the Vedas as the sole and sufficient fount of all knowledge and insight, it is not the intention of this paper to insist that whatever Gandhi had to say about public health is the last word on the subject. This paper, instead, is a naive attempt at historiography, on the one hand, and a defence of the Gandhian insight into health care, on the other.

The latter exercise is somewhat important in view of opinions that indict Gandhi for 'attacking modern civilization', imparting a 'serious setback' to the interest of the Congress in 'modern science' on account of his 'hostile indifference to modern science and technology'.[1]

Some of the premises on which this paper is based may be questioned by more sophisticated analysis; so it is fair to set them out unequivocally:

1. Gandhi's perception of the needs of the Indian people was realistic, compassionate and democratic.
2. Gandhi's style of political activity was not adversarial but conciliatory, so that demands concerning a whole range of issues were addressed equally to citizens and the state. The health

care sector was no exception to this generalization.

3. The solutions offered by Gandhi are deceptively simple in their statement, impeccable in their logic, yet frustratingly difficult to implement, in view of what is known of human behaviour. Nevertheless, they have immense capacity to enthuse us. In his own words, 'a way is not to be avoided because it is upward and therefore uphill.'[2]

4. Gandhi could revise opinions so far as to attain a stance diametrically opposite to a previous one. (This capacity of his shall be illustrated below through an example dealing with the treatment of malaria.) Thus, later opinions should be (and have been) construed as superseding earlier ones.

5. To an indeterminate, yet significant, extent, the freedom movement took serious note of Gandhi's opinions. The behaviour, pronouncements and actions of those engaged in the freedom struggle, therefore, were influenced strongly by Gandhi's attitudes.

Methodology

The *Collected Works of Mahatma Gandhi* (henceforth CW) represent a convenient, though admittedly not exhaustive, source for a limited enquiry into health care in India during the freedom movement. Gandhi's writings on infectious diseases, sanitation and nutrition relevant to public health have been culled mainly from keywords in the subject index to the CW. It must be confessed that despite the original intention, only volumes 50 to 90 (1933–48) have been covered with any degree of diligence.

A case is made out for evaluating Gandhi as a political thinker who appreciated not only the ethical need for the state to provide health care,[3] but also the strategic importance of including health care issues in grassroots politics, so that the people could be made aware of the importance of health care and of what they could do to help and empower themselves in order to improve public health status. One quotation should suffice to bolster the case that Gandhi was actually aware of the political nature of his programme on health care: 'Naturecure workers work for *Swaraj*.'[4] Another, though apparently professing an apolitical urgency, reveals the commitment that Gandhi felt for including nutrition, sanitation and health care in the agenda of the

Congress. Referring to the Constructive Programme of the Congress, which included village nutrition and sanitation work as a means of improving the health status, he said: 'The present programme is the foundation of an all-round improvement in the tottering condition of the seven lacs of India's villages. It is work that is long overdue. *It has to be done no matter what India's political condition is*[5] (emphasis added). I hope that this attempt to locate Gandhi, not merely as (but certainly also as!) a self-confessed 'crank, madman and faddist' or 'fanatic'[6] where matters of health are concerned, may also provide us with insights on health policies in the time of neo-liberal consensus.

An overview of the public health care system in British India is beyond the scope of the present work. One historian of medicine has pointed out that it is difficult to have 'a usable overview of a very long and complex set of changes (specially) in a study in development'.[7] Rather than attempting the heroic task, three sources have been used for additional information. The Bhore Committee Report[8] is an excellent source on the status and aims of the government's health care programme at that time. A little disappointingly, the contemporaneous report of the Congress's National Planning Committee[9] is more strident as well as sketchier. Roger Jeffery's work[10] is the source of almost all other information used in preparing this paper.

Nutrition

Gandhi has spoken and written about nutrition in the context of health with reference to famine and food shortage, as well as in normal times. Both kinds of writings reflect the style of politics referred to in the second premise listed above. Thus, the populace is implored to realize the benefits of a wholesome diet, and reminded that they need not look to the government for all they need. Congress workers are exhorted to spread awareness of simple measures that the people can adopt to improve diet, such as the use of pounded rather than polished rice, etc. Gandhi did seem to believe that the primary responsibility of good nutrition was in the hands of the people themselves, whatever the state may do to succour or deprive them.

Famine and food shortages were common occurrences during the British *Raj*. Then, as now, the role of nutrition in public health was considered only in passing by the government. Administrative exigency still continues to divide the work of 'Food and Civil Supplies' and 'Public Health', despite the growing realization that inter-sectoral cooperation is essential if any meaningful intervention in public health is to be made.

Gandhi's position on famine and food shortages can be easily summarized. It was obvious to him then, as it is to us in hindsight, that famine was (and is) a creation of the government.[11] The other important insight that he brought to this issue was that food shortages could be ameliorated if local produce was mobilized to supplement the diet.[12] Spelling out the role of government in creating famine, Gandhi has inculpated two aspects of agricultural production and distribution that are unfortunately still in practice. The first was the insistence on growing wheat and rice for the entire populace,[13] instead of a healthy mix of cereals like *jowar, bajra,* etc. The second was the procurement procedure, wherein all the produce is first transported to a central location and then painstakingly sent back to where it came from, after appropriating the amount required for urban consumption. With reference to the economics of local consumption of agricultural as well as cottage-industry production, he spelt out savings amounting to Rs 90 crore per annum in 1935, if 'the villagers are to be their own buyers. They will primarily consume what they produce. For they are ninety percent of the population.'5 When talking about the Constructive Programme of the Congress, he spelt out the '*khadi* mentality' thus: 'decentralization of the production and distribution of the necessaries [*sic*] of life'.[14] In 'olden times', he argued, every village had a granary and the populace had access to 'traditional means of agitation, insurrection and migration' when faced with a food shortage. The advent of rail transport disrupted this pattern of self-sufficient villages, and precipitated famine on a large scale.[11]

He holds the government responsible for famine, and refuses to offer appreciation for famine relief efforts, believing, no doubt, that tiding over famines using heroic measures would detract from the necessity of viewing their root cause. These views are consistently brought out when addressing the famine situation in Bengal (1943), where he asks the Congress not to cooperate with the government's effort at famine relief,[15] and with reference to famine in not only Bengal[16] but in several other areas.[17] Early expressions of these views can be encountered in references to famine in Orissa.[18]

The duty of the government, in happier times, lay merely in ensuring that its policies did not run counter to the needs of nutrition.

Even today, it is our demand of polished grain that results in loss of an extremely efficient source of micronutrients and fibre. Gandhi found the policy of encouraging mills for large-scale production of processed cereals worthy of comment. '(It is) incumbent on the government to see that at least the rice that is given to poor people has all its nutritive elements left in.'[19]

The Constructive Programme of the Congress, essentially Gandhi's brainchild, included 'Education in Health and Hygiene' in its agenda. Much of this education addressed nutrition. In addition to the Constructive Programme, the All-India Village Industries Association (AIVA) was expected to involve itself strongly in the work of nutrition. In a series of three articles in *Harijan,* Gandhi listed instructions to AIVA workers about implementing the use of un-polished rice, other common articles of food that were nutritious and locally available, and also regarding rural hygiene.[20] In discussing the 'meaning and place' of the Constructive Programme, Gandhi stressed the need to instill an appreciation of the importance of diet among the people.[21] Much earlier, addressing a meeting of the AIVA, he identified the 'triple malady' of Indian villages as comprising (1) want of corpo-rate sanitation, (2) deficient diet, and (3) inertia.[22]

Gandhi not only appreciated but repeatedly stressed the obvious: that nutrition is a prerequisite to health. References far too numerous to list here illustrate his concern for the diet of the common villager. This concern was firmly grounded on the perception of eco-nomic capacities. He once extolled a diet-chart prepared by Dr H.V. Tilak for the Bombay Baby and Health Week Association (!), and then proceeded to undo his praise by regretfully noting that it was not implementable in villages.[23] There are also numerous references to the need for better nutrition during pregnancy and lactation, but these are mostly derived from folk wisdom. Gandhi displays his fabled gender insensitivity in all of these writings, which I refrain from listing here.

The role of nutrition during states of disease was also spelt out in several instances. The 'Experiments in Dietetics' embodied in his autobiography, suggestions on diet to help a whole slew of ailments that his correspondents suffered from, and his own ill-informed attempts to give up animal proteins, I make bold to dismiss as unfortunate illustrations of his 'crankiness and faddism'. It is possible for a reader to experience extreme irritation at several of Gandhi's pon-tifications on the qualities of various articles of food. It is also tempting to speculate that such pronouncements could have antagonized or confused several of his followers, and strengthened the image of Gandhi as an irrational and impractical savant. The important thing, however, remains that Gandhi was ready to utter an opinion, however ingenuous it may have been, as soon as it was formed (at least as far as his experiments with health care are concerned). In this propensity at least, he was rather akin to present-day scientists like the present author, who rush to publish and propagate the results of every small experiment they undertake in their laboratory. Equally importantly, Gandhi's willingness to revise opinions, as stated earlier, in the light of new data, marks him out as a fellow-scientist with the required degree of open-mindedness. At least one such instance of revised opinion is worth describing here. The context is malaria. January 1935 has Gandhi declaring that 'quinine does seem to subdue malaria, but will not root it out.' He then suggests that the malaria patient 'must eschew starch, too much protein and live mainly on milk during convalescence'.[24] On 22 July 1935, he writes to Manilal and Sushila Gandhi, advising them to put malaria patients at the Segaon ashram under partial or complete fasting.[25] He goes on to describe with magisterial profundity a diet composed of this, that and the other, which is, by any standards, frugal and hardly likely to benefit a patient whose red blood cells are being destroyed by the malaria parasite. I could not trace what happened to those poor souls starved of nourishment when their reserves were already low,[26] but two years later, Gandhi himself blithely expounds to a journalist from *The Hindu*, the importance of a good diet during an attack of malaria.[27] He acknowledges admiration for quinine, but avers that 'administration of quinine is of no avail unless food is given to the people'. This instance is valuable in defence of Gandhi as a proponent of 'modern science and technology'. He comes across as 'scientifically minded' in a far better sense than someone who attaches more than due importance to the current scientific opinion. The criticism that he harboured 'hostile indifference to modern science and technology' is difficult to reconcile with the foregoing analysis.

It also probably needs to be pointed out that Gandhi was no proponent of vegetarianism where nutrition for the masses was concerned. There are numberless references to many non-vegetarians whom he saw as better proponents of non-violence than others who were vegetarian in diet but violent in thought, word and action.[28] More important, his writings and speeches in response to food shortages almost invariably ask people to use eggs, meat and fish to supplement their diets. A prosaic passage rendered poignant because of its date (29 January 1948) has Gandhi addressing a delegation from Madras that demanded rice and wheat from the Agriculture and Food Ministry of newly-independent India. He asks them to eat fish, which are 'available in plenty', and recalls a group of happy-go-lucky companions during the Dandi March, who used to hunt around for greens wherever the marchers stopped to camp, and cook them up in a stew for their meals.[12]

By far the most important thing, in Gandhi's view, was for the populace to be self-reliant in matters of nutrition as for other necessities. His model of 'real democracy' envisaged self-reliance and use of local material for food, 'leading to government action'.[12] It is evident that Gandhi expected the example of village communities that could demonstrate self-reliance, to steer policy adopted by the state. He was also able to appreciate the economic contribution of better nutrition, which he expected to ameliorate disease and improve the productivity of the people, as well as to result in savings on investment in health care. 'To provide nourishing food for the nation . . . is to give it both money and health.'[5]

The simplest solution that he had to offer for solving India's problems of nutrition can also be criticized on lines familiar to everyone who has ever been nonplussed by Gandhi's deceptively 'simple' ideas. 'Share your rations', he could say to partition refugees who had emerged from horror to confront squalor in the makeshift camp at Kurukshetra.[29] Utopian, perhaps, but how very ennobling as a vision of humankind behaving as it should instead of as it did!

Sanitation

Gandhi referred to sanitation, or the lack of it, with reference to health, in a huge number of documents. Of these, only 55 could be evaluated to arrive at the conclusions set out below. Once again, it is the populace that is the target of his address. As with nutrition, Gandhi places the onus for sanitation squarely on the people. There was no compromise with poverty being an extenuating circumstance for insanitation. 'Poverty is no bar to sanitation', he could proclaim, while acknowledging that 'chronic poverty and chronic breach of the laws of sanitation are equally to blame for (infectious) diseases'.[30] He could take no excuse, in fact, for uncleanliness, and there are several instances of him having spoken at civic receptions and addresses in his honour in a manner that was calculated to embarrass the organizers, perhaps to shame them into taking a greater interest in sanitation. He did this at Jamshedpur (to the discomfiture of the Tatas, one can imagine, telling them that 'the chain is only as strong as its weakest link'),[31] and at a whole host of other places including Ahmedabad, Allahabad, Goverdhan, Hardwar, Madras, etc.[32]

He has often gone so far as to dismiss all other health care programmes of various political and social formations as secondary to the problem of village sanitation. A group of Santiniketan students who had questions about the Constructive Programme was told that the conditions of the inhabitants of the villages would continue to 'be symbolized by the garbage dumps one finds in villages' 'so long as enough attention is not paid to village sanitation'.[33] Missionary ladies from Nagpur were dissuaded from setting up a dispensary to improve rural health—it would make 'no headway. . . . Tackling village sanitation is the only really substantial work.'[34] 'The intelligentsia—medical men and students' were told to do sanitation work in preference to practising medicine in villages.[20] His conception of the 'ideal Indian village' is one that 'will be so constructed as to lend itself to perfect sanitation'.[35]

To reiterate what has been said above, he was convinced, however, that no effort at improving sanitation would be worthwhile until it had popular support. Dear as the sanitation programme was to his heart, he was not willing to establish a fund apart from the Harijan Seva Sangh to further its activities. He was even opposed to attempts to collect money for sanitation work from outside the area where such work was planned. 'Let the work remain incomplete till the people themselves are prepared to pay for it', he wrote to Gangabehn Vaidya, who was engaged in sanitation work in (rural?) Bombay.[36]

It is in the matter of sanitation, however, that Gandhi can be observed to make clear and direct demands of the state. He has commented on the duty of the state to use revenue fairly: 'sanitary surroundings and fresh and wholesome water supply must form a first charge on the revenues of the villages as it affects the health of the people.'[19] Municipalities are encouraged to have 'bylaws requiring authorized receptacles, brooms, etc. . . . a simple working costume. Inspectors or overseers will be trained for humane sanitary work instead of being expected to extract work anyhow. The result of the present system is maximum insanitation and minimum work, plus bribery, corruption and bad manners.'[37] Still, on the issue of the duties of a municipal corporation, he wrote that 'the work and worth of the Corporation of Calcutta should be measured not by the number and beauty of its palaces, but by the condition of its slums'.[38] The individual Congress worker was suggested a course of action to make state bodies responsive to the needs of sanitation and sanitary workers, but at the same time reminded of the duties of the citizen. 'Corporations can lead the way . . . but they will not unless citizens insist. . . . Corporations have no soul that is apart from the souls of its citizens. . . . Concentrate his [Congress worker's] energy upon one single spot and there agitate, both among the people and their Corporation, for the much needed reform.'[39] For independent India, however, his advice is not to have a separate government department dedicated to promoting health-promoting lifestyles, regardless of the importance of the agenda. He felt that a government department would be an unnecessary expense, and the government would be 'delud(ing) itself and the gullible public that the greater the expense, the greater the utility'.[5]

The economic impact of insanitation was acutely appreciated by Gandhi, as was the case with nutritional deficiency. He also had comments on alleviating disease burden through sanitation, hoping that several diseases could be controlled through better sanitation. Much else of what he has said is difficult to dissect out from the next section. It may be important to state here that he realized the impact of insanitary conditions on the outbreak of a host of infectious diseases, including cholera, malaria, the plague and tuberculosis.

Infectious Diseases

Among the diseases that Gandhi addressed are cholera, jaundice, *kala-azar*, leprosy, malaria, the plague, smallpox and tuberculosis. While he was absolutely clear (as well as correct) on the issue of nutrition, sanitation and what has now come to be called 'community participation'[40] influencing outbreaks and outcomes, he was in a quandary (and is found to be wanting) in so far as his perceptions of appropriate therapy for these diseases is concerned. Sardar Patel undertook a relief campaign during a plague epidemic in Borsad during the summer of 1935. Gandhi's advice was to concentrate on scavenging, cleaning and rat-proofing dwellings, and distributing leaflets outlining preventive measures in order to 'create those conditions where rats and fleas can never flourish', without appeals for funds or volunteers from outside the area.[41] True to style, he appears reluctant to engage the state in demands for provision of health care.[42] Sardar Patel, engaged in grassroots work during the plague epidemic in Borsad, had apparently taken out a leaflet that might have been, among other things, critical of the government for its role in the epidemic. Gandhi wrote to him saying: 'I did not like the remark about the government or the local boards. Don't you think it is altogether importune at this time? In any case, it will certainly not help us.'[43] This reluctance is once again indicative of his propensities to conciliate rather than contend, and to expect the populace to be self-reliant rather than look to the state for help.

Gandhi's feelings for patients (rather, 'victims') of leprosy, indignation at the social stigmatization they incurred, and appreciation for Christian missionaries engaged in leprosy treatment are evident in several writings, but these do not easily yield any special understanding of his political agenda apart from *antyodaya.*

The rest of this section seeks to examine some of Gandhi's attitudes towards health care. It is also sought to be demonstrated that towards the end of his life, Gandhi accorded health care the foremost priority in his programme of action. The priority list in 1935 was 'removal of untouchability, khadi, village industries and plague work',[44] but by 1947, the plea was that 'the whole programme of village uplift [be pursued] together with nature cure'.[45] The story is best developed through an evaluation of his views on immunization, western medicine and nature cure.

Immunization

On the issue of immunization as a method of prophylaxis, his stand is clear but unjustifiable, in the light of epidemiologic experience since his time. He seems to have contracted an irrational dislike of the concept of vaccination, and plays disappointingly false to his robust sense of scientific enquiry when he condemns it out of hand. Something about the counter-intuitive nature of 'introduction of a disease in the guise of promoting health, such as the craze for various inoculations',[5] seems to have rubbed him the wrong way. He was 'convinced that vaccination has failed'[46] and 'disapprove[d] of it from every point of view',[47] even consoling a correspondent who had been given an 'injection of brandy' (!) that after all it was not 'as objectionable as a vaccine'.[48] The reproof is unmistakable in a letter to Jatindas M. Amin, who tried to go on fast to persuade inmates of Sevagram ashram to get inoculated against cholera. He is told to abandon his fast since 'we should make arrangements for those who wish to get inoculated, but we should not force those who are unwilling'. A day earlier he had written, apropos those inmates who did not wish to be inoculated: 'Let them die if they prefer to. They will have to be kept isolated if they contract cholera.'[49] The only conclusion possible is that Gandhi considered death preferable to immunization.

To be fair, however, he does warn other people of emulating him in this regard. He wrote to S.C. Das Gupta, a loved colleague (of whom more later): 'I don't know how far you are justified in avoiding vaccination (against smallpox). Of course, I am a fanatic about these matters. But I never like people to copy fanaticism.'[50] Again, to be fair, almost all quotations in the previous paragraph are blatantly out of context—a few words down the line, he would say something like 'our non-violent duty lies in either getting ourselves vaccinated or quitting the place. . . . I was asked . . . about the legislation concerning vaccination in Bombay and Madras [Presidencies, and said] that those who did not believe in vaccination should either leave the area or get themselves vaccinated.'[43] Or, he would reassure a concerned mother to get her children vaccinated, strangely, 'if you have no religious scruples'.[44] Even to Sardar Vallabhbhai Patel, he would admit that 'perhaps it would be safer to ignore my views regarding vaccination against the plague'.[51]

Pharmacotherapy, Outpatients and Institutional Care

Gandhi's views on therapeutic intervention in infectious disease were also novel, to say the least. He realized, of course, that modern medicine (he unfortunately refers to it most often as 'allopathy', after the fashion of most of our compatriots) was the most efficient in curing disease, and given certain reforms in aims and scope, 'an all-satisfying and inexpensive system'. However, he could still call it 'the concentrated essence of black magic'. This is one opinion he did not revise, and would allude to 'vivisection and other practices I call black' in 1933 as pejoratively as in 1947.[52, 53, 54]

He has written almost derisively of social workers who deliver 'medical aid' to the needy through distributing medicines, and instructs his workers to leave such work 'severely alone'.[55] Instead, his emphasis was always on educating people and searching for indigenous substitutes for common drugs. At Gandhi's behest, Satis Chandra Das Gupta undertook to produce a volume that could be used by village health workers, and also undertook several researches 'with a view to making drastic reductions in the number of [western] remedies, without diminishing their efficacy'.[56] This volume was started in 1933 and brought out in 1940 under the title of *Home and Village Doctor*, and received a rave-review from Gandhi.[57]

He was also sceptical about the scope of institutional care, although he collected funds for the Kamala Nehru Hospital and nurtured it with a view to make it 'primarily intended for the poor'.[58] In a significant letter to S. Ambujammal (Headmistress of Vidyodaya school, Madanapalle, and daughter of S. Srinivasa Iyengar), he explicitly stated that 'I do not expect a time when every villager who wishes can have good hospital treatment. But I do expect . . . [that] he can have at his door competent advice.'[59]

Despite his disillusionment with 'the false science'[60] of modern western medicine, Gandhi was no unqualified admirer of 'indigenous' (Ayurvedic, Unani) or 'alternative' (homeopathic) medicine. The criticism of *vaidyas* and *hakeems* for obscurantism and of homeopaths for inefficacy is nothing short of scathing.[61]

Gandhi's objections to modern medicine stemmed from his perception that it was:

1. Preoccupied with prolonging life and curing rather than preventing disease,
2. Expensive and not implementable in villages,
3. Reductionist and dismissive of traditional knowledge, and
4. Most often, the easiest way out for patients, not educating them about the cause of the disease they had, or equipping them with the wherewithal to resist diseases through their own initiatives.

Much of the criticism was and still is deserved, but Gandhi's attitude cannot be simply described as sufficiently reasoned. It is perplexing, for instance, that his fabled capacity for reconciliation could not be extended to reforming medicine and its practitioners along lines he thought appropriate. Instead, he seems to have preferred a clean and complete break with medicine, establishing the nature cure clinic at Uruli Kanchan.

Nature Cure

It is important to appreciate the background of events leading up to Gandhi's involvement in the grand enterprise of nature cure (NC). During 1944, Dr Dinshaw Mehta apparently got the idea of remodelling his clinic on Poona's Toddywala Road into an NC clinic, and thence to go on to establish a university dedicated to the study and development of principles of NC. At some point in 1944–45, he involved Gandhi in this project. Gandhi, probably at this very time, was himself contemplating an NC experiment on an ambitious scale. Writing to Mahavir Prasad Poddar inviting him to be a co-trustee in a trust comprising Gandhi himself, G.D. Birla, Dinshaw Mehta and Devdas Gandhi, he detailed his scheme. He wanted to take over about '1,000 acres' in an 'inaccessible village', where there would be no motorable roads but a well-planned settlement incorporating 'a swimming pool and gym' thriving on 'self-grown food'. NC (in all its glory) was to be practised there—including mud-packs, water therapy, the use of coloured cloth and bottles, sunlight, moonlight, air, etc. No modern methods or devices were to be employed. The emphasis, however, was to be on building up health: its 'preservation and improvement'. He hoped that this settlement would 'grow into an ideal village'.[62] The dynamic between Mehta and Gandhi is interesting in itself. Mehta seems to be keen on adopting some aspects of NC that may have been then prevalent in the west, and Gandhi replies, 'we should not use foreign things whether they are patent or not. We must make Sanatogen here.'[63] Gandhi suggests Nasik as a location for the proposed NC clinic, where the Birlas were 'willing to give land, etc.', but Mehta disagrees and the idea is dropped.[64] Nevertheless, a trust is formed with Gandhi, Mehta and Jahangir Patel as trustees in January–February 1946, and Gandhi sends a note to Mehta incorporating ten points on clinic administration on strictly democratic lines; examination, admission and treatment of patients through NC; and listing ailments that merit the clinic's attention. These include 'indigestion, fever, smallpox, constipation, headache, eczema, eruption, measles, chickenpox, itch, dysentery, such other ailments common among the villagers'.[65] However, the very next month, Gandhi begins to have misgivings about the project and, in a rather anguished confession published in the *Harijan*, shows disagreement with many facets of Dr Mehta's project. His concerns are that the project is not in consonance with his concept of NC being 'for the villager', 'near his cottage' and so on.[66] Very soon, he confides in Sardar Patel to the effect that 'nature cure is no longer a hobby with me. I must try it out in detail', and goes on to ask him to look for a suitable location for his own NC clinic.[67] Two days later, several prominent people from Uruli Kanchan, 30 kilometres from Pune on the Pune–Sholapur road, ask him to check out their village as a prospective site, and the decision to establish an ashram there is taken.

The therapeutic programme followed by the Uruli clinic would send shivers of disbelief and alarm down the spine of anyone acquainted with modern medicine, however prepared they may be to laud its objectives of providing affordable medical care using local remedies at the villagers' doorstep. It is disconcerting to realize that almost the entire British Pharmacopoeia was to be eschewed, no equipment, not even a microscope to be used and no 'present-day doctors' to be appointed at the clinic.[68] It is also with trepidation that one views the mystic's enthusiasm in propagating the recitation of *Rama nama* as 'the sovereign remedy', having 'no connection with superstition' and being 'nature's supreme law'.[69] However, there is much that is admirable, farsighted and innovative about the programme. As the manager of the ashram is told: 'when you develop nature cure to its highest potential, it will include village uplift work also.'[70] On this note, this paper had better end.

Acknowledgements are due to Anil Nauriya and the Amarpakshi Trust for having introduced me to Gandhiji, R.N. Misra for comments and criticism, and Saman Habib for help in preparing this paper. Prashant Kumar and Anupam Kumar, of Dastavez Prakashan, Lucknow, let me use their bookstore as a lending library.

Notes and References

[1] Jagdish N. Sinha, 'Science and the Indian National Congress', in Deepak Kumar (ed.), *Science and Empire*, New Delhi, 1991, pp. 161–81.

[2] M.K. Gandhi, *Collected Works of Mahatma Gandhi* (henceforth *CW*), 83, pp. 286–87 (19 March 1946), New Delhi, 1994

[3] *CW*, 62, p. 88 (2 November 1935).

[4] *CW*, 85, pp. 118–19 (3 August 1946). Also *Harijan*, 11 August 1946.

[5] *CW*, 60, p. 415. Also *Harijan*, 13 March 1935.

[6] *CW*, 90, pp. 268–69 (12 December 1947). Also, *Harijan*, 28 December 1947.

[See also *CW*, 53, p. 355 (19 February 1933) for the purpose of this citation but not subsequent ones.]

7 Joe Scott, 'Medicine and History in the SHP syllabus', in Michael Shortland and Andrew Warwick (eds), *Teaching the History of Science*, London, 1989.

8 *Report of the Health Survey and Development Committee*, Vols. I–IV, New Delhi, 1946.

9 *Report of the Subcommittee on Public Health*, National Planning Committee of the Indian National Congress, Bombay, 1946.

10 Roger Jeffery, *The Politics of Health in India*, London, 1988.

11 *CW*, 83, pp. 97–104, 286–87, 404 (March through May 1946). Also *Harijan*, 31 March 1946, 19 May 1946.

12 *CW*, 90, pp. 525–26, 530 (29 Januray 1948); *CW*, 86, p. 387 (24 January 1947). Also *Harijan*, 9 February 1947.

13 *CW*, 85, pp. 280, 350 (8 September 1946, 21 September 1946). Also *The Hindustan Times*, 9 September 1946, *Harijan*, 29 September 1946.

14 *CW*, 75, pp. 146–66 (13 December 1941).

15 *CW*, 77, p. 342 (29 June 1944).

16 Ibid., pp. 248, 344, 388; *CW*, 81, p. 453; *CW*, 82, p. 149; *CW*, 83, pp. 97, 123.

17 *CW*, 83, pp. 110–12, 123; *CW*, 85, p. 280.

18 *CW*, 18, p. 333.

19 *CW*, 70, pp. 34–40 (August 1939).

20 *CW*, 60, pp. 108–10, 150–51, 190–92 (*Harijan*, 25 January, 2 and 8 February 1935).

21 *CW*, 72, pp. 450–51 (14 September 1940), 378–81 (13 August 1940); *CW*, 75, pp. 146–66 (13 December 1941).

22 *CW*, 62, p. 379 (7 May 1936).

23 *CW*, 61, p. 379 and *Harijan* 31 August 1935.

24 *CW*, 60, p. 119 (28 January 1935).

25 *CW*, 61, p. 276 (22 July 1935).

26 A.H. Shankar, 'Nutritional modulation of malaria morbidity and mortality', *Journal of Infectious Diseases*,182 (Suppl. 1) 2000, S37–S53.

27 *CW*, 65, p. 35 (28 March 1937).

28 *CW*, 72, p. 387 (15 August 1940); *CW*, 62, p. 99 and elsewhere.

29 *CW*, 90, pp. 15–18 (12 November 1947).

30 *CW*, 86, p. 439 (6 February 1947). Also *Harijan*, 8 February 1947.

31 *CW*, 65, p. 299.

32 *CW*, 42, pp. 75, 179; *CW*, 56, p. 356 (January 1934); *CW*, 58, p. 18 (June 1934); *CW*, 84, p. 43 (April 1946).

33 *CW*, 87, pp. 229–30 (7 April 1947).

34 *CW*, 60, p. 324 (24 March 1935). Also *Harijan*, 29 March 1935.

35 *CW*, 64, p. 217. Also *Harijan*, 9 January 1937.

36 *CW*, 63, p. 162 (20 July 1936).

37 *CW*, 85, p. 401 (30 September 1946). Also *Harijan*, 6 October 1946.

38 *CW*, 62, p. 102. Also *Harijan*, 9 November 1935.

39 *CW*, 53, p. 268, Also *Harijan*, 11 February 1933.

40 V.P. Sharma (ed.), *Community Participation in Malaria Control*, Malaria

Research Centre, Indian Council of Medical Research, New Delhi, 1993. Also V.P. Sharma, Y.H. Bang, P. Rosenfield and C.P. Pant (eds), *Community Participation in Disease Vector Control*, Malaria Research Centre, Indian Council of Medical Research, New Delhi, 1986.

[41] *CW*, 61, p. 95. Also *Harijan*, 8 June 1935. *CW*, 60, pp. 420–21. Also *Harijan* 13 August 1935.

[42] *CW*, 85, pp. 122–24 (4 August 1946). Also *Harijan*, 11 August 1946.

[43] *CW*, 60, p. 336 (23 March 1935).

[44] Ibid., p. 361 (30 March 1935).

[45] *CW*, 87, p. 275 (13 April 1947).

[46] *CW*, 69, pp. 218–28 (6 May 1939).

[47] *CW*, 57, p. 222 (26 February 1934).

[48] *CW*, 56, p. 83 (11 October 1933).

[49] *CW*, 81, pp. 202, 212 (1 and 2 September 1945).

[50] *CW*, 53, p. 355 (19 February 1933).

[51] *CW*, 60, p. 372 (2 April 1935).

[52] *CW*, 65, p. 361 (3 July 1937).

[53] *CW*, 54, p. 305 (4 April 1933); *CW*, 85, pp. 122–24 (4 August 1946). Also *Harijan*, 11 August 1946.

[54] *CW*, 88, pp. 23–24, 386 (28 May and 21 July 1947).

[55] *CW*, 62, pp. 103–04. Also *Harijan*, 9 November 1935. *CW*, 60, p. 324 (22 March 1935); pp. 384–85. Also *Harijan*, 5 April 1935.

[56] *CW*, 60, pp. 384–85. Also *Harijan*, 5 April 1935.

[57] *CW*, 71, pp. 299–300 (4 March 1940). Also *Harijan*, 23 March 1940.

[58] *CW*, 70, pp. 365, 368 (19, 20 September 1939); *CW*, 73, p. 352 (28 February 1941).

[59] *CW*, 73, p. 272 (5 January 1941).

[60] *CW*, 88, pp. 23–24 (28 May 1947).

[61] *CW*, 90, p. 330 (31 December 1947); *CW*, 88, p. 386 (21 July 1947); *CW*, 85, pp. 457–58 (14 October 1946), pp. 122–24 (4 August 1946); *CW*, 78, pp. 350–51 (27 November 1944); *CW*, 77, p. 295 (27 May 1944); *CW*, 74, p. 281 (31 August 1941), p. 320 (September 1941); *CW*, 54, pp. 305–06 (4 April 1933).

[62] *CW*, 78, pp. 34–36 (17 August 1944).

[63] *CW*, 82, p. 75 (4 Novem,ber 1945).

[64] Ibid., p. 102 (21 November 1945).

[65] *CW*, 83, p. 94 (5 February 1946); *Harijan*, 10 February 1946; *CW*, 83, p. 157 (20 February 1946).

[66] *CW*, 83, pp. 217–19 (6 March 1946).

[67] Ibid., p. 288 (19 March 1946).

[68] *CW*, 87, pp. 275, 229–30 (13, 17 April 1947); *CW*, 85, pp. 105–06 (1 August 1946); *CW*, 84, p. 111 (6 May 1946).

[69] *CW*, 89, p. 470 (4 November 1947); *CW*, 88, pp. 23–24 (28 May 1947); *CW*, 87, p. 370 (27 April 1947); *CW*, 85, pp. 105–06 (1 August 1946); *CW*, 84, p. 125 (April–May 1946) and elsewhere.

[70] *CW*, 90, pp. 20–21 (12 November 1947).

Eliding History
The World Bank's Health Policies

Mohan Rao

One of the most remarkable things about the twentieth century has been the extraordinary improvement made in human health around the globe. India, for instance, commenced the century with a life expectation at birth of 22 years, the average life expectation of early agricultural societies and hunting and gathering ones. This was a terrible indictment of colonial rule and a reflection of the levels of hunger and infectious diseases—two of the horses of the apocalypse—that haunted us.

Today, of course, life expectations have vastly improved, and major famines and epidemics have been controlled. Average life expectation is in the early 60s, and infant mortality rates, considered a sensitive index of socio-economic development, have declined from around 200 in 1901 to around 62 in 2001.

Conventional wisdom is that this advance is a product of the rapid and dazzling progress made in medical technology. Wonderful new drugs, investigative techniques and their increasing access to the population at large, it is believed, are the 'magic bullets' that brought about this transformation, vanquishing those fearful enemies, germs. Such a germ-centric health history lies at the heart of public health both in India and the west. Contributing to this, developments in the field of psychology brought to the fore an individualistic and behavioural understanding of health and disease, wherein ill health was attributed to individual failings and proclivities.[1] At the same time, neo-classical economics, reinforcing the role of individuals as the sole movers of social events, reached its apogee.

These tendencies have largely influenced the understanding of public health across the globe. This paper argues that this approach is seriously misplaced and arises from a historiographic conflation of

265

the history of health with that of medicine. This historiography of medicine, however, seriously distorts an understanding of health and its determinants. As a consequence health policy planning not only limits its vision of intervention but also gravely undermines the possibilities of such intervention itself. This approach of uprooting health from its wider determinants finds its apogee in contemporary health policy initiatives of the World Bank.

I

A classic in the genre of the history of disease and health remains Zinsser's *Rats, Lice and History*.[2] Rich with epidemiological and historical insights, the work excavates the history of typhus, its impact on society and indeed on the tides of history, tracing the decline of this disease to a broad range of socio-economic factors. In contrast, McNeill's *Plagues and Peoples*[3] shrunk the epidemiological equation to the not unusual but nevertheless peculiar germ-centric focus characterizing much of the literature on the history of diseases.

The history of health is of course the history of the remarkable decline of infectious diseases. It involves tracing secular trends in consequences of exposure to diseases, the agent factors, and human resistance to infectious diseases, the host factors, in a changing, complex and dynamic environment. Together these interacting, complex, evolving systems constitute the epidemiological triad.

The power of the germ theory of disease is one factor underlying this shift of focus. Equally important is perhaps a shift in the concept of health itself, from one encompassing broadly social factors—availability of food, regularity and security of employment, wages, hours and conditions of work, the structure of the family and of work for women, leisure time, care for infants, and a more nebulous sense of social solidarity and well-being—to the absence of diseases.[4] In this broader view of health, a range of social factors interacting with the environment acted to predispose to diseases. In contrast, the Chadwickian revolution narrowed public health to water supply and sanitation, while the germ theory sharpened this narrow vision further. By restricting disease causation to a single cause, the social determinants of health were largely eclipsed. Together with the behavioural approach to health, these factors profoundly shaped how both public health workers and historians approached health.

Thomas McKeown, a medical doctor less well known than he

ought to be among both public health workers and historians, offered us startling new insights into the advances in human longevity and health.[5] Surveying the decline of the death rate in England and Wales during the registration period, he observed that significant and long-term declines in the death rate, commencing in the eighteenth century, had occurred due to a decline in infectious and communicable diseases, the quintessential diseases of poverty. More remarkably, by plotting the point on the declining curve at which effective medical technology became available, he concluded that medical technology had little to do with this decline of mortality, with the possible exception of smallpox.

Tuberculosis, that white plague of diseases, offers a striking McKeownite example. By the time the tubercle bacillus was identified by Thomas Koch, the giant of bacteriology and one of the architects of the germ theory in the 1860s, the death toll due to tuberculosis had shown a long-term secular decline. By the time effective chemotherapy was discovered in the 1940s, tuberculosis had ceased to be a major public health problem in the west. This is of course not to deny the important role of chemotherapy in the control of tuberculosis, but to highlight the importance of other factors all too frequently forgotten in technological hubris.

This remarkable decline in death rates was not restricted to tuberculosis alone, but to almost all the major infectious diseases: bronchitis, pneumonia, whooping cough, measles and so on. This decline in infectious diseases was unlikely to be related to changes in the virulence of the infectious agents over so short a period of time. Nor could it be attributed to salubrious changes in the environment, which had deteriorated due to industrialization and urbanization. Excluding these possible causes for the decline of infectious diseases, McKeown concluded that this dramatic decline could only have been a consequence of increased general resistance to infectious diseases through improvements in the nutritional status of the population, due to wide-ranging changes in the agrarian economy.

McKeown acknowledged that the public health revolution of the late nineteenth century played an important role in reducing exposure to water-borne diseases such as diarrhoea, dysentery and cholera. However, at the most, these could account for a quarter to a third of the mortality decline. Indeed, even in the case of this group of diseases, the underlying cause for the decline of lethality may well have been the

267

same, viz. increasing human resistance due to improvements in nutrition. Contributing to this, in the latter part of the nineteenth century, was an increase in real wages of the order of 66 per cent.[6]

This thesis has been a matter of some controversy, but has been strengthened by a number of studies noting that a host of other countries in the west had a similar health trajectory as living standards improved. The McKinleys reveal that modern medicine, both preventive and curative, accounted for a minor proportion of the mortality decline from infectious diseases in the United States.[7] Further, that while preventive health measures were largely undertaken in urban areas, the decline in the death rates extended to rural areas as well. At the same time, data from a number of European countries over this period indicate that there were increases in mean heights, along with a decrease in class differentials in heights, both attesting to improvements in the nutritional status of the population.[8] Indeed, Fogel concluded that improvements in the nutritional status, as indicated by stature and body mass index, accounted for a substantial proportion of the decline in mortality in England, France and Sweden between 1775 and 1875.[9]

When we turn, however, to India or to the other colonized countries, there is almost complete consensus that overpopulation was the cause of both poverty and diseases—Malthus resurrected in a new *avatar*—as the English nineteenth-century experience of rising income associated with increasing population is forgotten, as is the colonial (and continuing) drain of resources from these countries. The western experience is thus, it is maintained, not applicable to India, rendering the McKeownite model irrelevant. Solutions to the problems of ill health and disease are then sought in the domain of medical technology alone.

Kinsley Davis, the guru of modern demographers, set the trend in his classic, *The Population of India and Pakistan*, arguing that the 'gift of death control technologies' from the west was responsible for the decline in the death rate commencing in the 1920s.[10] He was referring of course to the role of DDT in the control of malaria. His primary argument, fuelled by Cold War concerns, was the urgent and critical need for birth-control technologies to control population growth. Perhaps picking up from Davis, the *Cambridge Economic History of India*, in its chapter on population, assumes that the post-1921 decline in the death rate was due to public health measures: while plague somewhat mysteriously subsided, cholera and smallpox were vanquished by public health intervention.[11] Indeed this technological determinism even colours the economic history of Bagchi, who observes that 'the fall in mortality . . . seems to have been caused by spectacular advances in medical technology for controlling such bacterial diseases [*sic*] as malaria, smallpox and cholera.'[12]

One significant problem with these avowals is that there is very little empirical data to substantiate them. Commencing in the 1920s, this decline in the death rate, a major proportion of which was due to a decline in deaths from malaria, preceded by at least three decades the launch of the malaria eradication programme in the 1950s. Further, over the same period, mortality due to a range of diseases, for which there were no preventive measures or specific therapies, also declined. These included diseases such as cholera and smallpox.[13]

Sumit Guha dismisses Davis's explanation as 'certainly not applicable to India between the Wars'.[14] He notes that income per capita and food availability both stagnated, but argues that the Indian population lived longer due to the munificence of the rain gods. This enabled the population to survive with a moderate level of malnutrition. While Guha's work traces the direction, begging many questions, it is to the work of Zurbrigg one must turn for convincing arguments and compelling empirical evidence.

Sheila Zurbrigg's work on hunger and epidemic mortality not only brings fresh insights challenging received wisdom, but also strengthens a McKeownite understanding of health history in India.[15] Studying malaria mortality in the Punjab between 1868 and 1940, Zurbrigg found a most extraordinary decline commencing around 1908. In the forty-one-year period between 1868 and 1908, malaria deaths were predicated upon not just rainfall, essential for malaria transmission, but foodgrain prices, soaring in years of soaring food grain prices. Malaria death rates dropped in the period between 1909 and 1941 to less than one-third of that earlier. This drop was accompanied neither by a decline in epidemiological indices of malaria transmission, in rainfall and flooding, nor in entomological indices. More significantly, there were no effective preventive and therapeutic measures widely applied. Indeed, per capita availability of quinine was so low as to make this explanation extremely implausible. What did change after 1908 was the incidence and severity of famine or epidemic hunger. While it is undoubtedly true that under the colonial regime per capita food availability declined, what Zurbrigg's work reveals is the critical importance of state intervention: the political exigencies which compelled the British government to haltingly, hesitantly, initiate steps to control famine. These did not reduce the prevalence of diseases or even their incidence; what they did do was to reduce excess deaths due to diseases induced by starvation, by lowering the lethality of the diseases.

The specific measure was the abandonment of the Malthusian policy of *laissez faire* in favour of purposive intervention through a changed famine code. This mandated public intervention through income support by employment generation in times of dearth and price rise. These steps did little to combat chronic hunger or endemic hunger. They did, nevertheless, leaven the excess deaths due to acute epidemic hunger and diseases that underlay the periodic subsistence crises of the period. In epidemiological terms, what changed was the lethality of diseases, in response to an altered epidemiological triad.[16]

It is this factor—organized public action—that lies at the heart of public health, in altering the outlay and impact of the web of factors that determine health. These include access to resources, employment, incomes and thus food. Equally important are other factors that offer a modicum of security to people's lives: conditions of work, access to water, sanitation and health facilities. This is not to undermine the importance of medical care or public health intervention, of which it forms a part, but to place it in a wider, pre-Chadwickian perspective.

II

Data on improvements in health in the twentieth century in England and Wales, however, also strengthen a McKeownite understanding of health improvement. The most marked improvement in life expectancy was in the decades of the two World Wars, despite the substantial losses of young lives (as revealed in Table 1). This, again, was due not to advances in health care but to increases in employment and, above all, food rationing.[17] It was also due to the more nebulous sense of social solidarity, which adds remarkably to well-being.

Substantiating these findings are data on more recent trends, as documented in the Black Report (as revealed in Table 2).[18] These showed a substantial increase in mortality differentials by class; the mortality rates among unskilled working-class men in 1981 were higher than they had ever been in the twentieth century, deteriorating

TABLE 1: *Longevity Expansion in England and Wales in the Twentieth Century: Increase in Life Expectancy per Decade*

Decade	Male	Female
1901–11	4.1	4.0
1911–21	6.6	6.5
1921–31	2.3	2.4
1931–40	1.2	1.5
1940–51	6.5	7.0
1951–60	2.4	3.2

Source: Jean Dreze and Amartya Sen, *Hunger and Public Action*, Delhi, 1993.

TABLE 2: *Mortality by Social Class 1911–81 (Men, 15–64 years, England and Wales)*

	Social Class				
Year	Professional	Managerial	Skilled manual and non-manual	Semi-skilled	Unskilled
	I	II	III	IV	V
1911	88	94	96	93	142
1921	82	94	95	101	125
1931	90	94	97	102	111
1951	86	92	101	104	118
1961[a]	76 (75)	81	100	103	143 (127)
1971[b]	77 (75)	81	104	114	137 (121)
1981[c]	66	76	103	116	166

Notes: [a] Figures are SMRs, which express age-adjusted mortality rates as a percentage of the national average at each date.

[b] To facilitate comparisons, figures shown in parentheses have been adjusted to the classification of occupations used in 1951.

[c] Men, 20–64 years, Great Britain.

Source: M.G. Marmot, 'Social Inequalities in Mortality: The Social Environment' in R.G. Wilkinson (ed.), *Class and Health: Research and Longitudinal Data*, London, 1986.

after 1971. Over this period, while diseases changed and technologies radically improved, while more was spent on medical care that was accessible to the entire population, what did not change were the social differentials in mortality. These were determined by prior factors affecting the health of the population. In other words, fresh evidence

271

that strengthens a McKeownite understanding of health.

These inequalities in health widened sharply during the Thatcher years.[19] Equally, class differences in heights among schoolchildren have again begun to widen. Substantial GDP growth, then, accompanied by greater inequality in wealth distribution and social hopelessness, clearly had a regressive effect on health.

Could this be a reflection of merely individual idiosyncrasies? Of smoking, drinking, lack of exercise, etc., choices exercised by individuals, and thus reflected in high incidence of coronary artery diseases, strokes and cancers? Or are there other, more fundamental, social factors? In other words, is the mortality load on a population merely natural, or does it reflect the social, economic and political arrangements of society? The answers to these questions is provided by a long-term study on mortality among British civil servants. The Whitehall Study convincingly proves the point that individual factors, while no doubt important, are not the primary causes of epidemiological patterns of diseases and deaths. Thus, so-called 'lifestyle' factors together accounted for merely a third of the differentials in death rates among the different social groups, a substantial proportion remaining unexplained.[20] In other words, there are more important underlying structural factors. These are factors affecting and governing economic, social and political inequalities.

The World Bank policies of individuating health, curtailing the role of the state, and focusing on advances in medical technology, clearly have elided any such reading of health history. This tendency to deal with disease and health merely at the individual level, to conceive of populations merely as aggregates of individuals, disregarding the social and economic context of diseases, has provoked a rich and heated debate in public health.[21]

It is abundantly clear that since the 1980s, inequalities across the globe and within countries have substantially increased. This has led to increasing levels of both absolute and relative poverty. As a result, advances in health made earlier in the twentieth century, accompanying the decolonization of third world countries and with the building of welfare states in the west, are being undermined. Indeed, in many countries across the globe, there have been increases in levels of infant and child mortality even as life expectancy has declined.[22]

Under the regime of globalization, liberalization and

privatization, while a small proportion of the world's population is becoming increasingly wealthier, unemployment, loss of assets and deprivation are growing in a widening share of the world's communities, including the poor in rich countries, profoundly shaping health. Expectation of life at birth has declined sharply in countries of the former Soviet Union, in large parts of Africa and in some parts of Latin America.[23] In Russia, innocuous diseases like measles, which had disappeared, have not only made a reappearance but have commenced taking a toll, riding on the back of increasing hunger, unemployment and the collapse of the welfare state. There has also been a resurgence of that disease of poverty and hopelessness, tuberculosis, albeit in a new and more lethal drug-resistant form.[24]

There is an imperative need to acknowledge that health improvement is less an outcome of medical technology than of living standards. Earlier efforts in India towards integrating health with overall development, albeit achieved in a limited manner, have been seriously undermined by new initiatives under the aegis of the Bank to drastically reduce the role and vision of public health to one based on technological hubris. At the same time the role of the state in the provision of the determinants of health is radically undermined. Health improvements based on narrow technical interventions are bound to be chimerical, as indeed has been the experience of India's malaria eradication programme. Health, then, holds a mirror to human civilization. What we see today is not very ennobling or dazzling.

As a public health worker and not an historian, I feel deeply honoured and profoundly humbled to have been invited to the Indian History Congress. I feel doubly honoured because both public health and history have been disciplines that have conventionally looked askance at each other, impoverishing both. I am grateful to the IHC and to Prof. Shireen Moosvi in particular.

Notes and References

[1] V.K. Yadavendu, 'Social Construction of Health: Changing Paradigms', *Economic and Political Weekly*, Vol. XXXVI, No. 29, 21 July 2001, pp. 2784–94.

[2] Hans Zinsser, *Rats, Lice and History*, Boston, 1935.

[3] W.H. McNeill, *Plagues and Peoples*, Harmondsworth, 1976.

[4] Christopher Hamlin, 'Predisposing Causes and Public Health in Early Nineteenth Century Medical Thought', *Bulletin of the Social History of Medicine*, Vol. 5, No. 1, 1992, pp. 43–70.

5 Thomas McKeown, *The Modern Rise of Population*, London, 1976.

6 David Blane, 'Real Wages, the Economic Cycle, and Mortality in England and Wales, 1870–1914', *International Journal of Health Services*, Vol. 20, No. 1, 1990, pp. 43–52.

7 J.B. McKinlay and S.M. McKinlay, 'The Questionable Contribution of Medical Measures to the Mortality Decline in the United States in the Twentieth Century', *Milbank Memorial Fund Quarterly*, Vol. 55, Summer, 1977, pp. 405–28.

8 Roderick Floud et al., *Height, Health and History: Nutritional Status in the United Kingdom, 1750–1980*, Cambridge, 1993, cited in Sheila Zurbrigg, 'The Hungry Rarely Write History and Historians Are Rarely Hungry: Reclaiming Hunger in the History of Health', unpublished paper, Department of History, Dalhousie University, Canada, 1994, pp. 1–23.

9 R. Fogel, 'Second Thoughts on the European Escape from Hunger: Famines, Chronic Malnutrition, and Mortality Rates', cited in Zurbrigg, ibid.

10 Kingsley Davis, *The Population of India and Pakistan*, Princeton, 1951.

11 Dharma Kumar (ed.), *The Cambridge Economic History of India*, Vol. II: c. 1757–c. 1970, Cambridge, 1983.

12 Amiya Kumar Bagchi, *The Political Economy of Underdevelopment*, Cambridge, 1982.

13 Christophe Guilmoto, 'Towards a New Demographic Equilibrium: The Inception of Demographic Transition in South India', *Indian Economic and Social History Review*, Vol. 29, No. 3, 1992, pp. 247–89.

14 Sumit Guha, *Health and Population in South Asia: From Earliest Times to the Present*, New Delhi, 2001.

15 Sheila Zurbrigg, 'Hunger and Epidemic Mortality in Punjab, 1869–1940', *Economic and Political Weekly*, Vol. XXVII, No. 4, 1992, pp. PE 2–26.

16 Sheila Zurbrigg, 'The Hungry Rarely Write History', pp. 1–23.

17 Jean Dreze and Amartya Sen, *Hunger and Public Action*, Delhi, 1993.

18 Peter Townsend and Nick Davidson (eds), 'The Black Report', in *Inequalities in Health*, Harmondsworth, 1992.

19 Margaret Whitehead, 'The Health Divide', in ibid.

20 M.G. Marmot, G. Davey Smith, S. Stansfield, C. Patel, F. North and J. Head, 'Health Inequalities among British Civil Servants: The Whitehall II Study', *Lancet*, 337, 1991, pp. 1387–93.

21 Neil Pearce, 'Traditional Epidemiology, Modern Epidemiology and Public Health', *The American Journal of Public Health*, Vol. 86, No. 5, 1996, pp. 678–83; Ann V. Diez Roux, 'Bringing Context Back into Epidemiology: Variables and Fallacies in Multilevel Analysis', *American Journal of Public Health*, Vol. 88, No. 2, 1998, pp. 1027–32; M. Susser, 'Does Risk Factor Epidemiology put Epidemiology at Risk?' *Journal of Epidemiology and Community Health*, 52, 1998, pp. 418–26, N. Kieger, 'Questioning Epidemiology: Objectivity, Advocacy and Socially Responsible Science', *American Journal of Epidemiology*, Vol. 89, No. 8, 1999, pp. 1151–53, among others.

22 Mohan Rao and Rene Loewenson, 'The Political Economy of the Assault on Health', *People's Health Assembly: Background Papers*, Dhaka, 2000.

23 G.A. Cornia, R. Jolly and F. Stewart (eds), *Adjustment with a Human Face: Country Case Studies*, Oxford, 1988.

24 Mark G. Field, David M. Kotz and Gene Bukhman, 'Neoliberal Economic Policy, "State Desertion" and the Russian Health Crisis', in Jim Yong Kim et al. (eds), *Dying for Growth: Global Inequality and the Health of the Poor*, Maine, 2000.

A Select Bibliography

Acharya, N.R. and S. Pandurang (eds) (1945), *Sushruta Samhita*, Bombay: Nirnay Sagar Press.

Allchin, Bridget and Raymond Allchin (1985), *The Rise of Civilization in India and Pakistan*, Cambridge: Cambridge University Press.

Anderson, Warwick (1998), 'Where is the Postcolonial History of Medicine?', *Bulletin of History of Medicine*, 72, pp. 522–30.

Annesley, James (1828), *Research into the Causes, and Treatment of the more Prevalent Diseases of India, and of Warm Climates more generally*, 2 vols, London: Longman, Reev, Orme, Brown & Green.

Arnold, David (ed.) (1989), *Imperial Medicine and Indigenous Societies*, Delhi: Oxford University Press.

——— (1996), *Warm Climates and Western Medicine: The Emergence of Tropical Medicine 1500–1900*, Amsterdam and Atlanta: Rodopi Press.

Arnold, David (1993), *Colonizing the Body: State Medicine and Epidemic Disease in Ninteenth Century India*, Berkeley: University of California Press.

——— (2000), *The New Cambridge History of India*, III (5): *Science, Technology and Medicine in Colonial India*, Cambridge: Cambridge Univrsity Press.

Askari, S.H. (1957), 'Medicines and Hospitals in Muslim India', *The Journal of the Bihar Research Society*, Vol. 43, Parts I and II, March–June.

Bala, Poonam (1991), *Imperialism and Medicine in Bengal: A Socio-Historical Perspective*, Delhi: Sage Publications.

Balfour, Francis (1808), 'Observations Representing the Remarkable

Effects of Sol-Lunar Influence in the Fever of India, with the Scheme of an Astronomical Ephemeris for the purposes of Medicine and Meteorology', *Asiatick Researches*, 8, pp. 1–34.

Balfour, Margaret and Ruth Young (1929), *The Work of Medical Women in India*, London: Oxford University Press.

Ballhatchet. K. (1980), *Race, Sex and Class under the Raj*, London: Weidenfeld.

Ballingall, George (1818), *Practical Observations on Fever, Dysentery, and Liver Complaints, as they occur amongst the European Troops in India*, Edinburgh: Brown and Constable.

Bang, B.G. (1973), 'Current concepts of the smallpox Goddess Sitala in parts of West Bengal', *Man in India*, 531, pp. 79–104.

Bayly, C.A. (1996), *Empire and Information: Intelligence Gathering and Social Communication in India, 1780–1870*, Cambridge: Cambridge University Press.

Bentley, A. Charles (1925), *Malaria and Agriculture in Bengal: How to Reduce Malaria in Bengal by Irrigations*, Calcutta.

Bell, Heather (1999), *Frontiers of Medicine in the Anglo-Egyptian Sudan, 1899–1940*, Oxford: Clarendon Press.

Bewell, Alan (1999), *Romanticism and Colonial Disease*, Baltimore: The Johns Hopkins University Press.

Bhardwaj, S.M. (1981), 'Homeopathy in India', in G.R. Gupta (ed.), *The Social and Cultural Context of Medicine in India*, Delhi: Vikas Publishing House, pp. 1–54.

Borthwick, Meredith (1984), *Changing Role of Women in Bengal, 1849–1905*, Princeton: Princeton University Press.

Bose, D.M. et al. (eds) (1971), *A Concise History of Science in India*, New Delhi: Indian National Science Academy.

Bourdillon, Hillary (1988), *Women as Healers: A History of Women and Medicine*, Cambridge: Cambridge University Press.

Brass, Paul. R (1972), 'The Politics of Ayurvedic Education: A Case Study of Revivalism and Modernization in India', in S.H. Rudoph and L.I. Rudolph (eds), *Education and Politics in India*, Delhi.

Brett, J.H. (1840), *A Practical Essay on some of the Principal Diseases of India*, Calcutta: W.Thacker and Co.

Bynum, W.F. (ed.) (1993), *Companion Encyclopedia of History of Medicine*, London: Routledge.

Bynum, W.F. and R. Porter (eds) (1987), *Medical fringe and medical orthodoxy 1750–1850*, London: Croom Helm.

Bynum, W.F. and V. Nutton (eds), 'Theories of fever from antiquity to the enlightenment', *Medical History*, Supplement No. 1, pp. 135–48.

Bynum, W.F. and Caroline Overy (eds) (1998), *The Beast in the Mosquito: The Correspondence of Ronald Ross and Patrick Manson*, Amsterdam and Atlanta: Rodopi.

Canguilhem, G. (1988), *Ideology and rationality in the history of the life sciences*, Cambridge, Massschussets: The MIT Press.

Cartwright, J.J. (1977), *A Social History of Medicine*, London: Longman.

Catanach, Ian (1983), 'Plague and the Indian Village 1896–1914', in P. Robb (ed.), *Rural India: Land, Power and Society under British Rule*, London: Curzon Press.

Chandpuri, Hakim Kausar (1960), *Atibba-i Ahad-i Mughaliya*, Karachi.

Chapman, Allan (1979), 'Astrological Medicine', in Webster (ed.), *Health, Medicine and Mortality in the Sixteenth Century*, Cambridge: Cambridge University Press.

Chattopadhyaya, D. (1977), *Science and Society in Ancient India*, Research India Publication, Calcutta.

Crawford, D.G. (1914), *A History of the Indian Medical Service, 1600–1913*, 2 vols. London: W. Thacker.

———— (1930), *Roll of the Indian Medical Service, 1615–1930*, London, Calcutta, Simla: W. Thacker.

Cunningham, A. and A. Bridie (eds) (1997), *Western Medicine as Contested Knowledge*. Manchester: Manchester University Press.

Curtin, Philip D. (1989), *Death by Migration: Europe's Encounter with the Tropical World in the Nineteenth Century*. Cambridge: Cambridge University Press.

———— (1998), *Disease and Empire: The Health of European Troops in the Conquest of Africa*, Cambridge: Cambridge University Press.

Deb, Radha K. (1831), 'Account of the tikadars', *Transactions of the Medical and Physical Society of Calcutta*, 5, pp. 416–18.

Davin, A. (1978), 'Imperialism and Motherhood', *History Workshop Journal*, 5.

Dharampal (1971), *Indian Science and Technology in the Eighteenth Century*, Delhi: Impex India.

———— (1987), *Some aspects of earlier Indian society and polity and their relevance to the present*, Pune: A New Quest Pamphlet.

Dimock, E.C. (1976), 'A theology of the repulsive: Some reflections on Sitala and other *Mangals*', in M. Davis (ed.), *Bengal studies in literature, society and history*, Michigan: Asian Studies Centre.

Dunn, L. Fredrick (1997), 'Traditional Asian Medicine and Cosmopolitan Medicine as Adaptive System', in Charles Leslie (ed.), *Asian Medical Systems: A Comparative Study*, Berkeley: University of California Press.

Dutt, U.C. and George King et al. (1922), *Materia Medica of the Hindus*, revised edn, Calcutta: Madan Gopal Dass.

Elgood, Cyril (1970), *Safavid Medical Practice or the Practice of Medicine, Surgery and Gynaecology in Persia between 1500 AD and 1750 AD*, London.

Engels, Dagmar (1996), *Beyond Purdah? Women in Bengal, 1890–1939*, Delhi: Oxford University Press.

Engels, D. and S. Marks (eds) (1994), *Contesting Colonial Hegemony: State and Society in Africa and India*. London: British Academic Press.

Ernst, Waltraud (1991), *Mad Tales from the Raj: The European Insane in British India, 1800–1858*, London and New York: Routledge.

Ernst, W. and B. Harris (eds) (1999), *Race, Science and Medicine, 1700–1960*, London: Routledge.

Fayrer, Joseph (1894), *Preservation of Health in India*, London: Macmillan.

Filliozat, Jean (1964), *The Classical Doctrine of Indian Medicine*, translated by Dev Raj Chanana, New Delhi: Munshiram Manoharlal.

Forbes, Geraldine (ed.) (2000), *The New Cambridge History of India*, IV (2): *Women in Modern India*, Cambridge: Cambridge University Press.

Forbes, Geraldine and Tapan Ray Chaudhuri (2000), *The Memoirs of Dr Haimabati Sen from Child Widow to Lady Doctor*, New Delhi: Lotus Collection.

Goodeve, H.H. (1837), 'A Sketch on the Progress of European Medicine in the East', *Quarterly Journal of the Calcutta Medical and Physical Society*, 2, pp. 124–56.

Grove, Richard (1999), *Green Imperialism: Colonial Expansion, Tropical Island Edens and the Origins of Environmentalism, 1600–1860*, Cambridge: Cambridge University Press.

Guha, Sumit (2001), *Health and Population in South Asia: From Earliest Times to the Present*, New Delhi: Permanent Black.

Gupta, Brahmanand (1976), 'Indigenous Medicine in Nineteenth and Twentieth Century Bengal', in Charles Leslie (ed.), *Asian Medical Systems: A Comparative Study*, pp. 368–78.

Gurumurthy, S. (1970), 'Medical Science and Dispensaries in Ancient South India as Gleaned from Epigraphy', *Indian Journal of History of Science*, 5, pp. 76–79.

Hamlin, C. (1998), *Public Health and Social Justice in the Age of Chadwik: Britain 1800–1854*, Cambridge: Cambridge University Press.

Harrison, M. (1994), *Public Health in British India: Anglo-Indian Preventive Medicine 1859–1914*, Cambridge: Cambridge University Press.

——— (1999), *Climates and Constitutions: Health, Race, Environment and British Imperialism in India 1600–1850*, Delhi: Oxford University Press.

Hart, E. (1894), 'The Medical Profession in India', Calcutta.

Hausman, G.J. (1996), *Siddhars, Alchemy and the Abyss of Tradition: 'Traditional' Tamil Medical Knowledge in 'Modern' Practice*, Ph.D. Thesis, University of Michigan.

Hehir, Patrick (1923), *The Medical Profession in India*, London.

Headrick, Daniel R. (1981), *Tools of Empire: Technology and European Imperialism in the Nineteenth Century*, New York: Oxford University Press.

——— (1988), *The Tentacles of Progress: Technology Transfer in the Age of Imperialism, 1850–1940*, Oxford and New York: Oxford University Press.

Hoggan, France Elizabeth (1882), 'Medical Women in India', *Contemporary Review*, 42.

Holwell, J.Z. (1970), 'The religious tenets of the Gentoos, Excerpted from J.Z. Holwell, 1767, Interesting Historical events relative to the province of Bengal and the empire of Indostan', in P.J.

Marshall (ed.), *The British Discovery of Hinduism in the Eighteenth Century*, Cambridge: Cambridge University Press, pp. 45–106.

———— (1983), 'An account of the manner of inoculating for the Smallpox in the East Indies', in Dharampal (ed.), *Indian Science and Technology in the Eighteenth Century: Some Contemporary British Accounts*, first edn 1971, Delhi: Impex India, pp. 195–218.

Hoodbhoy, Pervez (1991), *Islam and Science*, London: Zed Books.

Howard, Somerwel (1940), *The Knife and Life in India: History of Surgical Missionary of South Travancore*, London.

Hume, J.C. (1977), 'Rival Traditions: Western Medicine and Yunani-i Tibb in the Punjab, 1849–1889', *Bulletin of History of Medicine*, 51, pp. 214–31.

———— (1977), 'Medicine in the Punjab, 1849–1911: Ethnicity and Professionalisation in the Control of an Occupation', Ph.D. dissertation, Duke University.

———— (1986), 'Colonialism and Sanitary Medicine: The Development of Preventive Health Policy in the Punjab, 1860–1900', *Modern Asian Studies*, No. 20, pp. 703–24.

Hyam, Ronald (1991), *Empire and Sexuality: The British Experience*. Manchester: Manchester University Press.

Israili, A.H. (1980), 'Education of Unani Medicine during Mughal Period', *Studies in History of Medicine*, Vol. IV, No. 3, September.

Issacs, Jeremy D. (1998), 'D.D. Cunningham and the Aetiology of Cholera in British India, 1869–1897'. *Medical History*, No. 42, pp. 279–305.

Jalil, Abdul (1978), 'The Evolution and Development of Graeco-Arab Medical Education', *Studies in History of Medicine*, Vol. II, No. 3, September.

James, S.P. (1909), *Smallpox and vaccination in British India*, Calcutta: Thacker, Spink and Co.

Jardanova, Ludmilla (1989), *Sexual Vision: Image of Gender in Science and Medicine between the Eighteenth and Twentieth Century*, London: Harvester Westsheaf, 1989.

Jeffrey, Roger (1988), *The Politics of Health in India*, Berkeley, Los Angeles and London: University of California Press.

Jaggi, O.P. (1979), *History of Science, Technology and Medicine in India, XIII: Western Medicine in India: Medical Education and Research*, Delhi: Atma Ram, Delhi.

Jolly, Julius (1977), *Indian Medicine*, translated by G.G. Kashikar, second revised edn, New Delhi.

Kakkar, S. (1990), *Shamans, Mystics and Doctors*, Delhi: Oxford University Press.

Kakar, Sanjiv (1996), 'Leprosy in British India, 1860–1940: Colonial Policies and Missionary Medicine', *Medical History*, No. 40, pp. 215–30.

Kawashima, Koji (1998), *Missionaries and a Hindu State: Travancore 1858–1936*, Delhi: Oxford University Press.

Kennedy, Dane (1996), *The Magic Mountains: Hills Stations and the British Raj*, Berkeley: University of California Press.

Keshwani, N.H. (1974), *The Science of Medicine and Physiological Conception in Ancient and Medieval India*, New Delhi.

King, L.S. (1972), 'Medical Theory and Practice in the Beginning of the Eighteenth Century', *Bulletin of History of Medicine*, 46, pp. 1–15.

Klein, Ira (1972), 'Malaria and Mortality in Bengal, 1840–1921', *The Indian Economic and Social History Review*, Vol. IX, No. 2, June.

———— (1980), 'Cholera: Theory and Treatment in Nineteenth-Century India', *Journal of Indian History*, No. 58, pp. 35–51.

———— (1988), 'Plague, Policy and Popular Unrest in British India', *Modern Asian Studies*, No. 22, pp. 723–55.

Kosambi, Meera (1996), 'Anandibai Joshee: Retrieving a fragmented feminist image' *Economic and Political Weekly*, Vol XXXI, No. 49, 7 December, pp. 3189–97.

Kumar, Anil (1998), *Medicine and the Raj: British Medical Policy 1835–1911*, New Delhi: Sage Publications.

Kumar, Deepak (1995), *Science and the Raj: 1857–1905*, Delhi: Oxford University Press.

———— (1999), 'Colony under a Microscope: The Medical Works of W.M. Haffkine', *Science, Technology and Society*, IV, 2, pp. 239–71.

Kumar, Deepak (ed.) (1991), *Science and Empire: Essays in Indian Context (1700–1947)*, Delhi: Anamika Prakashan, Delhi.

A Select Bibliography

Kutumbiah, P. (1962), *Ancient Indian Medicine*, Madras: Orient Longman.

Lal, Maneesha (1994), 'The Politics of Gender and Medicine in Colonial India: The Countess of Dufferin's Fund', *Bulletin of History Medicine*, 68, pp. 29–66.

Lambert, Helen (1992), 'The Cultural Logic of Indian Medicine: Prognosis and Etiology in Rajasthan Popular Therapeutics', *Social Science and Medicine*, No. 34, pp. 1067–76.

Latour, B. (1993), *We have never been modern*, translated by Catherine Porter, New York: Harvester Wheatsheaf.

Leslie, Charles (ed,) (1977), *Asian Medical Systems: A Comparative Study*, California: California University Press.

Lifton, Robert Jay (1973), 'Popular beliefs about smallpox and other common infectious diseases in South India', *Tropical and Geographical Medicine*, 25, pp. 190–96.

Lindemann (1999), *Medicine and Society in Early Modern Europe*, Cambridge: Cambridge University Press.

Mackinnon, Kenneth (1848), 'A treatise on the Public Health, Climate Hygiene and Prevailing Disease of Bengal and the North West Provincess', Cawnpore.

MacLeod, R. (ed.) (2000), *Nature and Empire, OSIRIS*, Vol. 15.

MacLeod, R. and L. Milton (eds) (1988), *Disease, Medicine and Empire: Perspectives of Western Medicine and the Experiences of European Expansion*, London: Routledge.

Manderson, Lenore (1996), *Sickness and the State: Health and Illness in Colonial Malaya, 1870–1940*, Cambridge: Cambridge University Press.

Manucci, Niccolao (1966), *Storia Do Mogor*, translated with Introduction and Notes by Welkians Irvine, Calcutta.

Marglin, F.A. (1990), 'Smallpox in two systems of knowledge', in F.A. Marglin and S.A. Marglin (eds), *Dominating Knowledge, Development, Culture, and Resistance*, Oxford: Clarendon Press, pp. 102–44.

Marks, Shula (1997), 'What is Colonial about Colonial Medicine? And what has happened in Imperialism and Health', *Social History of Medicine*, 10, 2, August, pp. 205–19.

McAlpin, M.B. (1985), 'Families, Epidemics and Population Growth: The Case of India', in *Hunger and History: The Impact of*

Changing Food Production and Consumption Patterns on Society, edited by R.I. Robert and T.K. Rabb, Cambridge: Cambridge University Press, pp. 153–68.

Mehta, P.M. et al., *Introduction and Notes to Carak Samhita*, 6 vols, Jamnagar: Ayurvedic Society.

Metcalf, B.D. (1985), 'Nationalist Muslims in British India: The Case of Hakim Ajmal Khan', *Modern Asian Studies*, No. 19, pp. 1–28.

Meulenbeld, G.J. (1974), *The Madhavanidana and its Chief Commentary*, Leiden: E.J. Brill.

Mills, James (1997), 'The Lunatic Asylum in British India 1857 to 1880: Colonialism, Medicine and Power', Ph.D. dissertation, University of Edinburgh.

Mishra, K. (2000), 'Productivity of Crisis: Disease, Scientific Knowledge and State in India', *Economic and Political Weekly*, 28 October.

Mitra, Jyotir (1985), *A Critical Appraisal of Ayurvedic Material in Buddhist Literature*, Varanasi: The Jyotirlok Prakashan.

Moore, W.J. (1862), *Health in the Tropics or Sanitary Art Applied to Europeans in India*, London.

Mukherjee, G.N. (1913–14), *The Surgical Instruments of the Hindus*, 2 vols, Calcutta: Calcutta University Press.

———— (1922–29), *History of Indian Medicine*, 3 vols, Calcutta; rpt, Delhi: Orient Books, 1974.

Mukherjee, Sujata, 'Women, Medicine and Empire: Female Practitioners and Patterns of Health Care in Colonial Bengal', *Modern Historical Studies*, Vol. 2.

Mukhopadhyaya, Girindranath (1913), *The surgical instruments of the Hindus, with a comparative study of the surgical instruments of the Greek, Roman, Arab, and the modern Eouropean [sic] surgeons*, Calcutta: Calcutta University Press.

Muraleedharan, V.R. (1987), 'Rural Health Care in Madras Presidency 1919–39', *IESHR*, 24, pp . 324–34.

———— (1991), 'Malady in Madras: The Colonial Government's Response to Malaria in the Early Twentieth Century', in D. Kumar (ed.), *Science and Empire*, pp. 101–14.

Murti, Srinivasa (1948), *The Science and the Art of Indian Medicine*, Madras: Theosophical Pub.

Muthu, D.C. (1930), *The Antiquity of Hindu Medicine and Civilization,* London.

Nair, K.R. (2001), *Evolution of Modern Medicine in Kerala,* Trivandrum: TBS Pub.

Nahawandi, Abdul Baqi (1932), *Ma-asin-i-Rahimi,* edited by Hidayat Husain, Calcutta.

Naraindas, Harish (1996), 'Poisons, Putresence and the Weather: A Geneology of the Advent of Tropical Medicine', *Contributions to Indian Sociology,* (n.s.) 30, 1, pp. 1–35.

———— (1998), 'Care, welfare and treason: The advent of vaccination in the 19th century', *Contributions to Indian Sociology,* (n.s.) 32, 1.

Navarro (ed.) (1982), *Imperalism, Health and Medicine',* London: Pluto.

Neelmeghan, A. (1963), *Development of Medical Societies and Medical Periodicals in India 1780–1920,* Calcutta.

Nicholas, Ralph (1981), 'The Goddess Sitala and Epidemic Small Pox in Bengal', *The Journal of Asian Studies,* Vol. XLI, No. 1, November, pp. 21–44.

Nicholas, Ralph W. and Aditi N. Sarkar (1976), 'The fever demon and the census commission: Sitala mythology in eighteenth and nineteenth century Bengal', in M. Davis (ed.), *Bengal Studies in literature, society and history,* Michigan: Asian Studies Centre.

O'Malley, C.D. (ed.) (1968), *The History of Medical Education,* California.

Palladino, Paolo and Michael Worboys (1993), 'Science and Imperialism', *ISIS,* 84, pp. 91–102.

Panikkar, K.N. (1995), 'Indigenous Medicine and Cultural Hegemony', in K.N. Panikkar, *Culture, Ideology, Hegemony: Intelligence and Social Consciousness in Colonial India,* New Delhi: Tulika, pp. 145–75.

Pati, Biswamoy (1998), 'Siting the Body: Perspectives on Health and Medicine in Colonial Orissa', *Social Scientist,* 26, Nos 11–12, November–December, pp. 3–26.

Pati, Biswamoy and H. Mark (ed.) (2001), *Health, Medicine and Empire: Perspectives on Colonial India,* Hyderabad: Orient Longman.

Pearson, M.N. (1989), *Towards Superiority: European and Indian Medicine, 1500–1700*, Minneapolis.

———— (1995), 'The Thin End of the Wedge: Medical Relativities as a Paradigm of Early Modern Indian–European Relations', *Modern Asian Studies*, 29, pp. 141–70.

Philips, C.H. (1970), *Physician-Authors of Greco-Arab Medicine in India*, New Delhi.

Pickstone, John V. (1993), 'Ways of Knowing: Towards a Historical Sociology of Science, Technology and Medicine', *British Journal for the History of Science*, 26, pp. 433–59.

Pingree, David (1970–94), *A census of the exact sciences in Sanskrit*, 5 vols, Philadelphia: American Philosophical Society.

Pollock, Sheldon (1885), 'The Theory of Practice and the Practice of Theory in Indian Intellectual History', *Journal of the American Oriental Society*, 105, pp. 499–519.

Porter, Roy (1993), *Disease, Medicine and Society in England 1550–1860*, Cambridge: Cambridge University Press, 1993.

Power, Helen (1996), 'The Calcutta School of Tropical Medicine: Institutionalizing Medical Research in the Periphery', *Medical History*, 40, pp. 197–214.

Qaisar, A.J. (1982), *The Indian Response to European Technology and Culture (1498–1707)*, Delhi: Oxford University Press.

Rahman, A. et al. (1982), *Science and Technology in Medieval India: A Bibliography of Source Material in Sanskrit, Arabi and Persian*, New Delhi: Indian national Science Academy.

Ramanna, Mridula (1995), 'Indian Practitioners of Western Medicine: Grant Medical College, 1845–1885', *Radical Journal of Health*, (n.s.) No. 1, pp. 116–35.

———— (1996), 'Randchodlab Chotalal: Pioneer of Public Health in Ahmedabad', *Radical Journal of Health*, (n.s.) 11, pp. 99–111.

————, 'Western Medicine and Public Health in Colonial Bombay, 1845–1895', Hyderabad: Orient Longman (forthcoming).

Ramasubban, R. (1982), 'Public Health and Medical Research in India: Their Origins under the Impact of British Colonial Policy', *SAREC Report*, Stockholm.

———— (1988), 'Imperial Health in British India 1857–1900', in R. MacLeod and M. Lewis (eds), *Disease, Medicine and Empire: Perspectives on Western Medicine and the Experience of European Expansion*, London: Routledge, pp. 38–60.

Ranger, T. and P. Black (eds) (1992), *Epidemics and Ideas: Essays on the Historical Perception of Pestilence*, Cambridge: Cambridge University Press.

Ray, Kabita (1998), *History of Public Health: Colonial Bengal 1921–1947*, Calcutta: K.P. Bagchi & Sons.

Ray, P. and H. Gupta (1980), *Charak Samhita: A Scientific Synopsis*, New Helhi: Indian National Science Academy.

Ray, Priyadarajan et al. (eds) (1980), *Susruta samhita (a scientific symposis)*, New Delhi: Indian National Science Academy.

Reddy, D.V. Subba (ed.) (1966), *Western Epitomes of Indian Medicine*, Hyderabad.

Rezavi, S. Ali Nadeem (1983), 'Mutasaddis of the Port of Surat in the Seventeenth Century', *Proceedings of the Indian History Congress*, Burdwan.

Rezavi, Syed Ali (1992), 'An Aristocratic Surgeon of Mughal Empire: Muqarrab Khan', in Irfan Habib (ed.), *Medieval India*, Vol. I, New Delhi, pp. 154–67.

Riley, C. James (1987), *The Eighteenth Century Campaign to Avoid Disease*, London: Macmillan.

Robb, Peter (1993), *Society and Ideology: Essays in South Asia History*, Delhi: Oxford University Press.

Robb, Peter (ed.), *The Concept of Race in India*, New Delhi: Oxford University Press.

Rosen, George (1958), *A History of Public Health*, New York: MD Publications.

Ross, Ronald (1923), *Memoirs*, London: Murray.

Rupke, Nicolaas (ed.), *Medical Geography in Historical Perspective*, Atlanta: Rodopi Press (forthcoming).

Sachau, E. (1910), *Alberuni's India*, London.

Sangwan, Satpal (1991), *Science, Technology and Colonization: An Indian Experience 1757–1857*, New Delhi: Anamika Prakashan.

Sanyal, P.K. (1964), *A Story of Medicine and Pharmacy in India*, Calcutta.

Sharma, Shiva (1929), *The System of Ayurveda*; rpt, Delhi: Low Price Pub., 1993.

Sharma, P.V. (ed.) (1992), *History of Medicine in India*, New Delhi: Indian National Science Academy.

Shastri, K.A.N. (1960), 'Facets in the History of Indian Medicine', *Indian Journal of History of Medicine*, Vol. 5, No. 2.

Siddiqui, T. (1981), 'Unani Medicine in India', *Indian Journal of History of Science*, Vol. XVI, No. 1.

Siddiqui, M.Z. (1959), *Studies in Arabic and Persian Medical Literature*, Calcutta: University of Calcutta Press.

———— (1962), 'Medicine in Medieval India', *Indian Journal of History of Science*, Vol. VII, No. 1.

Sivin, Nathan (1988), 'Science and Medicine in Imperial China: The State of the Field', *Journal of Asian Studies*, 47, pp. 41–90.

Staal, J. Frits (1996), *Ritual and mantras: rules without meaning*, New Delhi: Motilal Banarsidass.

Steinthal, B.J. (1984), 'The Ayurvedic Revivalist Movement in Early Twentieth-Century British India', Master's dissertation, Harvard University.

Stepan, Nancy (1982), *The Idea of Race in Scientific: Greater Britain 1800–1900*, London: Macmillan.

Storey, C.A. (1971), *Persian Literature: A Bio-bibliographical Survey*, II, Part II: *Medicine*, London.

Subramanian, S.V. and V.R. Madhavan (eds) (1983), *Siddha Medicine*, Madras: IITS.

Sutphen, M. (1995), 'Imperial Hygiene in Calcutta, Cape Town, and Hong Kong: The Early Career of Sir William Simpson (1855–1931)', Ph.D. dissertation, Yale University.

Treacher, A. and P. Wright (eds) (1982), *The Probelm of Medical Knowledge: Examining the Social Construction of Medicine*, Edinburgh: Edinburgh University Press.

Turner, J. Howard (1999), *Science in Medieval Islam: An Illustrated Introduction*, Delhi: Oxford University Press.

Varghese, Benny (1993), 'Indigenous Health Care and Introduction of Western Medicine', M.Phil. dissertation, M.G. University, Kottayam.

Wadley, Susan S. (1980), 'Sitala: The Cool One', *Asian Folklore Studies*. 39, 1, pp. 33–62.

Watts, Sheldon (1999), *Epidemics and History: Disease, Power and Imperialism*, New Haven and London: Yale University Press.

Webster, Charles (1981), *Biology, Medicine and Society 1840–1940*, Cambridge: Cambridge University Press.

Webster, Charles (ed.) (1979), *Health, Medicine and Mortality in the Sixteenth Century*, Cambridge: Cambridge University Press.

Whitehead, Judy (1995), 'Bodies Clean and Unclean: Prostitution, Sanitary Legislation and Respectable Feminity in Colonial North India', *Gender and History*, Vol. 7, No. 1, April, pp. 41–63.

Wise, T.A. (1867), *Review of Hindoo Medicine*, 2 vols, London: Churchill.

Worboys, Michael (1977), 'The Emergence of Tropical Medicine: A Study in the Establishment of a Scientific Speciality', in G. Lemaine et al. (eds), *Perspectives on the Emergence of Scientific Disciplines*, The Hague: Mouton, pp. 76–98.

——— (1979), 'Science and British Colonial Imperialism (1895–1940)', D. Phil. thesis, University of Sussex.

——— (2000), *Spreading Germs: Disease Theories and Medical Practice in Britain, 1865–1900*, Cambridge: Cambridge University Press.

Wujastyk, Dominik (1998), *The Roots of Ayurveda*, New Delhi: Penguin.

Zimmer, H.R. (1948), *Hindu Medicine*, Baltimore: Johns Hopkins University Press.

Zimmerman, Francis (1987), *The Jungle and the Aroma of Meats: An Ecological Theme in Hindu Medicine*, Berkeley: University of California Press.

——— (1992), 'Gentle purge: the flower power of Ayurveda', in C. Leslie and A. Young (eds), *Paths to Asian Medical Knowledge*, Berkeley: University of California Press, pp. 209–23.

Zurbrigg, S. (1994), 'Re-thinking the "Human Factor" in Malaria Mortality: The Case of Punjab, 1868–1940', *Parassitologia*, No. 36, pp. 121–35.

Zysk, K.G. (1991), *Asceticism and Healing in India*, Delhi: Oxford University Press.

——— (1996), *Medicine in the Veda*, Delhi: Motilal Banarsidas.

Zysk, K.G., G.J.Meulenbeld and Dominik Wujastyk (eds) (1987), *Studies on Indian Medical History*, Groningen: Forsten.

Contributors

DEEPAK KUMAR teaches history of science, society and education at the Zakir Husain Centre for Education Studies, Jawaharlal Nehru University, New Delhi. He is the author of *Science and the Raj* (Delhi, 1995).

SURAJ BHAN, an eminent archaeologist, was Professor of Ancient Indian History and Archaeology at Kurukshetra University for several years.

VIJAY KUMAR THAKUR is Professor of Ancient Indian History at Patna University. He is known for his work on feudalism.

IQBAL GHANI KHAN teaches medieval Indian history and history of technology at Aligarh Muslim University, Aligarh.

S. ALI NADEEM REZAVI teaches at the Centre for Advanced Studies in History, Aligarh Muslim University, Aligarh.

SHIREEN MOOSVI is Professor of Medieval Indian History at Aligarh Muslim University, Aligarh. Her contributions to economic history of medieval India are well-known.

IRFAN HABIB taught history at Aligarh Muslim University, Aligarh for decades. His works inspire.

ISHRAT ALAM teaches history at Aligarh Muslim University, Aligarh. He is well versed with Dutch sources and archives.

HARISH NARAINDAS is a sociologist of medicine at the Department of Sociology, Delhi University.

IHTESHAM KAZI teaches history at the University of Dhaka, Bangladesh.

SIMKIE SARKAR teaches history at the University of Mumbai.

DHRUB KUMAR SINGH is a Ph.D. scholar at the Centre for Historical Studies, Jawaharlal Nehru University, New Delhi.

SABYA SACHI R. MISRA teaches history of science and technology at the Indian School of Mines, Dhanbad.

290

RAJ SEKHAR BASU teaches history at Rabindra Bharati University, Calcutta. He specializes in the history of missionary activities in south India.

SUJATA MUKHERJEE is a Reader at the History Department, Rabindra Bharati University, Calcutta.

SUNITHA B. NAIR is a research scholar at the Department of History, Mahatma Gandhi University, Kottayam.

MRIDULA RAMANNA has published on different aspects of history of medicine in western India. She teaches history at Mumbai University.

AMIT MISRA is a scientist at the Central Drug Research Institute, Lucknow.

MOHAN RAO specializes in health policy and teaches at the Centre for Social Medicine and Community Health, Jawaharlal Nehru University, New Delhi.

Index

Index

Index

Index

Index

Index

Index

Index

Shaikh Bhina, 50, 54
Shaikh Faizi, 45
Shaikh Mubarak, 67
Shaikh Muhammad Tahir, 54
Shalyatantra, 17
Sharaka Indianus, 16
sharbat (syrups), 51, 53
sharbat-i dig, 51
sharbat-i kaifnak, 54
sharbatkhanas, 41
Sharh-i Asbab, 41
shifakhanas, 47, 48
shiksha (phonetics), 15
Shiraz, 42
Shireen Moosvi, 124
shisha-i hajjam, 79
Shiva Das, 16
Shroff, E.D. (Dr), 243
Siddha, 226
Simon, John, 153, 155
Sind, 78, 147, 236
Singer, 33
Sitala (goddess), 86, 94, 95, 98
Sitala poetry, 95
Sitala worship, 95, 96
Sitalika, 86
skeletal evidence, at Harappa, 9; at Mohenjodaro, 9, 10
skin diseases, 207
Smallpox, 75–79, 94–119, 180, 184, 257; and Abstinence, 106–07; Cooling and Ventilating, 102–03; Diet and Intemperance, 103–04; Eighteenth-Century Tract on, 94–119; Practice, 104–06; Season and Diet, 101–02; Treatment, 85–93
Smallpox Inoculation, 75–79, 96, 97, 113
smallpox pustules, 78
Smilax China Linn, 73
Smilax Japonica, 73
Smith (Lt. Col.), 237
Smith, E.G. (Dr), 184
Smith, Pearl (Dr), 185
Snow, John, 145, 146, 147, 154, 155, 157, 159
Social Darwinism, 130

Social Resistance to Vaccination, 219–20
solar eclipse, 28
Soldier and the 'Scourge', 169–71
Somnath, 35
Soviet Union, 273
Spaniards, 75
specialized surgeons, 53
specialist of dog-bite, 50
Spectacles in India, 26–39
Spleen Census (1909), 133, 138
Srinivasa Ambirajan, xx
Srinivasa Iyengar, S., 267
Sri Ramakrishna Ashram Hospital, 225
Staffing of Institutions, 243–44
Stevorinus, 91
St Georges Hospital, 133, 234, 237, 238, 240, 244
Strachey, John, 172
Stri Dharma, 208
strokes, 272
sub-soil water theory, 162
Sucheendram, 220
sufuf, 51, 53
Surat Singh, 50
surgeries on women, 241
Surgery, 11, 18; in early India, 15–25
surgical instruments, 20
surgical operations, 20
Sushruta, 16, 17, 22, 23, 66, 85
Sushrutasamhita, 16, 17, 18, 20, 22, 85; surgical procedures, 22; operative extraction, 22
Swadeshi movement, 209
symptomatology, 53
Syphilis, 50, 71–75, 168–69; Medical Discourse on, 176–77; in Nineteenth-Century India, 166–79
Syuds, 78

Tabaqat al-Uman, xi
tabibs, 46, 53, 56
Tahrir al Manazir, 31
Talim-i Ilaj, xvi
Tanjore, 37
Tanqih al Manazir, 30
Tao Hongjing, 73

Index